LIFEPLAN

BY DONALD M. VICKERY, M.D.

YOUR OWN MASTER PLAN FOR
MAINTAINING HEALTH AND PREVENTING ILLNESS

Health Decisions, Inc.
2942 Highway 74, Suite 403
Evergreen, Colorado 80439
(303) 674-3200
Copyright 1990 by Donald M. Vickery, M.D.

Printed in the United States of America.

Library of Congress Catalog Card Number: 89-52083
ISBN 0-9625327-0-3
Second Edition

To my mother, Clarene
For giving, constant and selfless

PREFACE

Since *LifePlan* was first published in 1978, Americans have made some important changes in the way they care for their health. The percentage of people who smoke has dropped by about half. We eat more fish and chicken and less fatty meat and dairy products. Oat bran, which can lower cholesterol levels, has become the dominant factor in the purchase of cereals. These changes are proof that the average American is more conscious of preventing illness than ever before, and the results have been impressive: The death rates for stroke and heart disease have been just about cut in half.

The success of programs that help people make better choices is another sign of healthy change. For example, the Taking Care Program, of which *LifePlan* is a part, now brings health information and guidelines for medical decision-making to more than 1.5 million people. *Take Care of Yourself,* one of *LifePlan*'s companion volumes, has sold more than 5 million copies.

Underlying these changes has been an explosion in the amount of health information available to the public. Television, radio, magazines, newspapers—in fact, all forms of media—contain far more health information than ever before. And the supply has created a greater demand: Most Americans now want usable information on health and medical care.

These changes inspired me as I worked to revise *LifePlan.* But along with the inspiration, I have experienced frustration, because we still have a very long way to go. Health professionals and the public are only slowly recognizing the benefit of exercise; a recent national survey found that only 8 percent of adults exercised enough to make a real difference in their health. The drop in smoking has been uneven: Those with less than a high-school education continue to smoke at a high rate, and teenage girls are actually smoking more than in years past. And while the death rates for heart disease and stroke have declined, the cancer death rate is actually going up slightly. Finally, the way we use doctors and hospitals continues to suggest that many people overestimate the benefits of high-technology medical care and underestimate its risks and costs.

Arthur J. Barsky, M.D., associate professor of psychiatry at Harvard Medical School, states that modern medicine is better able to treat diseased organs than to address the problems of lifestyle and the environment that contribute to the leading causes of death in the United States. And, writes Barsky, "Medical interventions have a small impact upon the collective health of the whole society, because while they may be effective, the number of people saved by them is a small fraction of the total population."

In other words, when it comes to helping large numbers of people improve or maintain their health, people's habits and choices can do much more than the entire medical establishment. Yet as a nation, we still believe that medical care is the key to health. As long as we accept that myth, we will fail to invest in the personal actions that pay off in being healthier and feeling and looking better. Hardly a day goes by that some nationally recognized figure doesn't tell us that our improved health and life expectancy are due to modern medicine, when this simply is not true.

This edition of *LifePlan* acknowledges the many positive changes that have been made, but stresses that much remains to be done. For this reason, the new edition emphasizes *how* to make healthy changes, while it still explains thoroughly *why* those changes need to be made. Thus, the sections that provide the practical tools and information needed for leading a healthy life have been greatly expanded. To make room for this material, some sections dealing with specific diseases have been omitted. I hope that these changes will make it easier for you to put your personal LifePlan into action without delay.

Still, much of the book is devoted to helping you understand what affects health, and how to maintain and improve your health. Some readers may find this material too technical and detailed, at least at first. This information is important, however, because further progress depends on a clear understanding of the benefits and risks of both personal health decisions and professional medical care.

LifePlan is a tool to help you make and stick with healthy decisions about the way you live. If you make just one such decision, this book will have achieved its purpose. But there is no reason to limit your success. Healthy changes become easier as you make more of them. I hope you will choose success, and that *LifePlan* will help you make that choice.

ACKNOWLEDGMENTS

Those familiar with the first edition of *LifePlan* will note that this revision contains more new material than old. Much of this new material was contributed by Lydia Schindler and is evidence of her professionalism and expertise. I can say truthfully that without her help, this revision would not have come about.

Catherine Reef edited the entire manuscript and made original contributions as well. Her ability to turn my complicated prose into easily understood text has added immeasurably to the book's usefulness (and makes me wonder why I attempt writing at all).

Going far beyond the call of secretarial duty, Barbara Roland dealt with multiple contributors, my puzzling transcriptions and a myriad of other details to produce the manuscript and supervise book production. Thank you, Madam Publisher. And thanks to Charmaine Kershaw for her expert assistance.

I am indebted again to Lanie King for proofreading yet another manuscript, a task requiring many hours taken from family and friends. Thanks also to Mary Harris, Charlie Dodge, Carolyn Tubbs, Suzanne Hunt and Judy Harju for sharing this burden.

Elin Silveous was more than a vigorous and constructive manuscript reviewer. As our consultant on book design and layout, she often got us unstuck and moving forward.

Lynn Schenck, George Pfeiffer, Thomas Golaszewski, Ed.D., Robert Wilson and Allen Douma, M.D., cheerfully reviewed multiple drafts of the manuscript and provided valuable comments and suggestions. The careful review of the material on screening by Steven H. Woolf, M.D., M.P.H., resulted in important improvements.

The efforts of Richard Muringer and his colleagues at Chronicle Type & Design, who turned a sprawling manuscript into a book, are most appreciated.

Finally, as in the first edition, those leaders in the health field whose work inspired and contributed to this book must be recognized: Lester Breslow, M.D.; Rene Dubois, M.D.; Victor Fuchs, Ph.D.; Walsh McDermott; Thomas McKeown, M.D.; Lewis C. Robbins, M.D.; Ann Somers; and Lewis Thomas, M.D.

LIFEPLAN

SECTION IV: Prevention and the Doctor's Office

SECTION V: Defeating Major Diseases

SECTION VI: The LifePlan Record

INTRODUCTION

The purpose of *LifePlan* is simple: to help you unleash the power of prevention in your own life. This is not a simple task. Readers are different—different in the way they live, in their understanding of health and medical care, in their interest and willingness to make change. Fortunately, we know a good deal about the tools people need to make healthy changes, and I have attempted to include as many of those in *LifePlan* as the printed word will allow. You may need all of them or only a few. Here is how *LifePlan* can help you meet your needs.

Most of us need a way of relating the principles of prevention to our own lives. This is the purpose of Section I, LifeScore. LifeScore is a health risk appraisal, a self-test that can show you which of your habits are promoting good health and which could contribute to disease or disability. Based on factors known to influence health, the LifeScore questionnaire can also alert you to increased health risks based on your family history. Determining your LifeScore is the quickest way to find out how well you are doing—where you are strong, and where you need some improvement. If you do nothing else with *LifePlan*, calculate your LifeScore. It's interesting, it's easy, and it can change your life.

Section II, The Pursuit of Health and Happiness, provides the information that is the basis for our current understanding of health. I think that you will find this to be the most thorough discussion of this subject in any book intended for the general public. It is included here because I believe that we must understand why prevention is important. What's more, we must understand why it is more important to our health than medical care. It is not enough for experts and scientists to know this; it has been well accepted in the scientific community for over three decades, yet the average American feels more dependent on medical care than ever.

Understanding prevention as a whole is important, but the components of prevention must be understood and used in order to secure its benefits. In Section III, The Art and Science of Healthy Living, you will find out not only *why* each of the personal prevention practices is important, but also *how* to put these practices to use in your own life.

Immunizations and screening are specialized areas of prevention that involve the doctor's office or some other source of professional medical care. Each presents special concerns. Immunizations generally deserve their reputation as effective protection against disease, but more and more Americans are ignoring them. Screening, in contrast, tends to be overrated and enjoys increasing popularity. Your choices are important not only to secure the benefits of these procedures, but also to avoid unnecessary risks and costs. Using medicines wisely is another important way of avoiding unnecessary risk and cost. Each of these topics is covered in Section IV, Prevention and the Doctor's Office.

Strong enough prevention sometimes seems to be neglected because it is a "health" topic. The world continues to talk in terms of disease. Section V, Defeating Major Diseases, discusses the threat of the four major killer diseases. You will find that prevention is even more important when the topic is disease rather than health.

The LifePlan Personal Health Record, the last item in the book, is more than a personal medical chart. It allows you to track your progress toward health by recording your LifeScore from year to year. You will find that keeping track of your LifeScore will encourage you to make healthy choices.

Finally, enjoy. *LifePlan* is not something that has to be learned; it's not work, or something you "ought" to do. There is something interesting and entertaining in *LifePlan* for everyone. Use it whenever and however you like. Use it just for the fun of it.

SECTION I

WHAT'S
YOUR SCORE?

❑ LifeScore

WHAT'S YOUR SCORE?

*W*e have all made choices that have affected our health and happiness. Most of us would like to know how those choices have influenced our chances of a long and healthy life. We wonder whether further changes could improve our odds. This is where a health risk appraisal, such as LifeScore, can help.

Your LifeScore will tell you whether you are on the path to a long and vigorous life or heading down the road to ill health and unhappiness. It is the first step in developing a LifePlan that makes sense for you. You cannot achieve your goals unless you first know where you are, where you are heading and where you want to go.

Take a few minutes to compute your Life-Score now. I'm sure that you will find it revealing and useful.

LIFESCORE

INSTRUCTIONS

The LifeScore questionnaire awards you points for things that you do to improve or protect your health. If a certain behavior puts you at risk, you receive fewer points, or none, in that category, depending on the level of risk.

After you have scored all of the questions, transfer your scores to the chart on page 16 and calculate your LifeScore. This will give you an overall estimate of your health. Then, review the questions to learn your strengths and weaknesses. This is the first step in making changes that will turn the odds in your favor.

So that you will better understand the questions and answer them accurately, background information on each topic has been provided. References to other chapters in this book have been included as well.

EXERCISE

A complete exercise program improves or maintains endurance, strength and flexibility. It also includes light daily activity. (See Chapter 6 for more information on endurance, strength and flexibility, and for help with your exercise program.)

Endurance

Aerobic exercise increases endurance by conditioning the heart, lungs and blood vessels. Getting enough aerobic exercise on a regular basis can greatly reduce your risk of heart disease and stroke. Aerobic exercise can also help people with diseases such as arthritis and diabetes. It may even affect your chance of developing certain kinds of cancer. Certainly, aerobic exercise will increase your energy and enthusiasm and help you handle stress.

Aerobic exercise involves vigorous, continuous movement that raises your heart rate to at least 120 beats per minute. Activities that can be aerobic include jogging, running, fast walking, swimming, aerobic dancing, basketball, and fast non-stop games of tennis, squash or racquetball. Activities that usually do **not** raise endurance include baseball, bowling, golf, volleyball, and slow games of tennis, squash or racquetball.

How many minutes of aerobic exercise do you get each week?

	SCORE
Fewer than 15	= 0
15–29	= 3
30–44	= 7
45–74	=10
75–119	=13
120–179	=17
180 or more	=20
Your Score	

Strength

Medical science has not yet determined the influence of strength and flexibility exercises on life expectancy, but they are probably much less important than endurance in this respect. While they do not influence your LifeScore as much as aerobic exercise, strength and flexibility are necessary for full enjoyment of life. They become very important in preserving independence as you grow older.

Making muscles work very hard for relatively short periods increases strength. Weight lifting and calisthenics provide this benefit.

How many minutes of strengthening exercise do you get each week?

	SCORE
Fewer than 15	= 0
15–29	= 1
30–44	= 2
45–74	= 3
75–119	= 4
Your Score	

Flexibility

Stretching muscles to their maximal length improves flexibility. Moving joints through their full range of motion is helpful, too. Most stretching comes naturally; formal stretching exercises are part of yoga, some calisthenic routines and many Oriental forms of exercise. Always hold the stretch for a short period (15 to 30 seconds).

How many minutes of stretching exercise do you get each week?

	SCORE
Fewer than 15	= 0
15–29	= 1
30–44	= 2
45–74	= 3
75–119	= 4
Your Score	

Light Physical Activity

Light physical activity, such as gardening, walking, house cleaning or golf, is clearly good for your health, but we don't yet know to what degree. A few studies have suggested that light activity decreases the risk of heart problems as much as aerobic exercise; others suggest that this is not true. Certainly this lower level of activity does not produce as much conditioning or endurance as aerobic exercise. Could light activity protect in some other way? This is possible, but for now we'll have to credit light activity with less impact than aerobic exercise.

How many minutes of light physical activity do you get each week?

	SCORE
Fewer than 60	= 0
60–119 (one to two hours)	= 1
120–179 (two to three hours)	= 3
180–239 (three to four hours)	= 4
240–299 (four to five hours)	= 5
300 or more (five or more hours)	= 6
Your Score _____	

Your Total Exercise Score _____

BODY FAT

Questions about weight really should be replaced by questions about body fat. The fatter you are, the greater the risk to your life and, specifically, the greater your risk of heart disease, cancer, stroke, diabetes and arthritis (see Chapter 8).

Unfortunately, there is no easy, accurate way to determine how much of your weight is body fat. For a good estimate, use Table 1.1, and score yourself as follows:

MEN	WOMEN	SCORE
More than 25%	More than 30%	= 0
21–25%	26–30%	= 3
16–20%	21–25%	= 8
11–15%	16–20%	= 13
10% and below	15% and below	= 15
	Your Score _____	

Estimating Body Fat

Men should measure the waist exactly at the level of the navel, holding the tape measure perfectly horizontal. Then, use a ruler to connect your waist measurement with your body weight on the chart for men (right). Read your percentage of body fat where the ruler crosses the middle scale. For example, if you weigh 170 pounds and have a 34-inch waist, you are about 18 percent fat.

Table 1.1

Estimating Body Fat

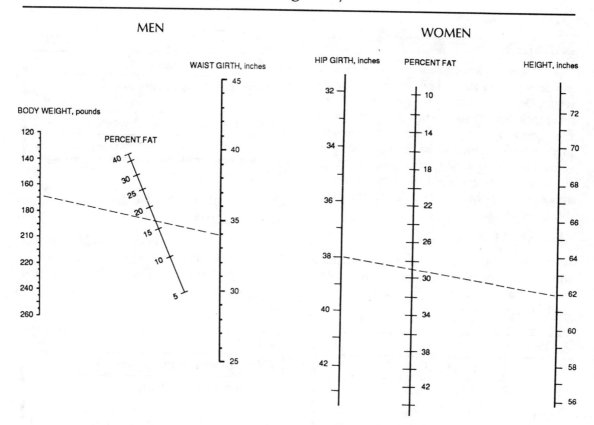

MEN

WOMEN

Source: *Sensible Fitness (Second Edition)* (p.30) by J. H. Wilmore, Ph.D., 1986, Champaign, IL: Human Kinetics Publishers. Reprinted by permission.

Women should measure the hips at their widest point. Use a straight edge to connect your hip measurement with your height, and then read your percentage of body fat on the middle scale. For example, if you are 5 feet 2 inches (62 inches) tall and have 38-inch hips, your body is approximately 29 percent fat.

Your Total
Body Fat
Score

_____

Sodium

How often do you eat foods high in sodium (salt), such as canned soups, hot dogs, pizza, chips, luncheon meats, pickles and TV dinners?

	SCORE
Often (several times a day)	= 0
Sometimes (once every day or so)	= 1
Seldom (once or twice a week)	= 2
Your Score	

NUTRITION

A low-fat, low-cholesterol, high-fiber diet will decrease your risk of heart disease, stroke and cancer. Diets high in beta carotene (vitamin A) and other antioxidants may also protect against cancer. It is also wise to limit sodium intake, although this may not be as helpful in avoiding high blood pressure as once thought: adequate calcium and potassium may be as important, perhaps even more important. (See Chapter 7 for help in making your diet a healthy one.)

Beta Carotene and Other Antioxidants

How often do you eat foods high in beta carotene and other antioxidants (vitamins C, E, polyphenols, lycopene)? These include yellow and dark green vegetables, such as carrots, squash and spinach.

	SCORE
Often (several times a day)	= 2
Sometimes (once every day or so)	= 1
Seldom (once or twice a week)	= 0
Your Score	

Saturated Fat

How often do you eat foods high in saturated fat or cholesterol, such as butter, cream, fatty meats, hot dogs, sausages, high-fat dairy products, candy, pastries and eggs?

	SCORE
Often (several times a day)	= 0
Sometimes (once every day or so)	= 5
Seldom (once or twice a week)	= 10
Your Score	

Fiber

How often do you eat foods high in fiber, such as bran cereals, bran muffins, beans, vegetables and fruits?

	SCORE
Often (several times a day)	= 6
Sometimes (once every day or so)	= 3
Seldom (once or twice a week)	= 0
Your Score	

Your Total Nutrition Score _____

SMOKING

Smoking is the number-one cause of unnecessary deaths. If you are a smoker, see Chapter 9 for help in overcoming this deadly addiction. Non-smokers should be concerned about inhaling other people's smoke (secondary smoking).

Cigarettes and Cigars

In terms of risk, one cigar is about equal to one cigarette.

How many cigarettes or cigars do you smoke each day?

	SCORE
0	= 18
1–9	= 10
10–19	= 8
20–29	= 6
30–39	= 4
40–49	= 2
50 or more	= 0
Your Score	_____

Pipes

Pipe smokers are at an increased risk, although their risk is not nearly that of cigarette smokers.

	SCORE
If you smoke only a pipe	= 0
Otherwise	= 3
Your Score	_____

Smoking and the Pill

Smoking and oral contraceptives cause a deadly interaction. (The risk may be lower for newer, low-dose contraceptives.)

For women only:

	SCORE
If you smoke and take birth control pills	= 0
Otherwise	= 6
Your Score	_____

Your Total Smoking Score

_____

ALCOHOL

Alcohol directly damages the liver, stomach and esophagus, the heart and other muscles, and the nervous system. It greatly increases the risk of all types of accidents, increases stress and impairs nutrition.

Several studies have shown that people who drink alcohol in moderation have a lower risk of heart attack than those who consume no alcohol at all. This has been disputed; what is certain is that going beyond moderation is deadly. (For information on helping yourself or someone else with an alcohol problem, see Chapter 10.)

For purposes of scoring, one drink is defined as a cocktail containing 1-1/2 ounces of liquor, a 12-ounce beer or 5 ounces of wine. If you drink "doubles," then double the number of these cocktails to obtain the number of drinks. If you drink 16-ounce beers, increase the number of beers by 1/3 to obtain the number of drinks.

How many drinks do you have each day, on average?

	SCORE
0	= 24
1	= 25
2–3	= 12
4–5	= 6
6–7	= 3
8 or more	= 0
Your Score _____	

Your Total Alcohol Score	_____

ACCIDENTS

The greatest risk factor for all types of accidents is alcohol use. The risk of car accidents, is also influenced by how much and how fast you drive and whether or not you wear a seat belt. A motorcycle is much less safe than a car. (For more information on preventing accidents, see Chapter 12.)

Alcohol

How many times in the last month did you drink and drive or ride with a driver who may have had too much to drink?

	SCORE
0	= 10
1	= 1
More than 1	= 0
Your Score _____	

Mileage (automobile)

In the next 12 months, how many thousands of miles will you travel by car, truck or van?

	SCORE
Fewer than 2,000	= 8
2,000–5,999	= 6
6,000–9,999	= 4
10,000–19,999	= 1
20,000 or more	= 0
Your Score _____	

Mileage (motorcycle)

In the next 12 months, how many miles will you travel by motorcycle?

	SCORE
None	= 12
Fewer than 2,000	= 8
2,000–5,999	= 2
6,000–9,999	= 1
10,000 or more	= 0
Your Score _____	

Safety Belts

What percentage of the time do you buckle your safety belt when driving or riding in a car?

	SCORE
0%–24%	= 0
25%–49%	= 2
50%–74%	= 4
75% or more	= 6
Your Score _____	

Speed

On average, how close to the speed limit do you usually drive?

	SCORE
Within 5 mph of the speed limit	= 4
6–10 mph over the limit	= 3
11–15 mph over the limit	= 1
More than 15 mph over the limit	= 0
Your Score _____	

Your Total
Accidents
Score   _____

MIND-BODY INTERACTION

Just about everyone agrees that the interaction between mind and body is very important to your health, but no one has developed a satisfactory way to measure this relationship. Three measures of stress are used here. The first, the Holmes scale, measures your exposure to stressful events. Of the three, this score is most directly associated with the risk of disease. Next, because satisfaction with life and ability to cope are also important, questions related to these areas are asked as well. Finally, studies have shown that the individual is perhaps a better judge of his or her health than doctors. The third measure is your own rating of your health. (For more information on understanding and dealing with stress, see Chapter 11.)

Change

The Holmes scale (below) lists 43 life events that have been shown to cause stress that can lead to disease. Each has been given a score. Add up the scores for all listed events that have happened to you in the last year or that you expect will occur in the near future.

THE HOLMES SCALE

(Check all items that happened to you in the last year or that you expect to occur in the near future.)

1. Death of a spouse	100	☐
2. Divorce	73	☐
3. Marital separation	65	☐
4. Jail term	63	☐
5. Death of a close family member	63	☐
6. Personal injury or illness	53	☐
7. Marriage	50	☐
8. Fired at work	47	☐
9. Marital reconciliation	45	☐
10. Retirement	45	☐
11. Change in health of family member	44	☐
12. Pregnancy	40	☐
13. Sex difficulties	39	☐
14. Gain of new family member	39	☐
15. Business readjustment	39	☐
16. Change in financial state	38	☐
17. Death of a close friend	37	☐
18. Change to different line of work	36	☐
19. Change in number of arguments with spouse	35	☐
20. Large mortgage	31	☐
21. Foreclosure of mortgage or loan	30	☐
22. Change in responsibilities at work	29	☐
23. Son or daughter leaving home	29	☐
24. Trouble with in-laws	29	☐
25. Outstanding personal achievement	28	☐
26. Spouse begins or stops work	26	☐
27. Begin or end school	25	☐
28. Change in living conditions	25	☐
29. Change in personal habits	24	☐
30. Trouble with boss	23	☐
31. Change in work hours or conditions	20	☐
32. Change in residence	20	☐
33. Change in schools	20	☐
34. Change in recreation	19	☐
35. Change in church activities	19	☐
36. Change in social activities	18	☐
37. Small mortgage or loan	17	☐
38. Change in sleeping habits	16	☐
39. Change in number of family get-togethers	15	☐
40. Change in eating habits	13	☐
41. Vacation	13	☐
42. Christmas	12	☐
43. Minor violations of the law	11	☐

Source: Thomas H. Holmes, M.D., Social Readjustment Rating Scale. Reprinted with permission.

If your total Holmes score is:

	SCORE
150 or less	= 6
151–250	= 3
251–300	= 1
More than 300	= 0
Your Score_____	

SATISFACTION

In general, how satisfied are you with your life?

	SCORE
Very satisfied	= 4
Satisfied	= 2
Not satisfied	= 0
Your Score_____	

In general, how satisfied are you with your work?

	SCORE
Very satisfied	= 3
Satisfied	= 2
Not satisfied	= 0
Your Score_____	

How often do you have a really good laugh and enjoy yourself?

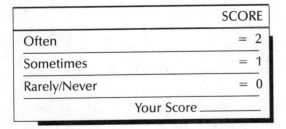

	SCORE
Often	= 2
Sometimes	= 1
Rarely/Never	= 0
Your Score_____	

COPING

How often do you try to change or eliminate the causes of stressful situations?

	SCORE
Often	= 2
Sometimes	= 1
Rarely/Never	= 0
Your Score_____	

How often do you try to change your perception of stressful situations?

	SCORE
Often	= 2
Sometimes	= 1
Rarely/Never	= 0
Your Score_____	

How often do you practice relaxation techniques, such as meditation, progressive muscle relaxation or the quieting reflex?

	SCORE
Often	= 2
Sometimes	= 1
Rarely/Never	= 0
Your Score_____	

How often do you use some form of physical activity or exercise to handle stress?

	SCORE
Often	= 2
Sometimes	= 1
Rarely/Never	= 0
Your Score_____	

How often do you talk over the stressful situations with others?

	SCORE
Often	= 2
Sometimes	= 1
Rarely/Never	= 0
Your Score	_____

In general, how strong are your ties with family and friends?

	SCORE
Very strong	= 2
About average	= 1
Weaker than average	= 0
Your Score	_____

RATING YOUR OWN HEALTH

Considering your age, how would you describe your overall physical health?

	SCORE
Excellent	= 6
Good	= 4
Fair	= 2
Poor	= 0
Your Score	_____

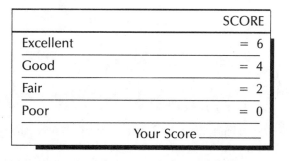

Your Total Mind-Body Score   _____

CHOLESTEROL AND BLOOD PRESSURE

High blood cholesterol levels and high blood pressure are often thought of as the most important risk factors for *atherosclerosis* (fatty deposits in the arteries) and, therefore, for heart disease and stroke. I prefer to think of these as secondary to the primary risk factors—smoking, a poor diet and lack of exercise—because high blood cholesterol levels and high blood pressure often result from these habits. However, when it comes to risk, blood pressure and cholesterol measurements give us more useful information than estimates from questions about habits. In other words, these numbers are easier to use and may be more reliable than questions about lifestyle. (For more information on cholesterol and blood pressure, see Chapter 18.)

Cholesterol

If you know *only* your total cholesterol, use Table A.

If you know your total cholesterol and your high-density lipoprotein cholesterol (HDL-C), calculate your total cholesterol: HDL-C ratio (great mental exercise!) and use Table B.

TABLE A

Total Cholesterol

	SCORE
Less than 180	= 18
180–200	= 16
201–225	= 10
226–250	= 4
Over 250	= 0

TABLE B

Total Cholesterol: HDL-C Ratio

	SCORE
Less than 2.5	= 18
2.5–3.5	= 16
3.6–4.5	= 10
4.6–5.5	= 4
More than 5.5	= 0

If you do not know your cholesterol measurement, score 10.

Your Cholesterol Score _____

Blood Pressure

Blood pressure is usually reported with the higher number, the *systolic blood pressure*, over the lower number, the *diastolic blood pressure*. The systolic blood pressure is measured while the heart contracts to pump blood. The diastolic pressure is measured while the heart is relaxed. A blood pressure reading of 120/80 is read as "120 over 80," and indicates a systolic blood pressure of 120 and a diastolic blood pressure of 80. Your total blood pressure score is based on separate scores for the systolic and diastolic blood pressures.

Systolic Blood Pressure

	SCORE
190 and above	= 0
160–189	= 1
140–159	= 3
120–139	= 6
Below 120	= 8
Your Score	_____

If you do not know your systolic blood pressure, score 4.

Diastolic Blood Pressure

	SCORE
115 and above	= 0
105–114	= 1
90–104	= 3
80–89	= 6
Below 80	= 8
Your Score	_____

If you do not know your diastolic blood pressure, score 4.

Your Total Cholesterol and Blood Pressure Score _____

FAMILY HEALTH

Heart disease, diabetes, breast cancer and many other diseases occur more frequently in some families than in others. It is not clear just how to measure the risk for each person, because the patterns of disease in families can vary greatly. However, the questions below will give a good indication of your risk of disease based on your family history. You can read about practical approaches to this risk in Chapters 18 (Heart Disease), 19 (Cancer), 20 (Stroke) and 21 (Diabetes).

Heart Disease

How many of your immediate family members (parents, brothers or sisters) experienced a heart attack, angina (heart pain), congestive heart failure (fluid build-up in the lungs and/or legs) or stroke before the age of 50?

	SCORE
None	= 6
One	= 3
Two or more	= 0
Your Score _____	

Diabetes

How many of your immediate family members developed diabetes before the age of 50?

	SCORE
None	= 4
One	= 2
Two or more	= 0
Your Score _____	

Breast Cancer

For women only:

How many of your immediate family members have had breast cancer?

	SCORE
None	= 4
One	= 2
Two or more	= 0
Your Score _____	

Your Total Family Health Score

_____

MEDICAL SCREENING TESTS

Following the screening recommendations in Chapter 15 will decrease your risk of several serious problems. Reward yourself according to the following schedule:

	SCORE
Blood pressure check every year	= 6
Cholesterol testing every three to five years	= 3

For women only:

	SCORE
Mammography and physician's examination of breasts every one to five years after age 50	= 4
Pap smear every one to three years after age 21 or whenever regular sexual activity begins	= 4
Your Score _____	

Your Total Screening Score

_____

FINDING YOUR LIFESCORE

Transfer the scores from each section to the columns below:

Exercise	_____
Body Fat	_____
Nutrition	_____
Smoking	_____
Alcohol	_____
Accidents	_____
Mind-Body Interaction	_____
Cholesterol and Blood Pressure	_____
Family Health	_____
Medical Screening Tests	_____
Total Points	_____

A LifeScore of 160 is about "average." If your score was above 175, you have a good chance of enjoying better-than-average health. A score of 200 or more means the odds of a healthy, long life are very much in your favor. A score below 125 means your probability of a healthy life is clearly decreased; below 100, you are heading for serious illness.

How long do you have? Another way of showing how your choices affect your health is to calculate their impact on your life expectancy. Use Table 1.2 to make a rough estimate of your life expectancy based on your LifeScore.

A WORD ABOUT THE QUESTIONS THAT LIFESCORE DID NOT ASK

LifeScore may not contain all of the questions that your knowledge of health and medicine or experience with other health risk appraisals led you to expect. There are three reasons for this. First, there are limits to the kinds of calculations that can be done in a self-scored health risk appraisal. Some questions were omitted simply because they required calculations that were more trouble than they were worth. For example, if you are a former smoker, your risk is influenced by how long and how much you smoked and how long ago you quit. But it is quite likely that the long series of calculations necessary to use this information would not change your overall score a great deal. We lost a little accuracy by omitting such questions, but not a lot. (LifeScore Plus, a computer-scored health risk appraisal that does these difficult calculations for you, is available from the Center for Corporate Health Promotion, 1850 Centennial Park Drive, Suite 520, Reston, Virginia 22091.)

Second, some conditions influence your risk in a very complex way, and there is no precise method for understanding the relationship. For instance, a chronic condition such as emphysema or heart disease could have an enormous impact if the disease were advanced, or it could have little impact if the progression of the disease had been halted at an early stage. Even if you were willing to answer many questions about the disease, there is no clear-cut way to estimate your risk or relate it to the other risks that LifeScore assesses.

Finally, many questions may seem important based on information in the media or in other health risk appraisals, but have no real bearing on your risk. Questions such as, "Do you drink diet sodas?" or, "Do you have headaches?" sound reasonable but, in fact, cannot be related to your overall risk of disease.

Table 1.2

Your Health	LifeScore	Estimated Life Expectancy	
		Men	**Women**
Excellent	Above 200	81 or more	85 or more
Good	176–200	78–80	82–84
Average	151–175	73–77	77–81
Below average	125–150	70–72	72–76
Poor	Less than 125	69 or less	71 or less

Don't worry about what is missing from LifeScore. When a relevant piece of information is missing, it is often taken care of by other questions that relate to the same risk. Most of all, use your good judgment and common sense. If you stopped smoking yesterday, you know that your risk is not exactly the same as that of someone who never smoked. But you also know that stopping was important and where to find more information about smoking within this book. And that's the point of LifeScore, after all.

AND NOW FOR THE GOOD PART

LifeScore measures your strengths and weaknesses with respect to health. The rest of LifePlan will tell you how to improve your weak points and capitalize on your strengths.

SECTION II

THE PURSUIT OF HEALTH AND HAPPINESS

- ❏ What Affects Health?
- ❏ Primary Prevention: Priority Number One
- ❏ The Promise and Problems of Screening
- ❏ Medical Care: The Double-Edged Sword

THE PURSUIT OF HEALTH AND HAPPINESS

*T*here are three ways to get healthy and stay that way:

1. Prevent disease and injury from happening. This is termed primary prevention, or simply *prevention*.
2. Detect and treat disease early, before it causes any symptoms. This means *screening*, or testing for diseases in people with no symptoms. It is sometimes referred to as secondary prevention.
3. If symptoms of disease have developed, obtain treatment to prevent disability or death and, if possible, cure the disease. Some people call this tertiary prevention, but all of us know it as *diagnosis and treatment*, or traditional medical care.

Which of these is most important? Is an ounce of prevention really worth a pound of cure? Read on to find out:

- What affects health.
- The importance of primary prevention.
- The benefits and drawbacks of screening.
- The powers and pitfalls of medical care.

WHAT AFFECTS HEALTH?

Myth: Health depends most on good medical care.

Fact: Factors that affect health are usually divided into four categories: heredity, environment, lifestyle and medical care. (Screening tests and immunizations are considered part of medical care.) The most widely accepted ranking of these categories is shown in Figure 2.1.

Figure 2.1

Factors that Influence an Individual's Chances of Surviving to Age 65

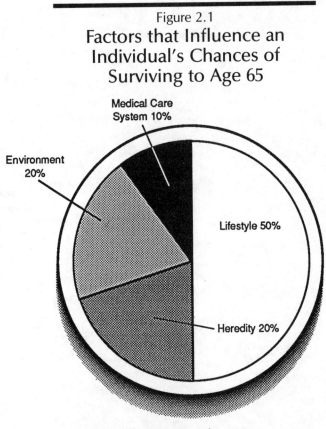

Source: Centers for Disease Control

It may be hard to believe that the environment and lifestyle are more important to your health than medical care. All of us have been raised hearing such statements as, "The miracles of modern medicine have given us the longest life expectancy the world has ever known." This is pure junk.

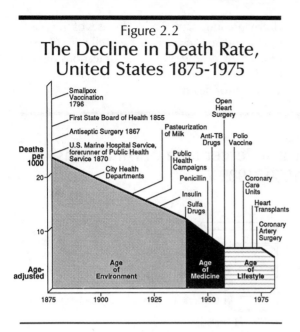

Figure 2.2
The Decline in Death Rate, United States 1875-1975

It's bad enough to make medicine divine, but it's worse to ignore the truth. (The United States ranks 18th in life expectancy—behind Costa Rica, Hong Kong and Cyprus, among others.) Such nonsense is believed to be "common knowledge" and is usually accepted without a second thought.

In reality, the nation's health began improving more than 200 years ago, long before the "miracles of modern medicine" existed. Most of this improvement did not involve medical care. Instead, three trends have influenced health over the past two centuries: environmental changes, medical advances and lifestyle improvements. Of the three, medical "wonders" played the least important role.

Figure 2.2 shows changes in the death rate in the United States over the last century. Death rates are the most frequently used measures of health, especially in attempts to understand the past. The graph also shows when major medical advances occurred.

Note the following points:
- By far, the greatest decline in death rate took place in the late 1800s and early 1900s. These were years of environmental

change, when cities installed sanitation systems and people had access to better food, shelter and clothing. This decline actually began in the 1700s and was largely due to fewer deaths from infectious disease.
- A brief period in the late 1930s and 1940s witnessed a more rapid decline in the death rate. During these years the most important advances in medical care—antibiotics and improved surgical techniques—became available.
- The trend of several centuries came to an end in the early 1950s when the death rate stopped declining. For the next 15 years there was no drop in death rate and no increase in life expectancy for the population as a whole. For middle-aged males, life expectancy actually decreased. This period of no progress saw the advent of high-technology medicine—coronary care units, heart surgery and all the rest. It also saw the beginning of the rapid rise in medical care costs.
- The death rate began to decline again in the early 1970s, largely due to fewer deaths from heart attacks and stroke. It coincided with such lifestyle improvements as reduced use of tobacco, less consumption of saturated fat and cholesterol, and increased exercise among Americans (see Chapter 18 for more on this).

THE DECLINE OF INFECTIOUS DISEASE: Who Gets the Credit?

There has been a remarkable shift in the major threats to our health over the last 200 years (see Figure 2.3). In 1850, infectious diseases accounted for seven of the 10 leading causes of death. Altogether, this amounted to more than 60 percent of all deaths. (The 1850 data are for England and Wales; such data are not available for the United States, but it appears that the situation was the same in this country. The data for 1900, 1950 and 1985 are for the United States.) By 1900, infectious diseases still accounted for half of the top 10 causes of death; however, a substantial decline in the infectious-disease death rate meant that diseases of the heart, cerebral vascular disease (stroke) and cancer would become leading causes of death. By 1950, non-infectious diseases were clearly predominant. Today diseases of the heart, cancer and stroke account for well over 60 percent of all deaths. Only one infectious-disease category, pneumonia and influenza, is in the top 10 causes of death.

Figure 2.3

The 10 Leading Causes of Death as a Percentage of All Deaths: 1850, 1900, 1950, 1985

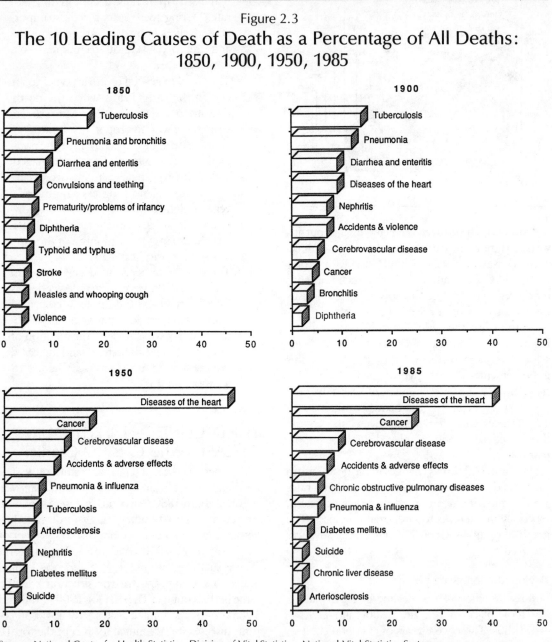

Source: National Center for Health Statistics, Division of Vital Statistics. National Vital Statistics System.

Most Americans believe that antibiotics and immunizations accounted for the decline in infectious disease. But consider the graphs in Figure 2.4. These are death rates for nine important infectious diseases. Each graph shows when an effective antibiotic or vaccine became available. With only one exception, poliomyelitis, these drugs or vaccines appeared after the death rate had completed most of its decline. The most important example is that of tuberculosis, the leading cause of death for hundreds of years prior to the mid-20th century. About 90 percent of the decline in the death rate from tuberculosis between 1900 and 1970 occurred before effective drug therapy was available.

Something other than medicine led to the decline in the death rate from infectious disease and, therefore, the decline in the overall death rate and improvement in health that occurred prior to the 1930s. That something else was a healthier environment—safer water supplies, improved sanitation, and so on. The age of environment saw real income increase dramatically, so that the amount and quality of food, clothing and shelter increased as well. Meanwhile, the number of persons living in close contact decreased, which was a major factor in the decline of infectious disease. The average number of persons living in each American household has gone from 5.4 in 1790 to 2.9 today.

In addition, great improvements in sanitation occurred in the 1800s and early 1900s. During this period, the federal government, every state government and most large cities formed agencies to promote sanitation and hygiene. Public health campaigns demonstrated that an awareness of the environment and sanitation measures could have a great effect. For example, a campaign to improve the general health of the residents of Framingham, Massachusetts, through better hygiene and sanitation was conducted between 1917 and 1923. As a result, the infant death rate dropped by more than one-third. Even more striking was the 70 percent decrease in the death rate due to tuberculosis. This death rate declined more than twice as fast in Framingham as in communities without such a campaign. And this occurred 30 years *before* anti-tuberculosis drugs were available.

Figure 2.4
Death Rates from Infectious Disease: 1900–1970

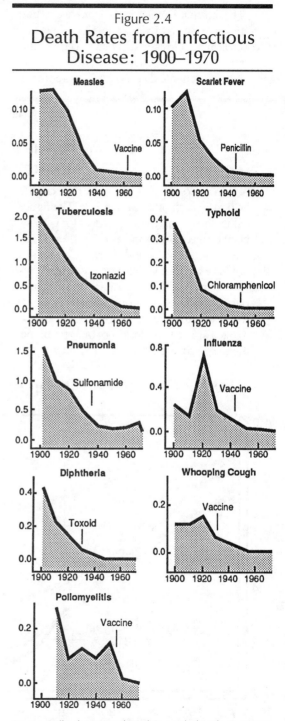

Source: *Milbank Memorial Fund Quarterly*, by John B. McKinlay and Sonja M. McKinlay (Summer 1977), pp. 405-429.

The fact that families no longer have to huddle together in overcrowded rooms has done more to control tuberculosis and other infections than antibiotics; clean water saves more lives than surgery; and an adequate diet has done more than all our hospitals put together. Things we take for granted, some of which we may regard as bureaucratic nuisances, are why we are healthier than our great-great-great-grandfathers, not those precious pills in our medicine cabinets.

Figure 2.5

THE IMPORTANCE OF SAFE WATER:
An American Example

Fairfax County and the City of Alexandria lie next to each other in Virginia. The figure below shows survivorship curves for persons born between 1800 and 1880 in these localities. During this period, Fairfax County did not have a public water system but used private wells. The City of Alexandria began a public water system around 1810. This system featured a large cistern-like filter; its use resulted in a very low incidence of water-borne diseases, such as typhoid and dysentery.

Survival for persons born in Fairfax County changed little during the period and is represented by a single line. Survival in Alexandria was quite different before and after installation of the public water system. After 1810, life expectancy was much better in Alexandria. It is thought that the public water system was responsible for a 30-year difference in life expectancies between the citizens of Fairfax County and those of the City of Alexandria.

Fairfax County vs. City of Alexandria Survivorship Curves

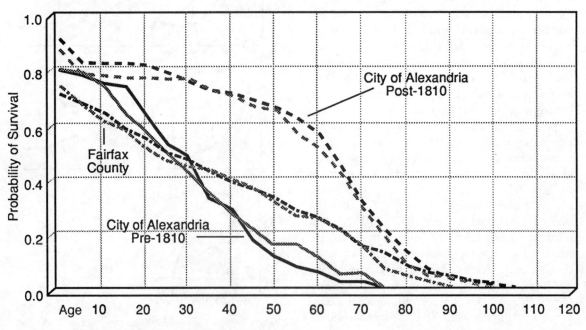

Source: Stuart D. Hubbard, Northern Virginia Heritage, June 1987

A NEW AGE: Lifestyle Determines Our Destiny

But what happened after 1954? The major improvements in the environment had already taken place; deterioration in the environment (air pollution, etc.) had begun, but had not yet greatly affected death rates or life expectancy. Advances in medical care were being made, and through Medicare, Medicaid and other programs, people had better access to medical care than ever before. Yet 1954 was the start of 15 years of no improvement in death rates for the population as a whole and increasing death rates for middle-aged men. Not until 1969 did the death rate resume its decline.

In 1954, we entered the age of lifestyle. Put simply, we have gotten just about all the help we can expect from the environment and medical care. We are now firmly in the grip of our own habits. Any great improvement or decline in health that we experience must now relate to how we live. This should come as good news. You are back in the driver's seat, with an opportunity to control your destiny to a very large degree.

You probably know that your habits are important, but do you know how important? In a well-known study, Dr. Victor Fuchs compared lifestyle habits and mortality in Utah and Nevada. Similarities between these states go beyond climate and geography. Their levels of income, education and medical care are just about the same. The most common lifestyles, however, are quite different. The influence of the non-smoking, non-drinking, family-oriented Mormons is felt throughout Utah. Nevada, in contrast, has high rates of smoking, alcohol consumption and divorce. (By the way, Nevada's statistics cannot be blamed solely on Las Vegas and Reno, for the pattern persists in all parts of the state.) Table 2.1 shows that Nevada's death rate is much higher than Utah's in all age groups. Most have from 35 percent to 70 percent more deaths. These differences are enormous. No epidemic can match them; the plague was a minor illness in comparison. When we look at deaths from two diseases due to habits—lung cancer and cirrhosis of the liver—things get totally out of hand. As Table 2.2 shows, almost six times as many

Table 2.1
Excess of Death Rates in Nevada Compared with Utah, Average for 1959–61 and 1966–68

Age Group	Males	Females
< 1	42%	35%
1–19	16%	26%
20–29	44%	42%
30–39	37%	42%
40–49	54%	69%
50–59	38%	28%
60–69	26%	17%
70–79	20%	6%

Table 2.2
Excess of Death Rates in Nevada Compared with Utah for Cirrhosis of the Liver and Lung Cancer, Average for 1966–68

Age	Males	Females
30–39	590%	443%
40–49	111%	296%
50–59	206%	205%
60–69	117%	227%

Source: Victor R. Fuchs, *Who Shall Live? Health, Economics, and Social Choice,* pp. 52, 54. © 1974 by Basic Books, Inc., Publishers, New York. Reprinted by permission.

young men die of these diseases in Nevada as in Utah.

In perhaps the most famous investigation of habits and health, Drs. Nedra Belloc and Lester Breslow studied the relationship between lifestyle and life expectancy in Alameda, California. They paid special attention to seven habits:

- Moderate exercise two or three times a week.
- Seven or eight hours of sleep each night.
- No smoking.
- Maintaining moderate weight.
- No alcohol or alcohol only in moderation.
- Breakfast every day.
- Three meals a day, avoiding snacks.

It was found that a 45-year-old man who practiced three of these habits had a life expectancy of 21.6 years—that is, he could expect to live to about age 67. But if he practiced six or seven of these habits, he could expect to live 33.1 years, or to age 78. In other words, an increase in life expectancy of more than 11 years was associated with the healthier lifestyle. This difference may be better appreciated if you realize that if we could prevent *all* deaths from cancer, life expectancy (at birth) would increase by only about two years. The 11-year difference associated with lifestyle is enormous. The study also found that a man who practiced six or seven of these habits was as healthy as a man *30 years younger* who practiced only one or two. How can you turn down being 30 years younger?

Follow-up in Alameda over the last 15 years suggests that two of the habits, three meals a day and breakfast every day, are less important than the others, but otherwise the results are the same.

Studies on deaths due to cancer also confirm the value of lifestyle. Mormons, who do not smoke, have a cancer death rate that is only 60 percent of that for the population as a whole. Seventh-day Adventists, many of whom do not smoke or drink and may be vegetarians, have a cancer death rate only 50 percent of that for the general population.

You do not have to choose between the benefits of lifestyle and medicine, but suppose for a moment that you did. What would your choice be? Consider this: Christian Scientists, who tend to have healthful lifestyles but avoid medical care, have greater life expectancies than the general population.

Environment, lifestyle, medical care—you now know something of their importance. Heredity, the fourth factor that affects health, must be considered least important for several reasons. First, it is very difficult to separate the effects of heredity from those of environment and lifestyle: It is just plain hard to say what is due to heredity alone. Second, even if we knew more, we couldn't do much about it. For the foreseeable future, genetic manipulation will remain a huge tangle of

scientific, ethical and legal questions without answers. Finally, we do not know the extent to which other factors can alter heredity's contribution. For example, the risk from a family history of hypertension (high blood pressure) may be very small if you are not overweight, have your blood pressure checked yearly, and treat hypertension should it occur.

In the past, environment was most important. As it improved, the effects of lifestyle became clear. While the achievements of medical science are significant and surely dramatic, medical care must rank behind these two. You are now in the age of lifestyle—your habits *are* your health.

Is Heredity More Important Than We Thought?

We may have to reassess the importance of heredity as we learn more about the causes of disease. Medical science is slowly defining the role of heredity in diseases such as diabetes, rheumatoid arthritis, cancer, alcoholism—even urinary-tract infections. In each case, it appears that inheriting certain genes does not make the disease certain but makes it much more likely than if the genes were not present. Still, it is unlikely that heredity will ever surpass lifestyle in importance, and the environment is threatening to make a comeback as a cause of disease. Heredity will remain the most difficult risk factor to alter.

A Healthy Future for Those Who Choose It

Could the age of lifestyle come to an end? Could prevention become less important? Anything is possible, of course. On the positive side, a series of medical discoveries could make it possible to cure heart disease, cancer, stroke and other major diseases, making medical therapy the major influence on health. On the negative side, we may pollute our habitat so much that we create a new age of environment, this time one that causes our

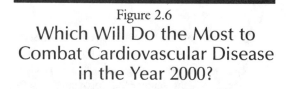

Figure 2.6
Which Will Do the Most to Combat Cardiovascular Disease in the Year 2000?

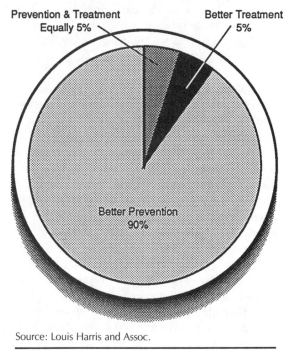

Prevention & Treatment
Equally 5%

Better Treatment
5%

Better Prevention
90%

Source: Louis Harris and Assoc.

remain dominant in combating these two disease categories, which account for almost 60 percent of all deaths in the United States. The forecast for stroke should be the same as for heart disease, because the principal cause of the problem, atherosclerosis, is the same. Indeed, with the possible exception of diabetes, we can expect prevention to

Figure 2.7
Which Will Do the Most to Combat Cancer in the Year 2000?

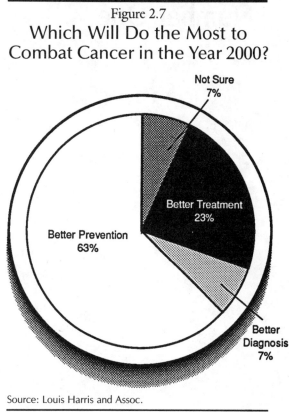

Not Sure
7%

Better Treatment
23%

Better Prevention
63%

Better
Diagnosis
7%

Source: Louis Harris and Assoc.

health to worsen. Or there could be an almost unthinkable catastrophe: global nuclear war, or a deadly infection that spreads rapidly and cannot be prevented or treated. These events and other far more incredible happenings are possible. But not likely. That's not to say that these aren't good questions.

Figures 2.6 and 2.7 show the responses of experts in science and medicine to just such questions. Figure 2.6 shows which factors experts think will be most important in controlling heart disease in the year 2000. Figure 2.7 shows their opinion concerning the most important way to combat cancer in the year 2000. (Prevention refers to primary prevention—in this case lifestyle change, because there is little indication of a role for immunization.) It is clear that prevention and lifestyle will

be most important with respect to every disease in the top 10 leading causes of death.

Medical science will advance, but usually it will not be able to undo what you have done to yourself. Lifestyle must be your top priority.

The bottom line is that you must take care of yourself, do your part to preserve and improve the environment and take advantage of what medicine has to offer. Helping you do this is the purpose of this book.

PRIMARY PREVENTION: Priority Number One

Now that we have seen why lifestyle and environment have the most impact on health, it seems clear that science has proven the wisdom of an old saying: An ounce of prevention really is better than a pound of cure. A beneficial lifestyle, a healthy environment and immunization are the primary means for preventing disease.

Much of prevention's importance comes from the relationship between lifestyle and disease. Lifestyle not only prevents many diseases, it can slow the progression of some and even reverse others. But this relationship is complex. It can be difficult or impossible to distinguish between preventing, slowing and reversing disease. The effect of lifestyle on atherosclerosis is a good example. *Atherosclerosis* is the clogging of arteries that is the main cause of heart disease, stroke and kidney disease (see Chapter 18, Heart Disease). It is quite likely that a rigorous program designed to eliminate risk factors would successfully prevent atherosclerosis if started early in life. Such a program would include a very-low-fat diet, a regular exercise program and no smoking. However, a somewhat less rigorous program might slow the development of atherosclerosis so much that there would be no signs or symptoms during the person's lifetime. Thus, while this lifestyle would only slow the development of atherosclerosis, it would prevent the resulting heart disease, stroke or kidney disease. Finally, we now know that a rigorous program begun after atherosclerosis is present can reverse the condition and, where tissue has not already been destroyed, reverse the effects on the heart, brain and kidneys. Many would view this as prevention of heart disease, stroke or kidney disease through reversal (cure!) of atherosclerosis.

Much of the fuzziness about whether lifestyle prevents, slows or cures disease depends on how you define the disease. For example, is atherosclerosis a disease before it causes coronary heart disease or some other problem? Similar confusion occurs with respect to aging. Most of what we have

Table 3.1
Kicking the Killers

Disease	Nutrition	Exercise	Immunization	Mind↔Body Interaction	Tobacco	Alcohol	Body Fat	Environmental Hazards
Atherosclerosis	○	○		○	●		●	
Cancer	○		○	?	●	●	●	●
Emphysema					●			
Cirrhosis				○		●		
Diabetes	○	○					●	
Accidents				○	●	●		●
Infection			○	○	●			●

○ = positive   ● = negative

called aging is actually chronic disease, such as heart disease or arthritis, and "disuse disease," the loss of some capability that was not used enough to retain it. Because lifestyle can prevent, slow or reverse much chronic and disuse disease, it may seem to prevent, slow or reverse many aspects of aging.

In contrast to chronic and disuse disease, true aging involves changes that occur with the passage of time and that cannot be prevented or reversed. However, it now seems that the rate at which these changes occur can be slowed by healthful lifestyles. Again, if we slow this change to the point that it does not become evident during a person's lifetime, this can be seen as preventing aging.

Common sense suggests a practical approach: Preventing disease from starting is best, but slowing its development should not be considered failure. We can all appreciate the benefit of delaying the onset of heart disease from age 40 to age 80. In short, we can recognize the value of preventive activities even when they do not prevent disease.

KICKING THE KILLERS

Prevention is the major means by which we have reduced the threat of the major causes of death. Table 3.1 lists the important preventive ac-

tivities for each cause.

A few lessons can be learned from the chart. First, a small number of preventive activities have enormous impact on a wide variety of diseases and on our health. In fact, the diseases listed account for over 90 percent of all deaths in the United States. Second, smoking causes many problems in addition to lung cancer. Indeed, smoking actually causes more deaths by contributing to heart disease. Finally, we are going out on a limb just a little bit by including mind-body interaction (stress, if you prefer) in the table, even though we have not developed a precise way to measure its impact and, therefore, be certain about its contribution. While we do not have as much evidence for stress's impact as we do for such activities as exercise or smoking, there is enough evidence to make it unwise to omit this important factor.

What About Cholesterol, Blood Pressure and Weight?

It's not that these measures are not important with respect to disease. It's just that we prefer to think of them as secondary to the factors listed in Table 3.1. This is in opposition to many scientists, who refer to these measures as primary risk factors. Our approach is based on the principle that, when

Table 3.2
Cholestrol and Blood Pressure Reflect Your Habits

Habit	Total or LDL ("Bad") Cholesterol	HDL ("Good") Cholesterol	Blood Pressure
Exercise	▼	▲	▼
Smoking	▲	▼	▲
Alcohol*	▼	▲	▼▲
Low-fat, high-fiber diet	▼	▲	▼
Fat control	▼	▲	▼

▲ = increase   ▼ = decrease

* Effects of alcohol on LDL and HDL cholesterol are relatively small. In moderate amounts, alcohol lowers blood pressure. With more than one or two drinks per day, blood pressure goes up in proportion to the amount consumed.

Table 3.3
Kicking the Killers: Atherosclerosis

Disease	Nutrition	Exercise	Mind↔Body Interaction	Tobacco	Alcohol	Body Fat
Heart Disease	♉	♉	♉	●	● ♉	●
Stroke	♉	♉	?	●		●
Kidney Disease	♉	♉	?	●		●

♉ = positive   ● = negative

it comes to preventing disease, lifestyle issues are primary. Their degree of success or failure is reflected in such measurements as blood pressure and cholesterol. Even though some of these measurements can be improved with medicine, the first and best approach is lifestyle.

Table 3.2 shows the relationships between cholesterol, blood pressure and lifestyle. These are probably just about what you expected. Putting this all together suggests the following:

- Your primary strategy should be to improve your lifestyle.
- Use the measurements to get motivated and to follow your progress.
- If cholesterol and blood pressure are still high after adopting a healthy lifestyle, then medications make sense.

- If body fat remains high, medications have little to offer. Further lifestyle changes are required.

Death from Clogged Arteries: Atherosclerosis

Atherosclerosis means clogged arteries. That means trouble anywhere in the body, but especially in the heart, brain and kidneys. By causing heart disease, stroke and kidney disease, atherosclerosis accounts for approximately 45 percent of all deaths. That is why much of lifestyle's power comes from its effect on atherosclerosis. Much of the importance of cholesterol, blood pressure and fat measurements is due to their relationship to atherosclerosis (see Tables 3.2 and 3.3). As a result,

Table 3.4
Kicking the Killers: Cancer

Type of Cancer	Nutrition	Exercise	Immunization	Tobacco	Alcohol	Body Fat	Environment
Lung	?			🍎			🍎
Breast	○					🍎	
Mouth	?			🍎	🍎		
Throat				🍎	🍎		
Larynx	?			🍎	🍎		
Esophagus	?		○	🍎	🍎		
Liver	?				🍎		🍎
Colon	○						
Pancreas	?			🍎			
Bladder	?			🍎			🍎
Prostate	○						
Uterus	○						

○ = positive   🍎 = negative

much of this book is directly or indirectly about atherosclerosis.

Deaths due to atherosclerosis have fallen by about 40 percent in the United States since 1963. At least 80 percent of this decline was achieved through lifestyle changes and, to a lesser extent, medical treatment of high blood pressure; less than 20 percent was due to improved medical treatment of heart disease. Now that we can devise lifestyle programs that can reverse atherosclerosis, it seems quite likely that we can make further decreases in the death rate due to this condition.

Death from Damaged Cells: Cancer

The cancer death rate is dominated by a single lifestyle factor: smoking (see Table 3.4). Lung cancer accounts for over 25 percent of all deaths due to cancer, and smoking accounts for 80 percent to 95 percent of all lung-cancer deaths. Smoking is also the major risk factor for cancer of the:

- Lips
- Throat
- Esophagus
- Kidneys
- Mouth
- Larynx (voice box)
- Pancreas
- Bladder

If Americans would stop smoking, we could cut cancer deaths by at least 25 percent. Instead, cancer death rates have actually increased somewhat over the last 20 years; we are losing the war on cancer. There are, of course, other important preventable causes. Exposure to radiation and certain chemicals in the environment may cause cancer (see page 301). For each of these substances, exposure to dangerous levels can be avoided.

Alcohol is a poison. The mouth, throat, larynx, esophagus and liver are most directly exposed to alcohol when we drink, so it is not surprising that alcohol use raises the risk of cancer in these organs. Last but not least, high-fat and low-fiber diets appear to be risk factors for breast and colon cancer, and diets high in beta carotene (vitamin A) appear to protect against cancer in general. Unfortunately, we cannot now determine the precise contribution of these factors or understand how far we might go in developing a diet that protects against cancer.

Some drugs may also cause cancer (see page 302.) Ironically, many of these are used to fight cancer. Finally, the hepatitis B and HTLV-1 viruses are known to cause liver cancer and leukemia, respectively. Hepatitis B infection can be prevented through immunization.

Death from Suffocation: Emphysema

The main problem in emphysema is that the lungs lose elastic tissue, and air cannot be expelled efficiently. Emphysema is almost always accompanied by bronchitis, in which the larger breathing tubes (bronchi) become clogged with mucus. This makes it more difficult to move air and contributes to the breakdown of the lungs' normal structure. The result is slow suffocation.

Smoking causes about 90 percent of emphysema. The rest is due to inherited defects, air pollution and other causes. Stopping smoking will not reverse emphysema, but it will prevent it from getting worse. Stopping will reverse bronchitis to some extent, so that smokers with emphysema and bronchitis who quit usually notice great improvement in their overall condition.

Death from Slow Poisoning: Cirrhosis

Alcohol is toxic to all cells in the body. The liver is the first stop for alcohol after it is absorbed in the stomach, and is the principal organ for metabolizing alcohol. As a result, it is a common site for injury from alcohol. Over time, alcohol kills liver cells, and they are replaced by scar tissue. Stopping drinking will stop the killing, but it will not reverse any damage that has been done. In fact, some of the problems caused by scarring may worsen even after someone stops drinking alcohol. This means that stopping alcohol use before much scarring occurs is necessary. While cirrhosis may result from other causes, such as viral infection (hepatitis), alcoholism accounts for about 75 percent of cirrhosis and the deaths that it causes.

Death from Overload: Diabetes

There are two types of diabetes, and in many ways they are separate diseases. Insulin-dependent diabetes mellitus (IDDM) is a severe disease of young people. It cannot be prevented by any known means, although lifestyle is important in its control. Non-insulin-dependent diabetes mellitus (NIDDM) usually occurs in middle age or later and is directly related to obesity and inactivity. In this condition, excess body fat makes insulin less effective. (This is called insulin resistance.) Losing fat helps to make insulin effective once more. Exercise also improves the effectiveness of insulin, and it helps to reduce fat. Finally, a diet that is low in fat and high in complex carbohydrates and fiber helps to reduce fat as well as to prevent the high levels of glucose (sugar) in the blood that may occur after eating food heavy in simple sugars or fats. (See Chapter 21 for a detailed discussion of diabetes.)

Death from Disregard: Trauma

Consider the following:

- Alcohol is involved in 50 percent of fatal automobile accidents.
- More than half of the deaths that occur during recreational activities (swimming, boating, fishing, hunting, etc.) are related to alcohol use.
- Alcohol plays a major role in deaths due to falls or drowning and injuries to pedestrians.
- Cigarette smoking is the cause of more than half of fatal house fires.
- The use of seat belts reduces the risk of death in automobile accidents by about half.
- Most accidental poisoning could be prevented if people kept toxins out of children's reach.

Need more be said? Probably not, but see Chapter 12 for more on preventing accidents.

Table 3.5
Immunization

Type of Infection	Immunization	Environmental Hazards
Polio	positive	
Mumps	positive	
Measles	positive	
Rubella (German measles)	positive	
Tetanus	positive	
Pertussis (whooping cough)	positive	
Diphtheria	positive	
Typhoid fever	positive	negative
Typhus	positive	negative
Yellow fever	positive	negative
Malaria		negative
Pneumonia	positive	
Cholera	positive	negative
Plague	positive	negative
Meningitis	positive	
Influenza	positive	
Hepatitis	positive	negative

positive = positive   negative = negative

Germs Can Still Kill

Infections were the leading threat to health right up until the middle of this century. A healthier environment, due to a higher standard of living and improved sanitation, was largely responsible for reducing this threat. However, you still need immunizations to protect against some diseases (See Table 3.5). Environmental measures are still important to reduce the risk of others. For example, destroying the breeding places of mosquitoes reduces the risk of malaria and yellow fever.

PREVENTING THE PAIN

Some problems don't kill, but they can be a major pain in the neck . . . or back . . . or foot . . . or some other portion of your anatomy. Table 3.6 lists some of these problems and factors that affect them. Note that factors under our control are not powerful enough to prevent these problems altogether, but they may go a long way toward making them less troublesome.

Muscles, Bones and Joints

Osteoarthritis, the most common form of arthritis, results when the cartilage within a joint wears down and bone spurs develop at the joint's edges. The result is pain, stiffness and, eventually, loss of movement. Osteoarthritis may affect any joint but usually causes problems in weight-bearing joints, such as the hips and knees. It often is visible as bumps on the last joint of the finger. Injury to a joint, obesity and lack of exercise all contribute to osteoarthritis. While the effect of an old injury cannot be changed, those of obesity and lack of exercise can.

Osteoporosis occurs when bones lose calcium and become brittle and weak. It becomes more common with advancing age and is most likely to be severe in women past the menopause. Exercise, along with adequate calcium and vitamin D in the diet, can prevent osteoporosis in almost everyone with the exception of women who have gone through the menopause. While exercise, increased calcium intake (1,500 milligrams per day) and adequate vitamin D are essential for these women, sometimes these measures are not enough. The addition of estrogen and perhaps fluoride may be useful. Also, please note that calcium is not well absorbed unless a demand for it is created through exercise.

Although both osteoarthritis and osteoporosis may cause *low back pain*, a far more common cause is muscle spasm. Occasionally, the infamous "slipped disc" really does cause back pain, but it is blamed more often than it should be. Pursuing a lifestyle that reduces the risk of osteoarthritis and

Table 3.6
Preventing Pain

Type of Pain	Exercise	Nutrition	Mind↔Body Interaction	Body Fat	Tobacco	Alcohol
Muscles, Bones and Joints						
Osteoarthritis	positive			negative		
Osteoporosis	positive	positive		negative		
Low back pain	positive			negative		
Hernia	positive			negative		
Pressure Problems						
Hemorrhoids	positive			negative		
Varicose veins	positive			negative	negative	
Thrombophlebitis	positive			negative	negative	
Gastrointestinal						
Gallbladder		positive		negative		
Ulcer		positive	positive		negative	negative
Spastic colon		positive	positive			
Diverticulitis		positive				
Infections						
Respiratory (colds, pneumonia)					negative	
Bladder		positive				
Dental Problems						
Tooth decay		positive				

○ = positive   ● = negative

osteoporosis—exercise, fat loss, and adequate calcium and vitamin D in the diet—also helps in back pain due to muscle spasm or disc problems. Keeping abdominal and back muscles strong and flexible helps in dealing with back pain due to muscle strain, so some of your exercise should be directed toward this goal. Maintaining the normal curve of the spine while sitting, sleeping, lifting, etc., is also important. And, while no study has actually proven that these lifestyle measures will prevent back pain altogether, it seems very likely that they will reduce the risk of very painful episodes.

It may seem strange to include *hernia* in a "musculoskeletal" section, but weak abdominal muscles and obesity increase the risk that tissue will bulge through the abdominal wall. Exercises for conditioning, as well as those that strengthen the abdominal muscles, are important preventive measures. They are also important for fat loss if obesity is a problem. Finally, stopping smoking will reduce coughing and remove this source of pressure on the abdominal wall.

Pressure on Veins

Hemorrhoids, varicose veins and thrombophlebitis all involve veins in which the flow of blood is no longer normal, and all may be affected by our lifestyle habits.

Hemorrhoids are veins that bulge into the rectum or through the anus. They have been a problem ever since man assumed an erect posture. This upright posture increases pressure inside the veins, which is enough to create hemorrhoids in some people. Anything that increases the pressure—obesity, lack of exercise, straining at the stool, sitting a lot—makes it more likely that hemorrhoids will occur. It seems logical that reversing these factors will help to prevent them. In addition, adequate fiber in the diet decreases pressure within the intestine and prevents straining to pass small, hard stools.

Varicose veins also result from pressure exceeding the tolerance of vein walls so that bulging occurs. Lack of exercise, prolonged standing and obesity all increase the risk of varicose veins.

Inflammation in veins, **thrombophlebitis,** is most likely when the flow of blood is sluggish, a situation that occurs when veins are bulging and under increased pressure. Clots often form in thrombophlebitis. These may break off and be carried to the lungs (pulmonary emboli) where they obstruct blood flow, a dangerous and sometimes fatal condition. Decreasing the risk of such bulging and slow blood flow also decreases the risk of thrombophlebitis. As you have guessed by now, exercise and fat loss are recommended. Note also that smoking is a risk factor for thrombophlebitis.

Gastrointestinal Pain

The **gallbladder** stores bile, which aids in digestion, for release into the intestine. The risk of gallbladder problems is greatest when the bile is heavy with fat and cholesterol, and its flow is sluggish. This is most likely to occur when the diet is high in saturated fat and the individual is obese. Obesity will also increase the risk of surgery should prevention fail.

Ulcers are often regarded as an example of the negative effect of mind upon body. We believe that mental distress can increase the risk of ulcer and improving the mind–body interaction lowers that risk. Smoking increases the risk of ulcer several-fold. Caffeine-containing drinks and food do not

seem to have as great an influence on the risk of ulcer as once thought. However, alcohol is a contributor, as are many drugs. Both corticosteroids — prednisone, cortisone, etc.—and so called non-steroidal anti-inflammatory agents — aspirin, ibuprofen, naproxyn (Naprosyn), piroxicam (Feldene), etc.—are most likely to cause a problem. These drugs should only be used when necessary.

Spastic colon and **diverticulitis** can both cause severe abdominal pain and are probably two stages of the same process. The basic problem is a lack of fiber in the diet, which results in a small amount of hard stool. This requires the colon (lower intestine) to work especially hard to pass the stool. The extra work results in spasms and increased pressure within the colon. Over time, this increased pressure pushes out small bulges in the colon wall, known as diverticula. Diverticula tend to become blocked, infected and inflamed, and this is known as diverticulitis. It appears that adequate fiber in the diet will help prevent both of these problems.

Infections

Smoking poisons the cells that fight infections within the lungs. It is not surprising that smokers have more minor infections (*colds*, and *flu*) and major infections (*pneumonia*) than do nonsmokers. Stopping smoking removes this unnecessary risk.

Bladder infections, a common problem for many women, are less common in men. The bacteria that cause these infections can literally be washed away if urine flow rates are high enough. Drinking lots of fluid produces frequent voidings of clear, colorless urine, which not only helps prevent bladder infections, but is also the mainstay of treatment. Antibiotics add little to this. Cranberry juice contains a natural antibiotic, so include some in your regimen. (A recent report suggests that there is a link between high fluid intake and bladder cancer. It is impossible to say at this time whether this will be confirmed or what it means, but it suggests that distention of the bladder might be harmful. Therefore, drink plenty of fluid, but don't hold it; there is nothing wrong, socially or physically, with frequent voidings.) Another preventive measure for women is to wipe with toilet paper from front to back so as to avoid transferring bacteria to the urinary opening (urethral meatus).

Dental Problems

The prevention of such dental problems as tooth decay and gum disease (gingivitis) is well understood, and you probably already know the basics:

- Flossing once a day.
- Brushing after meals with a fluoride-containing toothpaste.
- Using dental sealants for children.
- Eating foods that naturally help prevent tooth decay, such as popcorn, some cheeses and sugarless chewing gum.
- Avoiding foods that are sticky or contain refined sugar, which promotes tooth decay. These include caramels and other candies, sweetened soft drinks and raisins.
- Regular professional cleaning.

PREVENTION OF AGING

Our image of the aging is clear: slow, forgetful, tired, cantankerous, weak, sick, confused, idle, lonely. But however clear our image may be, it does not serve us well. An older American can be vigorous, vital and energetic. Indeed, his or her performance may easily surpass that of a person many years younger. Our distorted image obscures the fact that the effects commonly ascribed to aging are, in fact, due to three separate processes: disuse, chronic disease and cellular, or natural aging.

Disuse Degrades Life

The first process, disuse, refers to the decline in physical and mental faculties that results from failure to use them. "Use it or lose it" is not just a slogan, it is a fact of life, a biologic principle that applies to all ages. As Dr. Walter Bortz, president of the American Gerontological Association, has observed, "If you make an Olympic athlete stay in bed, you make an old man out of him." Thus, even in top athletes, the effects of inactivity are very

TEETH CLEANING: The Rule or the Exception?

Annual physicals and other routine visits to the doctor are often promoted as the same kind of routine maintenance that all complex machines require. In other words, your body needs a routine visit to the doctor just like your car needs a routine visit to the service station.

Yet there is no evidence that anything in medicine serves this kind of routine maintenance function. There is nothing that the doctor can do for your body that remotely resembles what changing the oil or getting lubricated does for your car. But there is in dentistry. Routine teeth cleaning and the use of sealants or fluoride treatments in children do help prevent tooth and gum disease. So you should have this kind of "servicing" done on a regular basis. At the same time, as noted in Chapter 15, there is no evidence that dental examinations to detect unsuspected problems are very useful. This is especially true of dental X-rays, which should be done much less often (perhaps once every five years) than on the every-year basis usually suggested. As a practical matter, the visual examination gets done along with the teeth cleaning; indeed, it would be hard to do the teeth cleaning without taking a look around.

similar to those we often ascribe to aging. With forced bed rest, world-class athletes become weak and have no endurance. They lose both muscle and bone mass and may even become anemic. Most strikingly, they are depressed and forgetful, and have trouble concentrating and performing simple mental tasks. If you would like to learn how it feels to be a sedentary 80-year-old, put yourself to bed for five days. You won't feel good.

Disuse degrades human performance. Quite simply, it makes you less able to live a full life. Declining physical performance has received the most attention, and endurance has been of special concern. Dr. Roy J. Shepard of the University of Toronto and many others have shown that endurance in older people can be greatly improved through aerobic exercise. As endurance improves, the tired and feeble image evaporates.

More and more, strength is being recognized as important to physical health and independence. For instance, older people often have difficulty getting out of a chair because they lack strength in their quadriceps. But the quadriceps can be strengthened through weight training. Dr. Everett Smith at the University of Wisconsin and others have shown that "pumping iron" can be safe and beneficial in older people. These older adults will never look like body builders, but they will be able to get out of a chair easily.

Flexibility can be maintained or improved through stretching, which is best done in combination with aerobic and resistance exercise. It is perhaps more surprising that older people can improve agility, as measured by reaction times. Research by Dr. W. W. Spirduso found that men and women aged 50 to 70 who regularly played racquet sports requiring quick reactions had reaction times similar to sedentary people aged 20 to 30. A second study showed that older runners also maintained quick reaction times, despite the fact that running is not usually thought of as a quick-reaction sport.

Measurements such as blood pressure and cholesterol are related to physical performance, of course.

It is ironic that many people consider declines in mental performance to be the most disturbing aspect of aging, yet improving mental performance has received much less attention than improving physical performance.

Intelligence has been measured in many ways, most often with "intelligence quotient" (IQ) tests. Numerous studies suggest that IQ scores may be improved in older adults through training programs or lifestyles that involve intellectual challenge. Most recently, Warner K. Schaie, Ph.D., at the Pennsylvania State University, reported that at least 50 percent of older people who had shown significant declines in IQ performed better after completing problem-solving exercises during five

Table 3.7
Improving Performances in Older Americans

Area of Improvement	Method
Physical	
Endurance	Aerobic exercise
	Decrease body fat
	Smoking cessation
Strength	Weight training
Flexibility	Stretching exercise
Agility	Games, exercise
Mental	
IQ	Intellectual challenges
Memory	Memory training
Wisdom	Experience

one-hour sessions. One-third returned to or exceeded their previous level of mental ability.

Problems with memory are perhaps the most frequently mentioned with respect to aging. Yet there are proven methods for improving memory through training—practicing the storage of information through concentration, repetition and association with other facts (mnemonic devices).

Finally, there is that elusive mental function called wisdom. Because we can't measure wisdom, we can't discuss its improvement in scientific terms. But I will suggest that wisdom is highly valued in this society, that it is related to experience, and that increased wisdom is an *advantage* of aging.

Chronic Disease

The second process that contributes to the common image of the aged person is chronic disease. Most of the effects that we ascribe to being old are actually the result of arthritis, heart disease, chronic obstructive lung disease, diabetes or some other chronic disease common to old age. Most important, inactivity is among the risk factors for these diseases, along with smoking and obesity. It is clear that disuse disease and chronic disease share roots in lifestyle: The border between the two is often blurred.

Cellular Aging

The third process is cellular aging, the natural aging that we can't do anything about, at least not at present. As an old professor of mine was fond of reminding those who got carried away with the idea of prevention, the death rate has never changed: It is still one per person.

Subtracting the effects of disuse disease and chronic disease from our image of aging leaves us with a somewhat strange—and short—list of effects for cellular aging. Changes in appearance receive much attention, and hope springs eternal that something will stop or reverse them.

Wrinkles are inevitable, if not forever: The value of cosmetic surgery or Retin-A is in the eye of the beholder. As for hair, despite publicity about the drug minoxidil and its ability to produce fuzz on balding scalps, most of us can only hope that we are left with something and then look to Grecian Formula 16 or some similar concoction if gray is not acceptable.

Table 3.8
Inevitable Changes

Hair loss	Graying
Loss of skin elasticity	Hardening of the arteries
Cataracts	Hearing loss

While external changes are not to be dismissed, internal changes have more impact. There is no question that aging decreases cell and organ functioning. Yet this decline does not appear to occur as quickly as once thought, perhaps because we have mistaken the effects of chronic or disuse disease for true aging. It is possible that the cellular processes of true aging have been altered in some people by a combination of factors, but not likely. We were probably just wrong about what older persons can do, and our earlier estimates were too pessimistic.

Our changing understanding of aging's effect on performance can be illustrated by a "peak

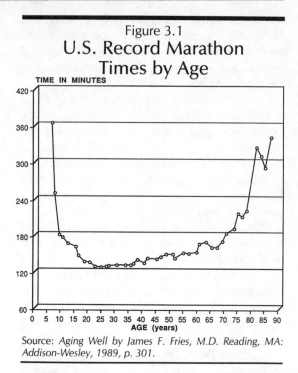

Figure 3.1
U.S. Record Marathon Times by Age

Source: *Aging Well* by James F. Fries, M.D. Reading, MA: Addison-Wesley, 1989, p. 301.

performance" measure, U.S. record marathon times for persons of different ages (see Figure 3.1). It seems clear that performance begins to decline around age 30. This is the inevitable part: The best 30-year-old in the country will always be able to perform better than the best 65-year-old. But now consider this: The current record time for 65-year-olds is lower than the winning marathon time in the 1908 Olympics. In other words, if we could enter today's 65-year-old record holder in the 1908 Olympics, he would beat the world's best—mostly men in their 20s—and do it rather easily. In 1908, it would have been absurd to suggest that a 65-year-old man could win the Olympics. Yet clearly it was possible.

As our expectations have changed, so have our estimates of the inevitable loss of capability that comes with aging. The gap between the peak performance of the young and the old continues to narrow. (Remember that, at age 37, the 1984 Olympic marathon champion was the oldest man in the race.) As training methods improve and more Americans use them, we will see a further narrowing of the gap for peak performance. But

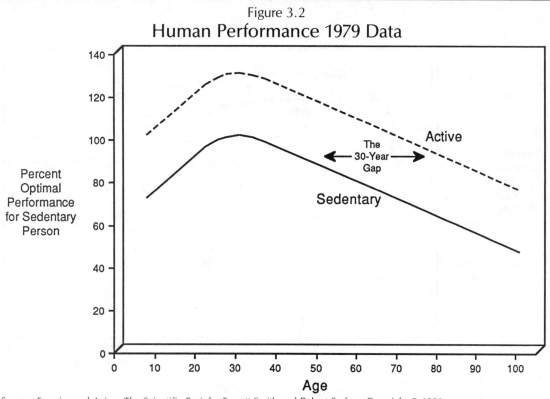

Figure 3.2
Human Performance 1979 Data

Source: *Exercise and Aging: The Scientific Basis* by Everett Smith and Robert Serfass. Copyright © 1981.
By permission of Enslow Publishers.

there will always be a gap, and there will always be a loss due to aging.

The Impact of Personal Health Promotion on Aging

Numerous studies have examined our ability to influence a wide variety of human-performance measures, both mental and physical, as we become older. Their results can be summarized in two curves that compare human performance for active and sedentary people (see Figure 3.2). This sometimes is referred to as the Euro-American curve, because studies on both sides of the Atlantic were used in its derivation. Simply put, for a wide variety of physical, physiologic and mental measures of human performance, there is a pattern of improvement until about age 30, followed by a continuing slow decline. However, while both active and sedentary people show curves with similar shapes, the

active person shows approximately a 25 percent increase in ability over a sedentary person. This difference is fairly constant at all ages.

This difference can be described another way: For any level of performance, there is a 30-year gap in the ages of active and sedentary people. That is, an active person has the performance characteristics of a sedentary person who is 30 years younger.

The 30-year gap is only a generalization, derived from many measures of human performance. Yet the same difference was detected in one of the most famous health studies of our time, the Alameda Study, in which Drs. Breslow and Belloc studied the impact of seven simple health habits—no smoking, exercise, normal weight, alcohol in moderation, eight hours of sleep, breakfast every day, and three meals a day—on life expectancy and health status (see Chapter 2). The researchers also

Figure 3.3
Human Performance

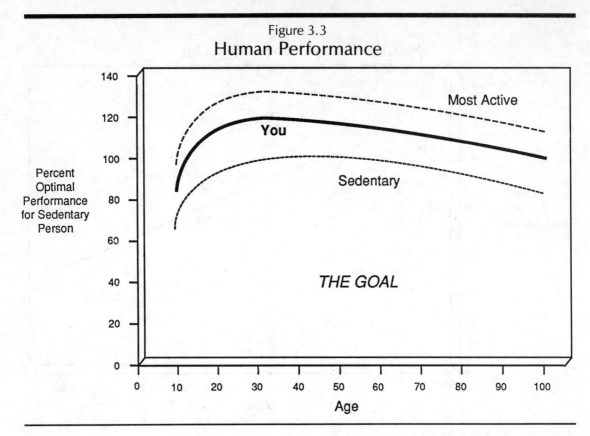

measured sick days and hospitalizations, and found a 30-year difference in health status between men who practiced six or seven of the good health habits and those who practiced no more than three. In other words, men who practiced the good health habits appeared to be as healthy as persons 30 years younger who do not.

Personal Best

Your goal should be to close the 30-year gap by reactivating any mental or physical function that you have been neglecting. When you do this, two miraculous things will happen:

- Your performance graph will shift toward that of the active people.
- Your performance will decline at a slower rate. This decreases the slope of the curve and flattens it out (see Figure 3.3).

Here is the miraculous part: Extend the end of your curve until you hit 100 years of age. At that point you will still have 100 percent of the optimal performance for the sedentary person at age 30. Voila! The 100-by-100 life!

Is this goal too ambitious? Perhaps. But clearly it is not impossible. I will even hazard a prediction: By the year 2001, many Americans will have lopped 15 years off the 30-year gap. In that year, these 75- to 80-year-olds will be as healthy and productive as 60- to 65-year-olds were in 1979.

Everything Can't Be Prevented

Prevention is powerful, but not all-powerful. While some diseases, such as lung cancer, can be avoided through changes in lifestyle and environment, at least part of the risk of many diseases is beyond our control. For example, you may inherit a tendency to develop diabetes or heart disease that can be modified by lifestyle changes but not completely eliminated. And, of course, there are many diseases for which no preventive measures are known. Table 3.9 lists some of these. We are still baffled as to what causes most of these diseases.

Table 3.9
Some Diseases with No Known Preventive Measures

Alzheimer's disease
Crohn's disease
Multiple sclerosis
Parkinson's disease
Rheumatoid arthritis
Systemic lupus erythematosus

We must be careful to take responsibility only for the things that we can control. People who believe strongly in prevention sometimes seem to be "blaming the victim," as if having a medical problem is a person's fault. This is not true. It's harmful, especially when you are the victim and you blame yourself.

Is It Hard to Get an "A" in Prevention?

Not as hard as you think. Undoubtedly, you have already gotten started in some areas, so you now have to focus only on a few. Odds are that you are not a smoker. Your immunizations are probably up to date; if not, one trip to the health department or your doctor's office will probably do the trick. Most likely, you don't need exotic environmental measures, such as mosquito control, and controlling your personal environment is largely a matter of common sense. In Chapter 7 we simplify good nutrition to the point that you may even be disappointed. An exercise program will go a long way toward controlling body fat. And you would want to pursue healthy mind–body interactions even if you didn't know their benefit, because they make you feel good. So if you don't go for an "A" in prevention, you must be afraid of either too much energy, satisfaction or fun, because it isn't too much work.

THE PROMISE AND PROBLEMS OF SCREENING

THE PROMISE

No one likes to think about, much less try to manage, a disease for which nothing can be done. Unfortunately, examples of such problems abound. Once cancer has spread, surgery or radiation therapy may make no sense; chemotherapy may be difficult and offer little. Once a stroke leaves someone paralyzed and unable to speak, little is gained by controlling blood pressure. Once a heart attack destroys heart muscle, no treatment will restore it.

When faced with these unpleasant truths, it is natural to hope that treatment might be effective if begun early in the disease's course. This would require detecting the disease in its *asymptomatic* phase, or before it caused any symptoms. Testing to detect asymptomatic diseases, better known as screening, is sometimes possible, as in the cases of high blood pressure, breast cancer and cervical cancer. But there are only a few such diseases—not nearly as many as you may have believed. And our desire to detect disease early is usually frustrated by problems that exist in the screening process itself.

THE PROBLEMS

The World Health Organization has adopted requirements for screening that have been accepted the world over. According to these guidelines, screening can only be worthwhile if these criteria are met:

- The disease must have a significant effect on the quality or length of life.
- Acceptable methods of treatment must be available.
- The disease must have an asymptomatic (symptom-free) phase during which detection and treatment greatly reduce disability and/or death.
- Treatment in the asymptomatic phase must be more effective than delaying treatment until symptoms appear.

- Tests that detect the condition in the asymptomatic phase must not be too costly.
- The condition must be common enough to justify the cost of screening.

What happens when we apply these standards to various screening tests? A few tests must be rejected because they are simply too dangerous or costly. A few more must be avoided because nothing seems to be lost by waiting for signs or symptoms to appear. By far the greatest number of proposed tests are rejected because they are not reliable when used for screening. Physicians and lay people alike often have trouble accepting this central fact: A test may be quite useful in diagnosing a disease in a patient *with* signs and symptoms but totally worthless in a patient *without* signs and symptoms.

We Americans do not like the idea that screening tests may not be a good thing. We like high-tech medicine, and we like the doctors who like tests. Several studies show that the number of tests ordered is most important in how we rate physicians. Doctors who order the most tests are given the highest compliment: They are called "thorough." (They are also prosperous.) However, most tests should not be used for screening. Here's why.

A laboratory test may be classified as to its sensitivity, specificity and predictive value.

Sensitivity refers to the test's ability to detect disease when it is present. In other words, sensitivity refers to the chance that the test will detect a disease that you have. A sensitivity of 95 percent is quite good, for it means that there is a 95 percent chance that the test will be positive if you have the disease. Put another way, if 100 people have the disease, the test will be positive in 95. In the other five, the test will be negative; these are *false negatives*, in which the disease will be missed.

Specificity refers to the test's ability to distinguish between people who have the disease and people who do not. A test will not be much good if it is often positive in those who do not have the disease as well as in those who do. Specificity can be defined as the chance that the test will be *negative* if you do *not* have the disease. Again, 95 percent would be an excellent specificity—it means that if you do not have the disease, there is a 95-percent chance that the test will be negative. Of 100 persons who do not have the disease, 95 will have negative tests. But five of every 100 persons without the disease will have a positive test. These are *false positives*, and they are important to keep tabs on, because they mean that the test shows there is disease when actually there is none.

Although sensitivity and specificity are important, they are not the most useful measures of a test's accuracy.

Predictive value is the real payoff of a laboratory test. What you (and your doctor) really want to know about any test is how accurately it will indicate the presence or absence of a disease when it is *not* known if you have it. *Negative predictive value* is the chance that a negative test means that you do not have the disease. *Positive predictive value* is the chance that a positive test means that you actually have the disease. For most screening tests, positive predictive value is much more of a problem than negative predictive value. For these tests, if your result is negative, there is a pretty good chance that you do *not* have the disease. Positive results are much less reliable. More often than not, a positive test is a false positive—a positive occurring although you do *not* have the disease. For this reason and for others, we will focus on positive predictive value.

To understand the importance of positive predictive value, imagine this hypothetical situation: A new test has been devised to detect brain tumors. If the test is negative, then nothing further will be done. But if the test is positive, you must have brain surgery to look for this cancer. The operation may kill or cripple you even if no cancer is found. The positive predictive value of this test is very important, because the last thing you want is to have this operation needlessly.

In order to determine positive predictive value, you must know the *prevalence* of a disease, or how many people in the group tested have the disease. You must also know the sensitivity and specificity of the laboratory test used to detect it.

Figure 4.1
How a Good Test Went Bad

100,000 individuals

10 with brain tumors
$\times$ .95 (sensitivity)
9.5 = ▶ 10 *true positives*

99,990 without brain tumors
$\times$ .05 (false positive rate)
4,999.5 = ▶ 5,000 *false positives*

$$\frac{\text{Predictive}}{\text{Value}} = \frac{\text{true positives}}{\text{total positives}} = \frac{10}{5,000 \text{ false positives} + 10 \text{ true positives}}$$

$= \dfrac{10}{5010}$ = .2% of positives are true positives, i.e., a 1 in 500 chance your positive is a true positive

Explanation:

In our example, we stated that brain tumors occur in roughly 10 out of every 100,000 persons. Let's assume that we test exactly 100,000 persons and there are exactly 10 people with brain tumors. Dealing with the people who have brain tumors first, we said that the sensitivity (the probability that the test will be positive when the disease is present) was 95 percent. On average, we would expect that 9.5 of the 10 persons with brain tumors would have a positive test. Let's be generous and round this off to 10, and credit the test with finding all 10 people with brain tumors.

Where we get into trouble is with the 99,990 people without brain tumors. We said that the specificity (the probability that the test will be negative when the disease is absent) was also 95 percent. But this means that 5 percent (1.00 minus .95) of the results in people without tumors will be false positives. Multiplying .05 times 99,990 gives us about 5,000 false-positive results. Comparing the 10 true positives with the 5,000 false-positives gives this horrifying result: There is a 0.2 percent chance that a positive test is a true positive—the positive predictive value is 0.2 percent. If you have the operation on the basis of a positive test, the odds are about 500-to-1 against the operation being necessary.

Let us assume that the test for brain tumors has excellent sensitivity and specificity, each at 95 percent. Brain tumors occur in roughly 10 out of every 100,000 persons. Now take a moment to figure out the predictive value of this test: If your test is positive, what are the chances that you actually have a brain tumor and that this dangerous operation will be worthwhile? If you're not good at figuring, then just take a guess based on your general feelings about the accuracy of laboratory tests.

If you came up with an answer of 0.2 percent, then you are both right and very unusual. Only one out of every 500 persons with a positive test would, in fact, have a brain tumor (see Figure 4.1). If surgery were done based on this test, then for every operation on a person with a brain tumor

there would be 500 on people without tumors. Therefore, in this example, the odds are 500-to-1 against the operation being necessary if you have a positive test. If the chance of dying from the operation were 1 in 10 (10 percent), then 51 people would die in order for 10 people with tumors to have the surgery. (One person with a tumor would die from the operation.)

Predictive value is very sensitive to prevalence—the probability that the disease is present. If you have the signs and symptoms of an illness, then a laboratory test may help to confirm or rule out the diagnosis, because these signs and symptoms make it more likely that you have the disease. For example, if there is a 50/50 chance that you have a disease because you have certain signs

Table 4.1
Effect of Occurrence on Predictive Value

Health Problem	Occurrence per 100,000	Predictive Value (%)
Smoking	35,000	91
Obesity	25,000	86
Hypertension (high blood pressure)	15,000	77
Alcoholism	4,200	45
Coronary artery disease (ischemic heart disease)	2,800	35
Diabetes (all types)	1,270	20
Glaucoma	360	6.4
Gonorrhea	285	5.2
Tuberculosis	80	1.5
Cancer of the breast	73*	1.4
Cancer of the colon and rectum	45	.85
Lung cancer	26	.49
Syphilis	11	.20
Bladder cancer	7	.14

*Occurrence is per 100,000 women.

Figure 4.2
False Positives in AIDS Testing
Percentage of Positive Test Results Likely to Be False Positive

Group	Ideal Testing Quality	Actual Testing Quality
High Risk (Urban gays, I.V. drug users)	0.04%	0.79%
Texas Marriage License Applicants	0.6	9.6
Males in Military	3.0	34.9
Females in Military	7.6	59.3
U.S. Blood Donors	11.1	69.0
Peoria, Ill., Blood Donors	33.3	89.9

Conclusion: The likelihood of a false-positive test result is greatest in groups with a low prevalence of AIDS infection.

Source: Office of Technology Assessment

and symptoms, and the test for that disease has a sensitivity and specificity of 95 percent, then both the positive and negative predictive value of the test is 95 percent. In other words, 95 percent of persons with a positive test will have the disease and 95 percent with negative tests will not have the disease. *Tests have most value when the chances are good that the disease is present. They are least useful when there is only a small chance, as is nearly always the case in screening programs.* Table 4.1 relates the occurrence of several major health problems to the positive predictive value of an excellent test. *The tests are hypothetical,* and each is given a sensitivity and specificity of 95 percent.

Unfortunately, few screening tests have such excellent sensitivity and specificity. Note that diagnosing three of the most common health problems (smoking, obesity and alcoholism) requires no laboratory test. Clearly, the odds are stacked against most screening simply because most diseases are not likely to be present when there are no symptoms.

The prevalence of a disease may be different in different groups, of course. This affects the predictive value and, therefore, the number of false positives. Figure 4.2 shows how the prevalence of AIDS affects the false positives in AIDS testing when the tests are done perfectly (Ideal Testing Quality) and how the problem is made worse because tests are not done perfectly in the real world (Actual Testing Quality). As you can see, where the prevalence is low (Peoria), almost all the positive tests are false positives.

Problems with false positives are worse when more tests are used. The more tests that are done, the more likely it is that a false positive will occur because each test will have the false-positive problem mentioned above. For example, if there are 25 tests and each has a specificity of 95 percent, your chance of having a false-positive result is about 75 percent. So even if you are perfectly normal, the chance that you can have an abnormal result is about three out of four.

Twenty-five tests may seem like a lot, but many executive physicals and screening programs approach this number and some exceed it. It is common to have 15 to 20 tests in a so-called blood chemistry panel alone (see Chapter 15). It is ironic that many of us have executive physicals or undergo batteries of tests in order to gain peace of mind. We have seen how the risk of false positives makes this a bad bet. When you are tempted to have a thorough physical or undergo a battery of tests, keep in mind that one inappropriate screening test is bad, but several are worse.

But what if you have already undergone a screening program containing inappropriate tests (usually a blood chemistry panel) and come up with a positive? A recent study confirms what many doctors have advised for some time.

1. The best thing to do is to ignore the result.
2. The next best thing is to repeat the test in hope that the second result will be normal.
3. The worst thing to do is to accept the test result as correct and order other tests or procedures to investigate the abnormality.

FOOLING OURSELVES

If so many screening tests are unreliable, why do we hear so much about them? Probably the most important reason is that we really want to do something about diseases that are hard to treat. Also, many medical education programs spend little or no time on screening, so that its problems simply are not known to many physicians. Finally, to conduct good scientific studies of screening, researchers must overcome several pitfalls. The list usually includes the following:

• **Lead time bias.** Screening may simply hasten the time of diagnosis without postponing the time of death. Lead time is an artificial increase in survival time that results from earlier-than-usual detection of disease rather than real prolonging of life.

• **Length bias.** A rapidly progressing disease, such as a fast-growing cancer, is more likely to create symptoms that cause it to be discovered. A slowly developing disease, such as a slow-growing cancer, takes longer to create symptoms. For this reason, it has a much greater chance of being detected through screening. Thus, screening may appear to increase the length of survival when it is simply detecting a slow-growing disease. Survival time will seem longer simply because of the slow growth even if treatment is not effective.

• **Patient selection bias.** People may seek screening because they have a greater-than-average risk of a certain disease. They may have a family history of the problem, its beginning symptoms or some other risk factor. Thus, screening may appear to de-

Figure 4.3

Cancer Screening/Survival Time Line

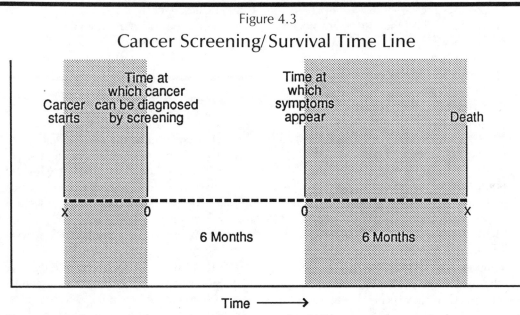

Without screening, survival appears to be six months. With screening, survival appears to be 12 months. But, treatment was of no help. The "increase" in survival is an illusion.

tect problems more effectively in these people than it would if it were applied to everyone.

Of all of these problems, lead time bias is the most important to understand, because it affects the judgment that you must make about the value of screening. To illustrate, let us assume there is a cancer that is always fatal six months after symptoms appear. Assume, too, that treatment is useless no matter when it is applied. Now suppose we devised a test that would detect this cancer six months before it caused symptoms. For those whose cancer was detected by screening, this is the time at which diagnosis would be made; otherwise, the diagnosis would be made when symptoms arose (see Figure 4.3). If the results of this screening program were reported, it would be said that patients whose cancer was detected by screening lived one year after diagnosis, while those diagnosed on the basis of symptoms alone survived only six months. It would seem logical to conclude that the combination of screening and treatment improved survival by six months. *But treatment was*

useless. We didn't add six months to the patient's life expectancy, we simply added six months to the time in which the cancer was known to exist.

Some would say that we robbed the patient of the last six months of normal life by telling him or her about the cancer six months earlier than he or she would have known otherwise. Is it a good thing to tell people that they have a disease if there is nothing to be done about it? You will have to form your own answer to this. And if nothing is lost by waiting for symptoms before starting treatment, there seems to be little point in undergoing costly and risky screening.

So What To Do?

Chapter 15 of this book discusses the most frequently advocated screening tests. The conclusions reached in that chapter can be summed up as follows:

A⁺ **A⁺**bsolutely recommended. As it turns out, there is only one test that receives the highest grade because it meets all of our criteria.

Blood pressure

A **A**cceptable. While these tests are not perfect, they are widely considered to be among the best.

Cholesterol (a special case)
Mammography
Pap smear
Physician examination of breasts

B **B**e selective. Generally speaking, these tests are not for everyone and should be used only when there is a higher-than-normal risk of the problem.

AIDS test
Gonorrhea, syphilis and chlamydia tests
Tuberculin skin tests

C **C**aution. These tests are borderline. They are low priority because it is uncertain whether their benefits outweigh their risks.

Breast self-examination
Dental examination
Hearing and vision tests
Occult blood in stool
Ophthalmoscopy and tonometry for glaucoma
Physical examination
Rectal examination
Sigmoidoscopy
Testicular self-examination

D **D**on't seek these. While these tests are often touted as part of a good "check-up," they create far more mischief than benefit.

Blood cell counts (including hematocrit, hemoglobin and complete blood count)
Blood chemistries (tests for liver or kidney function, gout, etc.)
Blood glucose
Urinalysis

F **F**orget these. Primarily because of problems with false positives, these pose a real threat to your health and should not be used for screening.

Carotid sonogram

Chest X-ray
Electrocardiogram, resting
Exercise stress test
Pulmonary (lung) function tests

Good Intentions, Bad Result

As an intern, I witnessed the sad end to what started out as the good intentions of doing a thorough annual physical. The patient was a well-known physicist who had immigrated from an area of China in which cancer of the mouth and nasal sinuses was quite common. Unfortunately, the patient's very active gag reflex prevented the physician from getting a good look at these areas, so it was decided that he should be placed under anesthesia in order to complete the examination. The patient was quite afraid of being put to sleep, so his blood pressure, which had been normal, became elevated. It was then decided that the high blood pressure should be investigated with an X-ray of the kidneys (intravenous pyelography). The patient had a reaction to a medicine used in this test, suffered cardiac arrest and died.

Each examination and test was justified as "playing it safe." Indeed, had this tragic event not occurred, everyone involved—physicians, patient, patient's family—would have agreed that they had been playing it safe and congratulated the doctor on being thorough. The truth is that none of them attempted to balance the benefits and risks of these procedures.

THE LAST-DITCH DEFENSE

We often hear screening tests defended because, "Even if they do no good, they do no harm." This is not true. Screening tests harm you in at least four ways:

1. The risk of false-positive test results is high. False positives expose you to the hazards of further testing and unnecessary treatment, and label you as "dis-

eased" when you are not. Moreover, the attempt to prove that an abnormal result is just a false positive may be costly, inconvenient and dangerous. Investigations of false-positive results have sometimes ended in disability or death.

2. Tests have inherent dangers. There really is radiation in those X-rays and, once in a great while, people really do have heart attacks during uncomfortable, stressful tests.

3. Screening programs may have indirect side effects. For example, Dr. Abraham Bergman studied the effects of screening programs for heart disease and sickle-cell anemia in children. In both cases, many of these children and their families acted as if the child had a disease when, in fact, he or she did not. For example, parents sometimes acted as if a harmless heart murmur (these are common in children) meant heart disease. These programs *created* more disease and disability than they detected.

4. Money spent on the useless cannot be spent on the useful. The cost of screening varies greatly, from $450 to $1,000 or more for the "executive physical" to about 75 cents for a single test of the stool for hidden blood. As a rule of thumb, the more expensive the test, the less likely it is to be worthwhile. Beware of those who try to get around this by saying that if many tests are done, the cost per test will decrease. If the test is useless, then doing one is bad, but doing many is worse.

The bottom line is that only a few screening tests are worthwhile. They do not need to be done often and they are not costly. Obtain the benefit of these tests by making them part of your LifePlan. And just as important, avoid tests that do more harm than good.

MEDICAL CARE: The Double-Edged Sword

*M*edical care cures, kills and costs. It can make you feel better, or make you feel worse. It can be the greatest bargain of your life, or it can bring financial disaster. So how can you win? Learn to play the game.

- **Know the rules**. You are the key decision maker about medical care, even though it may seem as if the doctor is in charge. Legally and ethically, no medical care can be given unless you give your *informed consent*. This means that you must choose among the treatment options that your physician presents to you.

- **Know the odds**. To make a good choice, you must balance the benefits of each option against its risks. Cost is important, too, but not as important as making sure that the benefit-versus-risk decision makes sense.

- **Play with a full deck**. You need to understand the benefits, risks and costs of all the options before you can make a good choice. Only you can determine how much the benefits are to be valued and the risks are to be feared.

DRUGS

Benefits

Drugs are medicine's most important tools. The last 60 years have seen the development of drugs that can treat a wide variety of disorders. These drugs have revolutionized the practice of medicine. Previously, there were perhaps a half-dozen drugs that could be prescribed and expected to work. This is not to say that other drugs were not used. On the contrary, useless and often dangerous concoctions abounded. Most were sold directly to customers who used them at their own risk. The risk was great, because drug testing was not required, nor were there any regulations to protect against contamination. A number of catastrophes, such as the death of 10 children due to contaminated tetanus toxoid vaccine, led to the demand that drugs be tested and their manufacture regulated.

In 1927, the Food and Drug Administration (FDA) became a separate agency empowered to oversee the testing of drugs. Most of this testing concerned new drugs, so that drugs in use before 1927 were exempt from many of the provisions established at that time. More importantly, the testing begun at this time was concerned with the *safety* of a drug, not whether it was *effective*. It was not until 1962, 35 years later, that the effectiveness of drugs became part of the FDA's concern.

We now have reached a point where you can be fairly sure that if the FDA has approved a drug as "effective" for a certain condition, the drug will most likely help at least some people with that problem. Note that effective in this case does not mean completely effective, nor does it mean that everyone will experience relief. A drug's effective-

AN AMERICAN MYTH: It is always vital to see the doctor as soon as a problem develops so that the disease may be treated early.

There is no question that this would make sense *if* we could easily diagnose and cure most diseases. We cannot. For most diseases, we lack either the ability to make an early diagnosis, an effective treatment or both.

Fortunately, with most illnesses your body will eventually cure itself. This is true for common viral problems, such as colds and the flu, a multitude of minor muscle pulls, strains and sprains, as well as a whole host of skin rashes that come and go on their own. (With regard to the latter, remember this piece of medical wisdom: "Only God can make a tree, but almost anything can make a rash.") The symptoms caused by these self-limited diseases can usually be treated without a visit to the doctor.

Also in your favor is the fact that many diseases can wait to be treated without causing irreparable harm. The allowable waiting period depends on the problem, but generally you have longer than you think. For example, even if there is a broken bone associated with that ankle sprain, you will not cause lasting damage if you don't get treated within the first few minutes or hours—if you know how to take care of yourself. On a much different scale, tuberculosis may stay hidden within the body for months or years before it causes problems. Even though we have a skin test (Tine or Purified Protein Derivative) to alert us to the possibility of tuberculosis, the actual diagnosis is often quite difficult. Therefore, the diagnosis may not be made until months or even years after the skin test turned positive. (Many people with positive skin tests never develop tuberculosis as far as we know.) Even with all these delays, we are able to treat tuberculosis effectively. It is very uncommon for this disease to have the severe effects that were so frequent before the turn of the century.

Finally, there are illnesses that can be neither cured nor controlled with treatment. In truth, the doctor has little to offer you if that cough is due to lung cancer. On the other hand, you could have lowered your chance of lung cancer to near zero by not smoking. Yet we find the notion of cure so desirable and changing our behavior so difficult that we deceive ourselves into thinking that everything would be curable if we could only catch it early enough. This can cost you money but, more importantly, it may cost you a chance to save your life.

So you, the key decision maker in health, have another decision to make. You can despair over the limits of medicine, or you can rejoice over the body's enormous power to make things right. Is there really any choice?

ness depends on the drug itself, the problem and the individual. For example, antibiotics are almost always prescribed for urinary tract (bladder) infections; these drugs are effective in that they will kill or retard the growth of the bacteria that cause these infections. However, studies have shown that antibiotics are *not* necessary to cure these infections. Simple measures, such as increasing fluid intake, may be more important for relief and recovery.

An effective drug does not always cure, either. This is usually the case with chronic diseases, such as arthritis. There are more than a dozen nonsteroidal anti-inflammatory drugs (NSAIDs) that are approved as effective for arthritis. All of them will relieve some pain and stiffness in many patients, but none will cure or stop the progress of the disease.

We are fortunate to have many effective drugs, and the benefit they offer can be very great. At the same time, you need to decide what effectiveness means for you each time that you consider taking a medicine. Your physician is the primary source of this information. Your pharmacist and various publications can provide information on side effects and drug interactions, but they are less apt to offer a judgment on how effective the drug is likely to be in your case.

Risks

Although FDA approval is often said to mean that the drug is "safe and effective," there is no drug that is completely safe. Risks vary greatly among drugs and must be weighed against the benefits. Thus, although it may be acceptable for an anti-cancer drug to have a high risk of serious side effects, this is not acceptable for something that treats athlete's foot.

There are three basic types of drug risks. The first consists of those effects directly due to the chemical itself, which are related to the amount taken. Every drug is a potential poison, and at some point the harmful effects of the chemical involved begin to outweigh its benefits. For example, aspirin irritates the stomach lining enough to cause some blood loss, but for most people this is not much of a problem unless the amount of aspirin taken is large.

The second type of risk is that of allergy. This is especially important, because allergic reactions are often unpredictable, and they can be severe even though only a small amount of drug has been taken.

Finally, there are several indirect or delayed side effects. For example, the more that antibiotics are used, the more likely it is that bacteria will become resistant to them. Infections due to resistant bacteria may be quite severe and tough to treat. Thus, treating a minor respiratory infection with penicillin runs the slight risk of helping to create a second infection (sometimes referred to as "superinfection") with bacteria resistant to penicillin. Superinfections are often severe and may be life-threatening. Resistant bacteria may also be passed from person to person; this is most likely to happen in the hospital and is a major hazard of hospitalization.

Drugs carry major risks. Consider the following:

- Dr. Leighton Cluff and his associates at Johns Hopkins Hospital followed 714 patients admitted to general medical beds. Five percent of these admissions were for drug reactions. The team found that 122 patients suffered 184 drug reactions while in the hospital. Six patients died from drug-related problems.
- A British survey found that 193 out of 731 patients (26 percent) admitted to a general medical hospital suffered harmful effects of drug therapy. Seventeen of the 67 deaths (25 percent) that occurred among these patients were due to drug reactions.
- Most drug reactions relate directly to the drug's chemical effect; only a small percentage (less than 10 percent) are due to drug allergy.
- It has been estimated that each drug prescribed has a 50 percent to 75 percent chance of being taken at the wrong time or in the wrong dosage, or is the wrong drug in the first place.

Drugs are mixed blessings. Those used most often (tranquilizers, decongestants, antihistamines and the like) are of uncertain value for many patients who take them. Those that can provide the greatest benefit can often cause great harm as well. They all present some risk to your health. Give them the respect they deserve.

Costs

While drugs account for only about 10 percent of the total amount spent on health care in the United States, they are far from cheap—as anyone who has had a prescription filled recently knows. There are three major factors that determine the price you pay for drugs:

1. **The availability of a generic drug.** As long as a drug is under patent, there are no generic versions available. Only one company can manufacture that drug. The price for such a "brand name" drug tends to be whatever the market will bear. Once the patent has expired and generics are available, there is competition. Prices for the generics are usually much lower than for the original brand.

2. **Obtaining a generic version.** Asking your physician to prescribe a generic version of the drug is always wise; however, for some drugs (digitalis, tricyclic antidepressants, thyroid medications and prednisone) the generic versions do not always deliver the same amount of drug as the original brand. This could result in less benefit or more risk of side effects. Therefore, do not be offended if your physician prefers to prescribe a brand-name product. Be sure that it is for this reason, not just because the generic version has been overlooked.

But even if your physician prescribes by brand name when a generic would be just as good, you may still be able to obtain the generic. All states now require physicians to indicate whether or not a generic can be substituted for a brand-name drug. However, there are impor-

tant differences in the way that this is done. In some states, the pharmacist can substitute a generic for a brand-name drug unless the physician indicates that this *cannot* be done. In other states, the physician must indicate that this *can* be done. This difference can have a great impact on the use of generic drugs.

Finally, even if your physician OKs a generic drug, the pharmacist need not provide one. The physician can make it possible to obtain the generic, but cannot guarantee it.

3. **The pricing policy of the pharmacy.** Studies show that the price of one drug may vary greatly between pharmacies in the same general area. Often prices are highest in the inner city and lowest in the suburbs. You are likely to find the best prices in areas where there is real competition between pharmacies. In any event, old-fashioned shopping by telephone to find the lowest price is wise. If you have a chronic disease that creates an ongoing need for medication, compare the prices of mail-order pharmacy programs available through some insurance companies, health care organizations, or membership organizations such as the American Association of Retired Persons.

SURGERY

Benefits

There can be little doubt that modern surgery can relieve pain, restore function and save lives. Cataract operations give sight to thousands who have become nearly blind. Artificial joints relieve pain and restore motion for arthritis sufferers. Heart operations may stop the crippling pain of angina when medicines no longer work. Emergency surgery saves the lives of accident victims.

Today, surgery is more effective than ever before. However, there is no agency like the FDA to approve operations or investigate their value and safety. In fact, there is no law stating that operations must be evaluated before they are used. We have only the commitment of physicians and the threat of lawsuits to encourage such evaluation. As a result, we know a good deal less about the benefits, risks and costs of surgery than we do about drugs. Doing controlled, scientific studies is much more difficult with surgery than with drugs, but avoiding such studies leads to an unacceptable situation—performing operations with unknown benefits, high risks and costs.

The history of surgery to relieve heart pain (angina) illustrates this point. Before coronary artery bypass grafting (CABG) became the rage, at least six operations were promoted for the relief of angina. All were claimed to relieve pain in 60 percent to 80 percent of patients. One of the most popular was internal mammary artery ligation. In this operation, two arteries in the chest wall were tied off so that more blood would flow into the blood vessels of the heart. This was a fairly simple and safe procedure that did not even require putting the patient to sleep. Originated in Italy, this operation spread like wildfire around the globe because it seemed safe, simple and effective. However, some American physicians doubted its value, and finally two controlled studies were performed. In each, one group of patients received the entire operation while a second group received a sham operation, in which the arteries were not actually tied off. In one study, 34 percent of the patients who had the entire operation and 42 percent of those who had the sham operation all reported improvement. In the second study, 10 of 13 patients who had the real procedure reported great improvement in their angina, but so did all five who had the sham operation. Thus, internal mammary artery ligation turned out to be nothing more than proof of the power in *believing* that surgery will help, or the power of surgery as a placebo.

Unfortunately, most operations are not as simple and safe as internal mammary artery ligation. This makes it harder to do a sham operation. But it also means that the harm done if the surgery is worthless is much greater. There have not been adequate studies of most surgical procedures. As a result, they have not been shown to be clearly good or bad. But all have risks and costs.

Here are a few points to ponder with respect to surgery:

- Dr. Robert H. Brook and his colleagues at the Rand Corporation and UCLA conducted a study of carotid endarterectomy (surgery to remove clotting from the carotid artery). They concluded that only 35 percent of patients had this risky surgery for appropriate reasons, 32 percent had it for questionable reasons, and 32 percent had it for the wrong reasons. From 1971 to 1985, the number of carotid endarterectomies performed yearly in the United States rose from 15,000 to 107,000. About 12 percent of the people have a severe stroke or heart attack, or die while undergoing this operation.

- Dr. Brook's research group performed a similar study of CABG and found that 56 percent of these operations were performed for appropriate reasons, 30 percent for questionable reasons, and 14 percent for the wrong reasons. In 1985 about 200,000 CABG procedures were performed in the United States, double the number performed in 1980.

- Caesarean sections increased from 5.5 percent of all births in 1972 to 24.4 percent in 1987. In 1988, Hialeah Hospital in Florida had the highest Caesarean-section rate in the country, 53.1 percent. Yet the best information suggests that the Caesarean rate should not exceed 12 percent.

- One study of hernia operations found that the procedure may increase the quality of life by avoiding the need for a truss (a supportive device worn to prevent enlargement of a hernia). But the procedure may decrease life expectancy, because the risk of death from the operation is greater than that from the hernia.

- A Seattle study revealed that less than one-third of tonsillectomies and adenoidectomies were performed for valid reasons. This means that there could be more than

500,000 needless operations of this type performed in the United States each year, with 25 children dying as a result.

- The reasons gynecologists give for doing hysterectomies range from relieving low back pain to treating cancer of the uterus. Again, there are no studies that demonstrate the value of hysterectomy, but there are conditions for which the best physicians would accept it as appropriate. Even so, it is likely that many hysterectomies are unnecessary. For example, the College of Physicians and Surgeons of Saskatchewan (Canada) found that, in some hospitals, up to 59 percent of hysterectomies were unjustified according to their criteria. For all of the hospitals together, about one-fourth of hysterectomies were unjustified. The rates for hysterectomy in the United States and Canada are twice that for Great Britain, where the financial incentive to operate is much lower.

Risks

Most people know that surgery is risky. Death rates for various operations are one sign of the risk involved, but they say nothing about the risk of disability or pain. For example, some operations offer little risk of death but a great risk of losing a limb or an eye, or of severe pain. Nevertheless, death rates are the best information we have on the risks of surgery. Table 5.1 lists death rates for some common operations.

Costs

The exact cost of all surgery is not known. In 1988, total spending for health care in the United States was about $560 billion. Perhaps 40 percent of that amount ($224 billion) was directly related to surgery. This estimate does not include the costs of disability or days lost from work. As anyone who has had surgery knows, the cost of a single operation is astounding. Table 5.2 shows some of these costs.

The reasons for these high costs are many, and include the way most hospitals are organized

---

Table 5.1
Death Rates for Common Surgical Procedures

Procedure	Deaths per 100,000 Procedures
Coronary artery bypass grafting	1,500
Cholecystectomy (gallbladder removal)	400
Radical mastectomy	400
Appendectomy	352
Tonsillectomy	5
All abortions	3.9
Abortions within the first three months of pregnancy	1.7

For comparison:
   Death rate for pregnancy and childbirth: 14.8 per 100,000 live births
   Death rate for general anesthesia (gas) *without* surgery: 2 per 100,000 procedures
   Death rate for cardiac catheterization and coronary angiography: 140 per 100,000 procedures

Source: Estimates based on information from various U.S. Government sources.

Table 5.2
Average Charges for Some Operations

Coronary artery bypass grafting	$30,500
Prostatectomy	10,400
Gallbladder removal	5,500
Cataract removal	5,400
Caesarean section	5,300
Appendectomy	5,090
Hernia repair	3,200

Charges are for the U.S. in 1986.
Source: *Statistical Bulletin*, Metropolitan Life Insurance Co., Vols. 67-70.

and how we pay for surgery. In addition, there is a financial incentive for both hospitals and surgeons to do more surgery rather than less. The bulk of most hospitals' income depends on the amount of surgery that is performed. Also, surgeons earn a good deal more than most non-surgeon physicians, including family practitioners, pediatricians and internists.

X-RAYS

Benefits

X-rays can be a very useful tool, and were one of the greatest advances in medicine. It is impossible to imagine modern diagnosis without them. X-rays are used to examine almost every portion of the body, and to investigate everything from arthritis to angina, and from head injuries to toe pain.

However, there is growing evidence that we have not been as accurate in determining the benefit of X-rays as we would like.

- A University of Washington School of Medicine study revealed that the X-rays of the skull that are routinely ordered following head trauma do not aid in diagnosis and treatment.
- In 120 patients with cough, Stanford University physicians reported that a chest X-ray affected treatment decisions in only two cases.
- Another study followed 495 patients who had X-rays of the upper gastrointestinal tract, often called the "upper GI series." About 70 percent of the X-rays were normal, and the X-rays changed therapy in only 7 percent.

Despite the fact that X-rays are routinely ordered upon hospital admission and as a part of medical and dental exams, their use in this fashion is of no proven value. And, with the exception of mammography, no X-ray has ever been shown to be a useful screening test (see Chapter 15). In general, X-rays are of greatest benefit in serious illnesses when the physician has a specific question in mind. They tend to be of least value when the illness is minor or when they are used as a screening tool.

Risks

It has long been known that X-rays can produce cancer (that they are oncogenic) and mutations in offspring (mutagenic). These effects are related to the amount of radiation in the X-ray and how much of that radiation reaches the ovaries and testes (gonads). It is not known what level of radiation is safe, or even whether there is a safe level. Radiation levels assumed to be safe in the past have proven not to be. For example, at one time many children with large tonsils or adenoids, acne, or ringworm of the scalp were treated with X-rays to these areas. Now, 20 to 30 years later, we are seeing the effects: cancer of the thyroid and mouth.

The best information we have indicates that there is no absolutely safe level and that the effects of radiation tend to add up. Thus, the best policy is to avoid X-rays unless they are necessary. Note also that the amount of radiation in X-rays varies greatly. There is a good deal less radiation involved in an X-ray of a limb for a possible fracture, or even in a single chest X-ray, than there is in a series of X-rays of the upper or lower gastrointestinal tract (upper GI or barium enema).

Costs

X-ray equipment is expensive, and radiologists are well paid. As a result, X-rays themselves are costly. Also, there is a powerful financial incentive to use X-ray facilities in order to recover their cost. X-ray units are usually quite profitable for hospitals as well as for radiologists practicing outside hospitals. The cost of X-rays makes up a large portion of the cost of hospital care and physicians' services.

A very important reason for the increased use of X-rays is the fact that many patients (66 percent in one survey) believe that ordering many X-rays is a sign of an excellent physician. This attitude is reflected in the decisions of courts and juries, who have often viewed the performance of an X-ray as evidence that a physician was conscientious and thorough. This is a major reason why skull X-rays are done for every bump on the head, why every bruised limb gets X-rayed, why every hospitalized patient has a chest X-ray, and so on. The overuse of X-rays is a classic example of patients and physicians overestimating benefits and underestimating risks.

Hospitals

Benefits

Hospitals offer non-surgical services to patients with problems of varying severity who need many different diagnostic procedures and treatments. Thus, evaluating the benefits of hospitalization is not easy. Yet while there are no studies that place a specific value on the hospital's role, the hospital is necessary for the best care of many patients. At the same time, the benefits of the hospital —and of its specialized units in particular—need careful consideration:

- Most Americans regard the coronary care unit (CCU) as necessary for treating persons with heart attacks (myocardial infarction). Yet studies from Great Britain have found that many patients do as well with home care as with CCU care, and that some heart-attack patients (older patients without complications) do better at home.

- Dr. Paul Griner of the University of Rochester found that patients with congestive heart failure did as well on the general medical ward as in the CCU.

- When the CCU first appeared in the 1960s, some people predicted it would prevent up to 50 percent of deaths due to heart attacks. It now appears that the CCU's major effect is to postpone a small number of deaths until after discharge from the hospital. Thus, the CCU's effect on surviving for six months, one year or five years after a heart attack is very small. However, this should not surprise us. Persons who have heart attacks have severe disease, which the CCU does nothing to remedy.

- Like the CCU, the intensive care unit (ICU) is an area of high technology and highly trained personnel. A study of 226 patients admitted to the ICU at the Massachusetts General Hospital yielded these startling results: At the end of one month, 123 patients (54 percent) were dead, 72 were still hospitalized, and 31 were home. One of the 103 survivors had fully recovered. At the end of 12 months, 165 patients (73 percent) were dead, 10 were still hospitalized, and 51 were home. Only 27 (12 percent) of the original 226 patients had fully recovered.

- Using standardized criteria, a series of studies found that most hospitals are used for the wrong reasons 20 percent to 44 percent of the time. This was true for both children and adult patients.

Risks

A study from Yale illustrates the risks associated with hospitalization. It involved 1,014 patients admitted to the university medical service over eight months. All complications and problems were recorded as "episodes." All episodes that were due to human error were *excluded*, so the study only gave information on the risks of excellent hospital care. Here are the results:

- There were 240 episodes in 198 patients.
- 110 episodes were short and subsided without special treatment.
- 82 episodes required significant treatment or prolonged hospitalization.
- 48 episodes were life threatening or contributed to death.
- 16 episodes ended in death. Of these deaths four were reactions to diagnostic procedures (two occurred during barium enemas), six were due to infections acquired in the hospital, four involved reactions to drugs, and two resulted from treatment procedures.

The death rate associated with hospitalization was 1.6 percent. This means that entering the hospital for diagnosis and therapy may be as risky as many major operations.

It is often said that doctors are the worst

patients. Maybe yes and maybe no, but they do avoid the hospital unless there is no other choice. They know that the hospital is a hazardous place. Working there has its risks, but they are nothing like those of being a patient. The hazards that the doctor fears may be hidden to most patients. As you ponder hospitalization, open up your eyes to the *terrible* I's: infection, inactivity, inherent risks and incorrect actions.

Infection

One of the earliest and most important studies of infectious disease found that hospitalization greatly increased the risk of infection. The Hungarian obstetrician Ignaz Semmelweis noted more than 100 years ago that many more mothers died during childbirth in the hospital than during childbirth at home. These deaths were due to childbed fever (puerperal sepsis). He later proved that the risk could be reduced by simply having doctors and nurses wash their hands before and after deliveries.

But the risk could not be completely eliminated by hand washing then, and it hasn't been eliminated today by antibiotics or other modern medical practices. Hospital infections are still a major problem for the following reasons:

1. There are a lot of "bugs" in the hospital. Patients, visitors and staff all bring their own complement of bacteria and viruses into the hospital. And, of course, some patients are admitted because they already have infections. The simple fact is that you have a greater chance of bumping into a new bug in the hospital than in almost any other place.

2. The widespread use of antibiotics in the hospital causes some of the bugs to become very nasty—they become resistant to antibiotics. Infections caused by such bacteria may be hard to treat.

3. Hospital routines expose people to infection. Patients are cared for by a staff that is also caring for others, which means that the spread of infection is a constant threat. Further, routine procedures such

as shots or I.V. therapy often breach the body's first line of defense, the skin.

4. A 1985 study of hospital infections concluded that they are a major threat, and that the biggest problem was *still* getting doctors and nurses to wash their hands!

Hospital staffs know all these risks, of course, and take steps to minimize them. But the risks cannot be eliminated, and some hospitals do a better job of minimizing them than others.

Inactivity

One of the most harmful myths of our time is that rest is good for what ails you. We now know that putting someone to bed as a form of treatment is to be avoided. **The body requires activity to remain healthy**. Hospital routines make it hard to stay active even if you have not been told to stay in bed.

Inactivity creates a number of problems:

1. It raises the risk of infection, especially in the lungs.

2. It robs you of conditioning, making you less able to deal with the stress of hospitalization and any procedures that you may undergo.

3. It contributes to depression and malaise.

Most importantly, a healthy circulatory system requires exercise and activity. Bed rest increases the risk of inflammation within veins (thrombophlebitis), especially in the legs. Thrombophlebitis may cause swelling and severe pain, but its greatest hazard lies in the formation of blood clots that can break free and be carried to the lungs (pulmonary emboli). We now know that pulmonary emboli are fairly common. Small ones may cause few symptoms and are rarely diagnosed. But if the clots are large or there are many of them, they may seriously impede the flow of blood to the lungs and cause severe problems, including death.

You will have to work at being active in the hospital.

1. Walk, walk, walk!

2. Do whatever else (bending, push-ups, etc.) that your condition permits. Stay as active as you can within the limits of your

medical problem. It can save your life.

One final note: Elastic stockings are sometimes used to try to prevent thrombophlebitis and, therefore, pulmonary embolism. They are controversial and, if used improperly, actually may increase the risk of thrombophlebitis. Do not put faith in these stockings. They are no substitute for activity.

Inherent Risks

All of medicine's tools—drugs, X-rays and surgery—carry built-in risks, as you know from reading this chapter. Hospitalization means that more of these tools will be used, and the risks will increase accordingly.

Incorrect Actions

The people who work in hospitals use powerful tools—tools that can hurt as well as help. Sometimes, people make mistakes. You have heard the horror stories—the wrong patient operated on, the wrong leg amputated, the good eye removed, the wrong drug injected. In many of these cases, there is reason to believe that negligence may have played a role. But this is not always so. There are such things as honest mistakes, and the best doctors, nurses and hospital staffs can make them.

Finally, the hospital is infamous for the stress it places on the patient. It is noisy, the food often leaves a lot to be desired, and it comes equipped with roommates whose habits are totally different from yours. Its routine seems strange, as if devised by persons who used to plan schedules for boot camps. Sometimes it seems that the staff is required to barge in when you are trying to sleep and be on the other side of the building when you want them. Here, *many* things go bump in the night.

Costs

Hospital costs are simply incredible. The average charge for a single day in the hospital is well over $700, and the cost of an average hospital stay is well over $5,000. Use of a specialized unit, such as the ICU or CCU will just about double the charge. In 1988, Americans spent about $224 billion on hospital care, or about $1,000 for every man, woman and child in the country. Even with

---

The Peculiar Way We Use Medical Care

- In one study, physicians judged that only 17 percent of patients' visits were for serious problems while almost 50 percent were for problems that were not serious at all.
- The most common reasons for visiting the physician are routine physical examinations, colds and the flu, yet there is no evidence that patients benefit from visiting the doctor for these reasons.
- Only 10 percent of visits to the emergency room are for true emergencies.
- Twenty-five percent to 50 percent of all patients never take any of the medicine prescribed for them.
- Less than 20 percent of patients who receive penicillin for strep throat (streptococcal pharyngitis) take the medicine as directed.

---

good insurance, a prolonged hospital stay can be a major burden. Without such insurance, it is a financial disaster for many Americans.

YOU BE THE JUDGE

Medical care is neither always good nor always bad. Good or bad isn't even the issue. Medical care always has benefits, risks and costs. As the patient, only you can determine the degree to which the benefits are to be valued and the risks are to be feared. It's your choice. Obtaining the most reliable information you can is the best way to make that choice. This is no guarantee that you will always obtain medicine's benefit and avoid its complications. Nothing can do that. But it's your best chance that medical care will help more than it hurts.

SECTION III

THE ART AND SCIENCE OF HEALTHY LIVING

- ❑ Exercise: The Very Best
- ❑ Food for Life
- ❑ Fat Control
- ❑ Smoking: The Black Cloud
- ❑ Putting Alcohol In Its Place
- ❑ Mind ↔ Body
- ❑ Safe and Sound
- ❑ Dealing with Drug Abuse
- ❑ Creating a Healthy Environment

EXERCISE:
The Very Best

Remar Sutton was not a happy man. His mirror revealed someone who was fat, flabby and 40. It was time, he decided, for drastic measures. Sutton headed for the Bahamas to revamp his lifestyle. He exercised regularly and ate wisely. And he chronicled his progress weekly in *The Washington Post*.

Gradually the pounds dropped off, the flab hardened to muscle, and a fitness crusader was born. Sutton was soon recruiting non-athletic *Post* readers to join him in a 1988 Bahamas "Concha-thon"—a one-mile swim, 10-mile bike ride and four-mile run. Four hundred people, most over 40, signed on. They trained seriously, competed good naturedly and felt wonderful about what they had accomplished—not only crossing the finish line, but also recharging their lifestyles.

It's a sure bet these "Fit Over 40s" also improved their health—physical as well as mental—and lengthened their life expectancy. Exercise works wonders: It may well be the single best thing you can do if you want to live a long and healthy life. Studies of people who lived to a great age—into their 90s and beyond—show they have at least one thing in common: regular, vigorous exercise.

Exercise helps people live better as well as longer. Again and again, studies show that people who exercise regularly enjoy a sense of well-being. They feel and look younger than non-exercisers. They have more energy, and they don't feel tired out—thanks to better muscle tone and circulation. Routine, vigorous exercise is also one of the best ways known to reduce stress of all kinds; it can even outperform drugs in the treatment of mild to moderate depression.

Besides boosting the psyche, exercise provides countless health benefits. It prevents heart disease, strengthens bones and reduces the risk of high blood pressure. It raises levels of the "good" cholesterol, combats obesity and provides energy.

Studies documenting the benefits of exercise abound. Researchers have found that:

- Among 17,000 Harvard graduates between the ages of 35 and 74, those who burned more than 2,000 calories a week in exercise increased their life expectancy by an average of two years, reduced their risk of a heart attack by a third, and reduced their death rate from all causes by more than one-fourth.
- Even moderate activity helps. Researchers at the University of Minnesota studied more than 12,000 middle-aged men at high risk for coronary heart disease. They found that those who spent an average of 47 minutes a day in such leisure activities as yard work, walking, golfing or hunting had a 37 percent lower risk of heart disease and sudden death and a 30 percent drop in overall mortality compared with men who were active only 15 minutes a day.
- Similarly, a 1989 report in the journal *Circulation* described a group of more than 3,000 railroad workers who were observed for periods lasting 17 to 20 years. The men with higher levels of leisure-time activity had lower levels of heart disease. Death rates from heart disease were lowest for men who burned 1,000 calories or more a week in activity, but men who reported burning just 250 calories a week—a small amount—were much better off than men who were sedentary. It would take 10 minutes a day of walking at three miles an hour to burn 250 calories in a week.
- In 1987, the Centers for Disease Control reviewed 43 studies on exercise and health. It was found that regular exercise could do as much for heart health as quitting smoking, lowering blood cholesterol or controlling blood pressure.
- Postal workers who carried mailbags had fewer heart attacks than their peers who sat behind desks. If they did have a heart attack, they were less likely to die or be seriously disabled.
- Middle-aged men doing heavy physical work had less heart disease and developed

Time Required to Burn 2,000 Calories in Exercise*

Exercise	Time
Running at 7 mph	2 hours 51 minutes
Cross-country skiing at 5 mph	2 hours 51 minutes
Swimming (crawl, 20 yards/minute)	6 hours 40 minutes
Bicycling on level ground at 5 mph	8 hours 10 minutes

*For a person weighing 154 lbs.

it later in life than men whose jobs required little or no physical activity. At autopsy, their hearts showed the same signs of heart disease as inactive men 10 to 15 years younger.

- Men who walked to work—even when the walk took less than 10 minutes—showed less evidence of heart disease on electrocardiograms than men who rode buses or drove. (The automobile may be killing more of us by replacing exercise than by dismembering us on the highway.)

Exercise staves off heart disease in part because it alters other risk factors (see Chapter 18). Regular exercisers are much less likely to be overweight; exercise not only burns calories, it appears to suppress appetite. Exercise reduces blood pressure; in fact, exercise combined with weight loss can often control high blood pressure without medication. Smokers who start exercise programs often quit smoking. And aerobic exercise—specifically jogging—has been shown to raise levels of HDL cholesterol, which protects against heart disease, while lowering LDL cholesterol, which is associated with a greater risk of heart disease. (See Chapter 18 for more on the "good" and "bad" types of cholesterol.)

What's more, the effects of exercise may outweigh the effects of diet. When researchers compared 600 Irish-Americans who had lived in Boston for at least 10 years with their brothers who had never left Ireland, they found that the Irishmen ate 500 calories a day more than their American

Table 6.1
Calories Expended with Exercise
Per Hour by Activity

Activity	Calories expended (per hour) by person weighing:		
	110 lbs.	154 lbs.	198 lbs.
Brick Laying	160	205	250
Calisthenics	235	300	365
Car Repair	180	230	280
Carpentry or Farm Chores	180	230	280
Chopping Wood	355	450	550
Cleaning Windows	180	230	280
Dancing			
Moderate	350	445	540
Vigorous	515	655	795
Fox Trot	195	250	305
Rhumba	215	300	365
Square	330	420	510
Waltz	195	250	305
Driving	130	180	235
Floor			
Mopping	195	275	355
Sweeping	160	225	290
Gardening	155	215	280
Gardening and Weeding	250	315	380
Hill Climbing	470	600	730
Hoeing, Raking and Planting	205	285	370
House Painting	165	210	255
Housework	175	245	320
Motorcycling	165	205	250
Mountain Climbing	470	600	730
Mowing Grass			
Power, self-propelled	195	250	305
Not self-propelled	210	270	325
Office Work	115	145	175
Pick and Shovel Work	315	400	490
Sawing Wood	180	230	280
Shoveling Snow	475	610	745
Walking			
2 mph	145	185	225
4.5 mph	325	450	550
Downstairs	355	450	550
Upstairs	720	920	1120
Yard Work	155	215	275

Adapted from Charles T. Kuntzleman, *Diet Free*: Arbor Press, Spring Arbor, MI.

Table 6.1
Calories Expended with Exercise, continued
Per Hour by Activity

Activity	Calories expended (per hour) by person weighing:		
	110 lbs.	154 lbs.	198 lbs.
Sports			
Archery	245	315	380
Baseball/Softball			
Infield/Outfield	220	280	340
Pitching	305	390	475
Basketball			
Moderate	435	555	675
Vigorous	585	750	910
Bicycling (on level ground)			
5.5 mph	190	245	295
13 mph	515	655	790
Bowling (non-stop)	210	270	325
Canoeing (4 mph)	490	625	765
Golf			
Twosome	295	380	460
Foursome	210	270	325
Handball/Racquetball	610	775	945
Rowing (20 strokes/min)	515	655	795
Running			
5.5 mph	515	655	795
7 mph	550	700	850
9 mph	720	920	1120
Sailing (calm water)	120	155	190
Skating (ice)			
Moderate	275	350	425
Vigorous	485	620	755
Skiing			
Downhill	465	595	720
Cross-Country (5 mph)	550	700	950
Soccer	470	600	730
Swimming			
Backstroke (20 yds/min)	165	235	305
Breaststroke (20 yds/min)	210	295	380
Butterfly (per hour)	490	630	760
Crawl (20 yds/min)	235	300	365
Sidestroke (per hour)	230	320	420
Tennis			
Moderate	335	425	520
Vigorous	470	600	730
Volleyball (moderate)	275	350	425
Waterskiing	335	475	610

brothers and almost twice as many eggs. Nonetheless, the Irish brothers weighed less, had lower cholesterol levels, and had only half the incidence of high blood pressure. The likeliest explanation is that the Irishmen were more active, thanks largely to frequent biking and walking.

Exercise also strengthens bones. Without exercise, bones lose their calcium and grow brittle. This happens most rapidly with bed rest (and it's one reason patients are urged to get out of bed as soon as possible, even after major surgery or heart attacks). Calcium loss has been observed in astronauts returning from space, where zero gravity can rob exercise of its value.

Weak and brittle bones due to lack of exercise are common in the aged. For older people, the upshot is more than a broken bone. Almost everyone has seen an older friend or relative break a hip and then go rapidly downhill. Too often fractures in older people mean the end of an active and useful life.

Finally, regular exercisers are more productive. A study at the Taking Care Center, a state-of-the-art fitness facility at The Travelers Companies' headquarters in Hartford, Connecticut, showed that employees taking part in a fitness program missed significantly fewer workdays than they had the year before. Another study, this one at the University of Connecticut, found that aerobic training is linked not only to decreased lost work days, but also to improved job satisfaction, attitude toward work and quality of work. And at Tenneco, in a group of 3,000 white-collar workers who had the option of joining a fitness program, those who were highly ranked in job performance tended to be those who exercised most. Don't forget, too, that being in shape adds to your image as a productive worker. The boss may find it difficult to promote someone who is flabby and seems to be out of breath with the least exertion.

So What's Your Excuse?

Surveys show the American public can come up with lots of lame excuses for not exercising:

- **"No time."** Many people can't find the time in their "busy" schedules. First of all,

exercise doesn't have to take a lot of time. Second, think about the time people spend watching TV: It's a matter of priorities. Third, the extra energy you derive from exercise will provide you with more time for everything. Dr. George Sheehan, cardiologist and fitness expert, puts it this way: "One hour of good exercise will give you back two hours for other activities. The busier you are, the more you *need* to exercise."

- **"Too tired."** Many people leave work exhausted and feel they have no energy left for exercise. Yet when you're out of shape, you tire more easily. Then you don't exercise because you're tired, and it becomes a vicious circle. Regular exercisers have more energy for the things they *like* to do as well as for the things they *have* to do. And they feel less tired.

- **"I get enough exercise."** Many Americans cling to the belief that they get enough exercise in their daily routines. Unfortunately most jobs, including housework, do not provide enough exercise to keep the body fit. Most people need to introduce fitness into their way of life. More than half of all Americans do not make this effort.

Before You Start

Isn't it risky to start an exercise program without first having a complete physical and an exercise stress test? After all, endurance improves when the body becomes strong in response to physical *stress*.

It is unlikely that you need an exercise stress test before starting to exercise for several reasons. First, exercise is less stressful than many other activities, including the exercise stress test. Dr. Roy Shepard puts it this way: If you are at high risk for a heart attack, the chances of having one can be increased by any number of activities. (See Table 6.2.)

To avoid all stress, you should refrain from skiing. But you will also have to give up sex, never run to catch a bus, and—above all—never submit to a stress test. You must also avoid arguments

Table 6.2
Risk of Heart Attack

Risk Factor	Activity
1	Rest
3–4	Cross-country skiing
5	Sexual intercourse
6–12	Unaccustomed, severe exercise
30–60	Exercise stress test

with your spouse, conflicts with the boss, cheering your favorite team, and anything else that might rev you up. The point is, of course, that none of us can lead a stress-free life. And exercise *decreases* the overall odds of a heart attack. Which of your other stressors will do that?

It may seem strange to talk about increasing the risk of a heart attack through exercise while advocating exercise to decrease the risk of a heart attack. Let's be clear on the basics. First, exercise does decrease your overall risk of heart attack, so someone who works out regularly is at less risk than someone who doesn't.

It is true that if you compare a minute of rest to a minute of exercise, the minute of exercise carries more risk. But remember, most exercisers work out for an hour a day or less, so the real issue is the risk of the 23 hours or so of non-exercising minutes. Because exercise greatly lowers the risk for all those non-exercising minutes, the exerciser comes out far ahead overall.

Second, the exercise stress test is not a very useful indicator of heart disease, especially in people without symptoms. As you will see in Chapter 15, most positive stress tests are *false* positives, showing that disease is present when it is not.

To determine whether you should have a medical evaluation before you begin exercising, answer the following questions:

- Do you have chest pains when you exert yourself?
- Do you get short of breath with mild exertion?
- Do you have pain in your legs when you walk that disappears with rest?

- Do you regularly have ankle swelling (not associated with the menstrual cycle in women)?
- Has your doctor ever told you that you have heart disease, high blood pressure, arthritis or some other serious disease?
- Do you have a family history of heart attacks and sudden death before age 50?
- Do you have a musculoskeletal problem such as low back pain?

If you answered "yes" to any of these questions, call your doctor before starting your program. The odds are still against the need for a physical, and you may be able to clear up the problem over the phone. Usually the only real question is whether your exercise should be medically supervised. For someone known to have heart disease, this may be wise, at least at the start.

The most important safety factor is how you exercise, not getting a physical or stress test beforehand. *Common sense says to start slowly and increase the amount of exercise gradually*. You don't need a doctor to tell you that you are asking for trouble if you haven't exercised in years and then run a three-mile race. You have months, years if you like, to reach your goals. Take your time. Forget about "no pain, no gain." Sweating, heavy breathing, yes. Pain, no. If symptoms such as chest pain occur during exercise, that's the time to see your doctor.

Finally, assume you *do* have heart disease and are at risk of a heart attack. What now? You can sit back and wait for it to happen, or you can begin to exercise and to shift the odds in your favor.

ON YOUR MARK

The chief goals of exercise are to condition the heart and circulation (so-called cardiovascular conditioning); to build endurance; to improve flexibility in muscles and joints; and to strengthen muscles, especially in the legs, back and abdomen.

- **Endurance.** Endurance underlies most of the physical and mental health benefits we've been talking about. To build endurance—in other words, to achieve cardiovascular conditioning—exercise must be *aerobic* (that is, "with oxygen"). Aerobic exercise makes the heart a stronger muscle, and readies the heart and lungs for prolonged work.

Aerobic exercise involves non-stop motion that increases breathing and causes the heart to pump vigorously. Rhythmic, continuous exercises are the best—things like jogging, swimming, riding a bike, jumping rope and aerobic dancing. Short sprints are not likely to help, but fast-paced sports, such as basketball, racquetball, squash, soccer and handball, can be aerobic if the motion is continuous.

The value of many activities—tennis, for instance—depends on how you play the game. If you are moving all the time—chasing down balls, avoiding breaks between points—then you are getting worthwhile exercise. On the other hand, it is possible to play a pretty decent game of tennis while nearly standing still. If you learn to win without moving, you will lose in the long run. As a rule, golf, bowling, volleyball and baseball don't provide aerobic exercise.

- **Flexibility.** Flexibility, which refers to the range of motion within a joint, is the key to remaining able to function as you grow older. It is influenced by the condition of the ligaments, tendons and muscles that support and move the joint. You can lose flexibility through disuse; older people often suffer such loss. Limited flexibility makes muscles less efficient and leaves a person open to injury.

You can maintain flexibility through stretching exercises. The warmer the muscles, tendons and ligaments are, the more flexible they are; so to get the most out of stretching, do it *after* you have warmed up.

- **Strength.** Although most studies of exercise's health benefits have focused on aerobic exercise, we can be pretty certain that strength exercises provide real health benefits, too. Strength is essential for preventing many of the frailties associated with aging. (And aging starts in the 30s, if not

Seniors Go for Power

In a study at Tufts University, 12 men (ages 60 to 72) volunteered for a 12-week strength-training program (three days per week) for the thigh muscles. At the program's end, the muscles in the front of the thigh (the quadriceps) had increased in strength by 107 percent while the muscles in the back of the thigh (the hamstrings) had increased their strength by 227 percent. Their muscles had increased in size by about 10 percent, too. Rumor has it that they will have their own section at Muscle Beach for "bulking up" this summer.

the 20s.) Strength exercises also aid in fat control, because they build muscle. And a body with more muscle is better at burning calories.

Most children naturally put their bodies through a challenging range of activities; as people get older, they lose the habit. By the time people reach older life, they have gone so long without building strong muscles that they have trouble getting around. Many older people lose strength in their thigh muscles and find it hard to get up from a chair. They try less often to stand, or they rely on their arms to boost themselves up. Some even resort to a motorized chair that thrusts them out. As a result they lose even more strength. Many older people move slowly not because their joints hurt, but because they're afraid of what will happen if they move fast. The unsteadiness, shakiness or slowed motion we attribute to arthritis, nerve problems or poor balance is too often evidence of weak muscles that cannot make fine adjustments.

Strength results when muscles work against resistance. The resistance may be provided by free weights, such as barbells or dumbbells, by weight machines, such as Universal or Nautilus machines, or by body weight, as in sit-ups or push-ups. For the average person, body weight exercises are enough, but weight lifting or weight machines can also be useful and safe.

GET SET

In planning to exercise, choose an activity that you are likely to keep doing. It is often said that you can't stick with exercise until you find something that is fun. This is nonsense. Your chosen form of exercise need not fill you with joy from start to finish. Exercise isn't always fun, especially at the start. Lots of people—myself included—do things that don't leave them giggling with delight. The running, the bicycling, the weight machines —they wouldn't be so compelling if I were not getting something very worthwhile out of the effort. More important than fun is the satisfaction you derive afterwards—feeling better, looking better, having more energy and being less stressed. When those rewards kick in, they make people want to continue.

There's a lot of talk about which type of aerobic exercise is best. Some people favor walking; others tout cross-country skiing. In choosing an activity, here are some things to think about. Exercise that uses all of your body, not just your legs—cross-country skiing or swimming, for example—are good choices. So are exercises that don't put a lot of wear and tear on joints—swimming or other water exercises, or bicycling, either outdoors or on a stationary cycle.

Many exercisers find enjoyment in the setting: Some—long distance runners, for instance —enjoy the chance to be alone with their thoughts, while others prefer to walk, swim or jog with a buddy. Some folks like to socialize in the locker room or over lunch afterwards, while others enjoy competition: Sports often provide that extra enjoyment that keeps them going. If you like the structure of formal programs, you may opt for calisthenics like those outlined in the Canadian Air Force exercises or for an aerobic-dance class.

Varying your activities can also help to make you a regular exerciser. Run one day, bike another, swim the next. Do calisthenics, or take up a recre-

Is Walking the Best Exercise?

Just plain walking has a lot going for it. It doesn't require a lot of equipment or any instruction. It can be done almost anywhere, and it encourages good thoughts and good talks. Done regularly, it will reduce the risk of heart disease. On the other hand, it doesn't really qualify as an aerobic activity and will not do as much to condition your heart and blood vessels. (Aerobic, or power, walking does provide this conditioning; see below.) All of us would benefit from doing it more often, but walking alone will not produce the kind of physical fitness that most of us should attain.

ational sport, such as tennis or squash. Cross-training, as this is called, not only adds spice, but uses different muscles and contributes to all-around fitness.

Exercise should not require a heroic sacrifice of time or convenience; choose activities that can be worked into your schedule. Taking up swimming when the only pool is 40 miles away dooms you to failure, no matter how much you like to swim. You would be wiser to bike or jog to work or take an exercise class during your lunch hour. And make exercise part of your daily routine— don't ride when you can walk; take the stairs instead of the elevator.

Setting challenging yet realistic goals gives purpose and focus to your program. For example, during your first six weeks you may decide to run the equivalent of the Boston Marathon or the length of the Grand Canyon. Your long-term goal may be to run the length of the Great Wall of China. (See Table 6.3.)

GO

Your exercise program should include both aerobic and strengthening exercises, preceded by a warm-up and stretching, and followed by a cooldown. Three to five vigorous sessions of aerobic exercise a week is ideal; working out every other

Table 6.3
Exercise Equivalents/Goal Setting
(Six Weeks or Longer)

Walking or Running

Boston Marathon	26 miles, 385 yards
Length of the Grand Canyon	217 miles
Length of the Great Wall of China	1,500 miles
New York City to San Francisco	2,930 miles
Establish your own _____	

Stair Climbing

Sears Tower Building, Chicago (tallest office building in the world)	1,454 ft.
River to South Rim of Grand Canyon	4,460 ft.
Base camp to peak of Mt. Everest	16,000 ft.
Establish your own _____	

Aerobic Exercise/Dance

Dance at each of New York City's dance schools	14 schools/sessions
Complete professional team training camp	24 sessions and make the team
Establish your own _____	

Swimming

From Alcatraz to freedom	1 1/2 miles
English Channel (Dover to Calais)	21 miles
Establish your own _____	

Bicycling

Los Angeles to San Francisco	387 miles
Tour de France	2,500 miles
Establish your own _____	

Weight Lifting

Lift an African elephant	16,000 lbs.
Lift a Sherman tank	94,000 lbs.
Lift a blue whale	240,000 lbs.
Lift the Queen Mary oceanliner	162,474,000 lbs!
Establish your own _____	

Choose a Goal from One of Those Listed Above or Design Your Own.

day is a natural schedule. More than five sessions doesn't add enough conditioning to offset such risks as sore or pulled muscles or a twisted ankle. Strength-building exercises can be performed at the end of an aerobic session or scheduled on alternate days.

When you start your aerobic-exercise program, alternate periods of activity and rest—walk in the middle of jogging, hold onto the edge in the swimming pool for a bit. Work up to exercising for the full time without stopping.

THE WARM-UP

To prevent injuries and keep from overstressing the heart, always warm up before exercise. The idea is to raise body temperature and oxygen demand gradually with a few minutes of easy activities. If your chosen form of exercise is a repetitive one, such as walking or biking, you can simply do it at a slow pace. If you have chosen an active sport like racquetball, warm up by jogging or biking to the court or by running in place. Allow five to 10 minutes for warming up.

Use the chart below to describe your goal, identify its equivalent and promise yourself a reward, perhaps a new warm-up suit. Then, record each workout and shade in the bar graph to track your progress toward your goal.

A Six-Week Challenge

Select an exercise activity that you will enjoy for the next six weeks to get into shape and feel better. The total amount of exercise that you achieve will equal a rather impressive accomplishment. Select your preferred exercise and a realistic, yet challenging, goal from Table 6.3. Then, establish a reward for eventually reaching your goal.

1) I Will _____ .
   (Name of exercise, activity and total distance or amount to be accomplished.)

2) In the next six weeks, my accomplishment will be equal to
   _____ .

3) I will reward myself with _____ .

Daily Record of Distance Covered/Amount or Step Accomplished

Week One	Week Two	Week Three
M _____	M _____	M _____
T _____	T _____	T _____
W _____	W _____	W _____
Th _____	Th _____	Th _____
F _____	F _____	F _____

Week Four	Week Five	Week Six
M _____	M _____	M _____
T _____	T _____	T _____
W _____	W _____	W _____
Th _____	Th _____	Th _____
F _____	F _____	F _____

Total accomplishment _____

Shade in the portion of your goal achieved.

10%   20%   30%   40%   50%   60%   70%   80%   90%   100%

Celebration—
Deserved Pride
of Accomplishment

"I've Got What it Takes to Go the Distance."

_____   _____
Signature   Date

_____   _____
Witness   Date

STRETCHING

Next, slowly stretch the major muscles used in your activity, such as those in the legs and back.

Stretching helps prevent injuries, feels good and improves posture and muscle tone.

Your Stretching Program

The following stretching exercises are designed to: (1) increase the range of motion in your muscles and joints, (2) help prevent soft-tissue injury, and (3) help minimize post-exercise soreness.

Before stretching, it's important to warm up first. Your muscles are more easily stretched once blood flow is increased. Warm up for a few minutes through slow jogging, brisk walking or calisthenics such as jumping jacks. Hold each stretch for 15 seconds. Don't bounce or jerk through the movement. Repeat these exercises during your cooldown.

(1) Side Stretch

Feet should be wider apart than shoulder width. Turn your right foot out with your left foot turned slightly in. Slowly slide your right hand down the back of your leg to a point of tension. Stop and hold for 15 seconds. Your left arm should be perpendicular to the ground. Repeat two or three times on each leg.

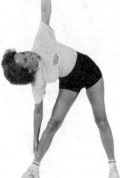

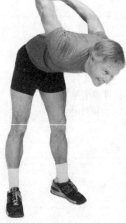

(2) Swimmer's Stretch

While standing, place one hand under the other, palms facing up. Position your hands behind your neck, and slowly stretch your arms overhead, keeping your hands together. Hold the stretch for 15 seconds. Repeat three times.

(3) Hip Stretch

Lying flat on your back, bring your left knee up toward your chest. Interlock your fingers and grasp behind the knee. Keep your right leg straight and your head on the floor. Hold for 15 seconds. Repeat two to three times on each leg.

(4) Shoulder Stretch

Place your right hand behind your head, reaching toward the middle of your back. Place your left hand on your right elbow. Push your right arm slowly down your back. Hold for 15 to 30 seconds. Repeat with each arm.

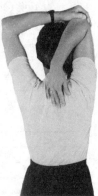

(5) Calf Stretch

Stand an arm's length from a wall or tree. Keep your feet together, heels flat, and lean forward, using your arms for support. Hold this position for 30 seconds. Next, bend your knees while maintaining the leaning position. Hold for 30 seconds. This helps stretch the muscles deep in your calf.

Repeat these stretches after cooling down.

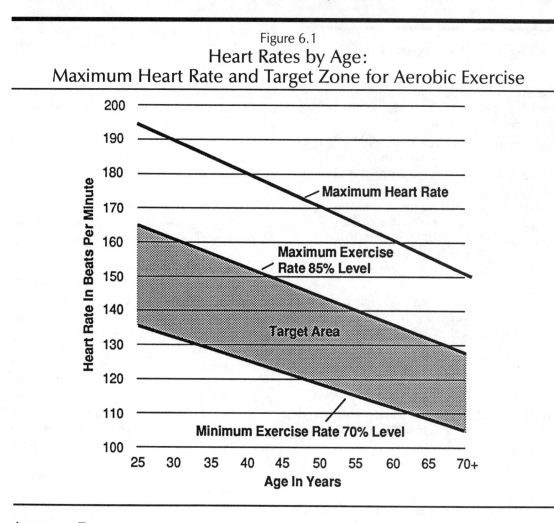

Figure 6.1
Heart Rates by Age:
Maximum Heart Rate and Target Zone for Aerobic Exercise

AEROBIC EXERCISE

A typical exercise session should allow 15 to 60 minutes for aerobic exercise—rhythmic, continuous movement that speeds up your heart rate and breathing. Popular aerobic exercises include walking, jogging, swimming, cycling, jumping rope, cross-country skiing and aerobic dancing.

The traditional way to tell if the exercise is benefiting your heart and lungs is to take your pulse before, during and after the workout. You can find your pulse by lightly placing the tips of your first two fingers on either the radial artery in the wrist or the carotid artery on the side of the neck. Count the beats for 10 seconds (the first beat counts as "zero"), and then multiply this number by six to get your heart rate per minute.

Most adults have resting heart rates of 60 to 75 beats per minute. During exercise, your heart rate should fall into the target zone for your exercise heart rate, between 70 percent and 85 percent of your maximum heart rate, which is 220 minus your age. For example, if you are 50 years old, your maximum heart rate is 170, and your target zone would be between 119 (70 percent) and 144 (85 percent) beats per minute. For a quick fix on your target zone, consult Figure 6.1.

While the target zone helps define an effective level of aerobic exercise and limit the risk of

Ensure the Proper F.I.T.T.

To be safe, effective and beneficial, your exercise program should comply with the F.I.T.T. principle. Pay attention to these four factors:

- **Frequency**: To gain a "training" effect, you need to exercise three to five times a week, with adequate rest between sessions.
- **Intensity**: An effective workout requires some sweat and heavy breathing, but not pain. Use your heart rate as a guide.
- **Time**: Each workout should last 30 to 60 minutes. Your goal is to gradually work up to the point where you can maintain a continuous, steady pace.
- **Type**: The core of any adult fitness program is aerobic exercise, but stretching and strengthening "fitt" in easily and naturally.

injury, there is nothing magic about it. If your heart rate is at 65 percent of maximum, you do not lose all the benefit of exercise. And if you should go over 85 percent of maximum, you do not face immediate, unavoidable collapse. When you exercise at lower levels, the impact on conditioning is less, but so is the risk of injury; at higher levels of exercise, the opposite is true.

Don't let the target zone become a burden. You don't need to check your pulse often during exercise; once halfway through your workout is plenty. Also, don't worry about exact numbers. An easy rule of thumb is that a heart rate over 120 beats per minute puts you into the vigorous-exercise category. Again, don't fret if your heart rate is 100 or 110. This is still a worthwhile effort, and you can increase the intensity of your workout later on.

Exercising too hard is usually a problem only when starting out. Poor conditioning may allow the heart rate to rise rapidly at this time, so you may want to watch your heart rate to avoid overdoing it. As exercise becomes routine, most people settle into a pattern in which the heart rate is in the lower or middle range of the target zone. Checking the

heart rate becomes unnecessary, and people can gauge the intensity of their exercise by how it feels.

Exercise should be strenuous but not agonizing. If you push yourself too hard, you greatly increase the risk of injury or illness. Remember that exercise should not leave you too out of breath to talk. Start out slowly, in terms of both time and effort, and increase gradually.

If you feel pain, walk around for a while and end your exercise session gradually. If you injure a knee, ankle or other joint, rest it until the pain is gone and don't exercise it until it heals.

Three of the most popular aerobic exercises are power walking, jogging and aerobic dancing.

Power Walking

Almost anyone can walk. It requires little in the way of equipment or special facilities. And it doesn't stress the joints or legs much. With the aging of America, walking is becoming the aerobic activity of choice for many people.

Walking slowly has benefits, but it will not produce much improvement in endurance unless you are really out of shape. Aerobic or power walking raises your heart rate to at least 120 beats per minute. Like other exercises, power walking should be accompanied by a warm-up and cool-down. You should start slowly and gradually increase your distance and pace. When you reach a fitness level at which walking no longer raises your heart rate enough, you can make your body work harder by wearing a weight belt, walking uphill or trying the increasingly popular race walking. (To learn how to race walk properly, work with a coach, perhaps someone from a local recreation center or university.)

Walking can let you lose fat without eating less; studies show that women can achieve significant fat loss by walking 40 minutes a day. And walking is relaxing; a recent report in the *Journal of the American Medical Association* stated that 40 minutes of vigorous walking can reduce anxiety and tension and improve mood for two hours or more.

Many people have found that walking with a partner or joining a walking club is a good way to

Table 6.4
Sample Walking Program
Beginner Program

Week	Mileage	Pace (mph)	Heart Rate (% of maximum)	Frequency (times per week)
1	1.5	3.0	70	5
2	1.5	3.0	70	5
3	1.75	3.0	70	5
4	1.75	3.0	70	5
5	2.0	3.0	70	5
6	2.0	3.0	70	5
7	2.0	3.5	70	5
8	2.25	3.5	70	5
9	2.25	3.5	70	5
10	2.5	3.5	70	5
11	2.5	3.5	70	5
12	2.5	3.5	70	5
13	2.75	3.5	70	5
14	2.75	4.0	70–80	5
15	3.0	4.0	70–80	5
16	3.0	4.0	70–80	5
17	3.25	4.0	70–80	5
18	3.25	4.0	70–80	5
19	3.5	4.0	70–80	5
20	3.5	4.0	70–80	5

At the end of this 20-week fitness walking protocol you may either stay at this schedule or increase your pace and distance.

Adapted from: *Rockport's Fitness Walking* by Robert Sweetgall, The Putnam Publishing Group, New York, NY, 1985. Printed with permission.

make exercise a social event. Walking in the protected environment of a shopping mall is popular with older adults, but you don't have to be senior to enjoy it. There are more than 1,000 mall-walking groups nationwide.

For proper power walking:

- Purchase walking shoes that provide enough support (see box).

- Walk erect, but stay relaxed.

- Foot contact should be heel to toe, with the stepping leg straight as you go into your next step.

- Hold your arms at a 90-degree angle and swing them back and forth to help maintain momentum. Don't cross your arms in front of your chest.

Walking Shoes

1. All parts of your foot must be able to fit comfortably into the walking shoe.
2. The shoe must be flexible in the sole and the top to assist in the walking motion.
3. A cushioned sole is mandatory for walking long distances.
4. There should be good support at the heel and arch.
5. The upper part of the shoe should be made of material that will allow the shoe to breathe.
6. Whenever possible, shoes should be lightweight.
7. The ideal walking shoe should have a curved sole.

Jogging

Jogging is more demanding than walking and is often the next step up from a walking program. People who are obese, for instance, should not start out by jogging, but should embark on a regular walking program until they lose some body fat and develop some conditioning.

Persons graduating from a walking program should view the first three weeks of jogging as a conditioning period that readies the joints and cardiovascular system for added stress. The beginning jogger can make the greatest progress by slowly increasing the workout period while keeping his or her heart rate in the same range. In other words, you want to work longer, not harder. (See Table 6.5.)

Getting Off on the Right Foot

You don't need fancy equipment, it's true, but you do need *proper* equipment. Don't try to be a runner in tennis shoes or a walker in loafers, just as you wouldn't try to play tennis without a racquet. Thanks to the fitness boom, good exercise shoes are widely available. You usually can't go wrong if you stick to the major brands. The key points are fit and comfort.

For proper running or jogging:

- Purchase shoes that provide appropriate support (see box at right).
- Maintain an upright posture, so that an imaginary plumb line would pass through your earlobe, shoulder, hip, knee and ankle.
- Think of your upper body as "going for a ride" as it sits on your hips. Let your legs propel you forward.
- Use your arms for balance; bend them at a 90-degree angle and hold your hands at chest height. Touch your forefingers to your thumbs, and swing your arms gently back and forth. Avoid a side-to-side motion.
- Plant your foot heel to toe. Touch the ground with the front of the heel, and then roll to the toes.
- Plant your foot directly below the knee, not in front, where it would break your momentum.
- While you are running, fix your eye on a point on the horizon at eye level; if it appears to be bouncing a lot, you are taking too long a stride. Shorten your stride until the bouncing diminishes.
- Breathe naturally, through your mouth.

Table 6.5

Sample Jogging Program

Week	Workout Period (Jogging)	Recovery Period (Walking)	Number of Repetitions
1–3	1 minute	1 minute	20
4	2 minutes	2 minutes	10
5	3 minutes	2 minutes	7
6–7	5 minutes	2 minutes	4
8–10	7 minutes	2 minutes	2
11–12	10 minutes	2 minutes	2

How to Buy Athletic Shoes

Here are some guidelines developed by Dr. Lloyd Nesbitt of the Canadian Podiatric Sports Medicine Academy that you can follow to put your best foot forward:

- When buying shoes for exercise, have both feet measured in athletic socks. (One foot is generally larger than the other.) Shop for shoes in the late afternoon, when your feet are most likely to be somewhat swollen—just as they will be after a workout.
- For walking shoes, look for a shoe that's lightweight, flexible and roomy enough for your toes to wiggle, with a well-cushioned, curved sole; good support at the heel; and an upper part made of a material that "breathes" (allows air in and out).
- A running shoe should be strongest in the areas of cushioning, support and stability while still being soft, flexible and lightweight. The sole should be durable on the outside, with a moderately soft layer in the midsole of sufficient flexibility that you can bend it easily by hand. Without this flexibility, you may stress your Achilles tendon and calf muscles as you propel off the ball of your foot into your next step.
- Look for adequate cushioning under the ball of your foot. The insole should be firm but provide adequate shock absorption. Running and particularly sprinting exert a great deal of pressure in this area.
- The shoe should have a solid, but not a snug, heel cup. The heel counter should be firm and well padded to prevent too much side-to-side motion. The heel itself has to absorb the shock of impact with the ground. A slightly elevated heel lessens the strain on the back of your legs.
- You should be able to wiggle your toes easily, but the front of your foot shouldn't slide from side to side, which could cause blisters. Your toes shouldn't touch the end of the shoe, because your feet will swell with activity. Allow about half an inch from the longest toe to the tip of the shoe.
- The tongue and upper sole should be well padded and fashioned to stay in place as you run. The shank area, under the arch of the shoe, needs to be rigid and lie flush with the ground. If it buckles at foot contact, it may cause heel and arch injuries. As a test, try bending the shoe in this area. If it flexes easily, it may not offer enough support.
- For racquetball shoes, look for reinforcement at the toe for protection during foot drag. The sole should allow minimal slippage. There should be some heel elevation to lessen strain on the back of the leg and Achilles tendon. The shoe should have a long "throat" to ensure greater control by the laces.
- For tennis shoes, look for reinforcement of the toe. The sole at the ball of the foot should be well padded, because that's where most pressure is exerted. The sides of the shoe should be sturdy, for stability during continuous side-to-side motions. The toe box should allow ample room and some cushioning at the tips. A long throat ensures greater control by the laces.
- Don't wear wet shoes for training. Let them air dry, because a heater will cause them to stiffen or shrink. Use powder in your shoes to absorb moisture, lessen friction and prevent fungal infections. Break in new shoes for several days before wearing them for a long-distance run or a competition.

Aerobic Dancing

Some 23 million Americans take part in aerobic-dance classes, but aerobic dance can be strenuous, and injuries are a concern. Most of these injuries occur below the knee, the result of repeated impact of the feet on hard surfaces. Shin splints are a common complaint: The membrane around the shinbone becomes inflamed, causing pain, tenderness and sometimes swelling. Symptoms usually clear up in a week to 10 days if the leg is rested. Aerobic dance can also aggravate old injuries to the ankles, knees or back.

Most of the injuries triggered by aerobic dancing are not serious, and they can be avoided. It is important to:

- Exercise on proper surfaces. The ideal surface is neither too hard nor too soft and provides shock absorption and stability. The safest surfaces are heavily padded carpeted floors, foam mats and newly developed hardwood-over-airspace floors. The most dangerous surfaces are carpeting over concrete and tile-covered concrete.
- Wear the right shoes. It's a mistake to use running shoes for aerobic dance—they are designed for forward movement, whereas aerobic dance involves many side-to-side motions. Aerobic-dance shoes should provide ample flexibility in the ball of the foot, heel cushioning, lateral support and a slightly raised heel to take force off the Achilles tendon.
- Perform adequate warm-up and cool-down exercises. It is important to stretch the key muscle groups in the legs, hips, shoulders and arms.
- "Train, not strain." No one should exercise too long or too hard. As with any aerobic activity, it takes time to build up endurance. Don't try too much too soon, or attempt to progress too quickly.
  Here are some other helpful tips:
- If traditional aerobic-dance movements cause you trouble, switch to low-impact techniques. These eliminate hard jumping but still provide a training effect.
- To avoid overuse injuries, alternate aerobic-dance workouts with other aerobic activities or resistance (strengthening) exercises.
- If you are injured, you need not halt your exercising. Substitute another activity, such as bicycling or swimming, which won't stress an injured leg or foot.
- Work with a qualified aerobic-dance instructor. An able instructor will know about safety factors and how to screen people for their suitability for a program. He or she is likely to be certified by a reputable professional organization, such as the American College of Sports Medicine, the International Dance and Exercise Association or the Aerobics and Fitness Association of America.

THE COOL DOWN

After exercise, you need to readjust the body by following a regular cool-down routine. Walk slowly for three to five minutes and stretch the major muscle groups once again. This is a good time for stretching, because muscles and joints are warm and flexible. Following the proper warm-up and cool-down procedures reduces soft-tissue injury, increases flexibility and minimizes post-exercise soreness.

In terms of safety, cooling down is the most important thing you can do. Stopping suddenly can disturb the rhythms of the heart. Statistically, the end of exercise is when most heart problems occur.

TOPPING OUT

You have little to gain in terms of conditioning after you reach a level of 60 minutes of aerobic exercise three to four times a week. The important thing is not to do more, but to stick with it. Marathons and triathlons are about challenge, mastery and companionship—in other words, mental, rather than physical, fitness. If you want to run a marathon for that reason, that's fine. But it is not a part of becoming physically fit.

Exercises that Strengthen

Muscular strength can be defined as the amount of weight a person can move or lift at one time. Strengthening exercises, which can be performed using free weights, such as barbells or dumbbells; weight machines, such as Nautilus or Cybex Eagle; or body weight, as you would with sit-ups or push-ups, should be done at most three times a week. You can alternate the days you do strengthening exercises with the days you do aerobic exercises or tack these moves on to the end of three of your aerobic sessions, for 10 or 15 minutes. However, strengthening exercises always require a day of rest between sessions. In fact, a day of rest is not a bad idea for most kinds of exercise, if you're doing just one kind. On the whole, it is better for your body if you vary your activity from day to day.

Weight exercises may increase blood pressure and decrease blood flow to the heart. This is especially true for those known as *isometrics*, which require a good deal of muscle tension but little or no motion. Improper breathing during exercise makes things even worse. This may pose a hazard for people with heart problems; for those with normal hearts, it is not usually a cause of concern.

For the average adult, muscular endurance is more important than muscular power, because the activities of daily living—house cleaning, lifting, climbing stairs, yard work—as well as most leisure sports require repetitive motions. Muscular endurance refers to the amount of repetitive work that can be performed before fatigue.

The following exercises are designed to develop endurance and improve strength through more repetitions with a low resistance.

There are a few basic rules to observe:

- All exercises should take muscles through their full range of motion.
- All exercises should be performed slowly and rhythmically.
- Don't hold your breath; breathe naturally, exhaling whenever you contract your muscles.
- Do 15 to 20 repetitions at a time. (Such a cluster of repetitions is known as a "set.")
- Allow two to three minutes between each set.
- When using hand weights such as dumbbells, select a weight that is comfortable; don't try to lift a weight that is too heavy for you. As you build endurance and strength, you can increase the weight as well as the number of repetitions and sets.

Strength Exercises

Using Body Weight As Resistance

1. Abdominal Curls
A. Lie on your back with your arms crossed on your chest and chin tucked to your chest.
B. The legs are to be bent, with heels flat on the floor. The feet should be six to 12 inches from the buttocks. The lower back should be flat on the floor.
C. Sit up slowly, raising the shoulder blades six inches from the floor, but keeping the small of the back on the floor. Exhale as you come up. Don't hold your breath!
D. Lower the upper body slowly to the floor.
E. Complete 15 to 20 repetitions for a set.

F. Eventual goal: two to three sets. (If you have difficulty performing this exercise with your arms crossed on your chest, keep your hands on your thighs, and slide them to your kneecaps as you come up.)

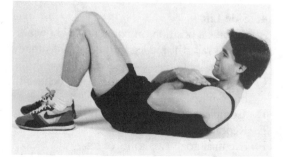

STRENGTH EXERCISES
Using Body Weight as Resistance

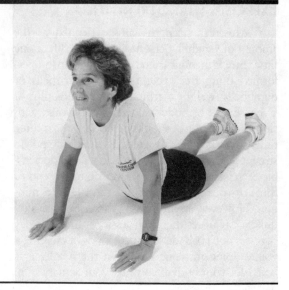

2. Trunk Extension
A. Lie on your stomach with your hands under your shoulders.
B. Your feet should be six inches apart.
C. Slowly extend your arms, raising your head and chest from the floor but keeping the hips, hands, legs and feet on the floor.
D. Exhale as you come up.
E. Slowly lower your body to the floor.
F. Complete 15 to 20 repetitions for a set.
G. Eventual goal: two to three sets.

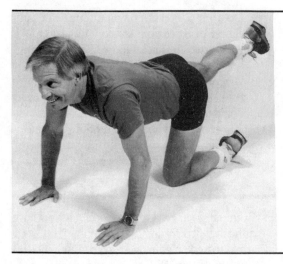

3. Back Leg Lift
A. Assume a position on your hands and knees as shown.
B. Keep your head up and look ahead.
C. Extend your right leg back with your toe on the floor. Slowly lift the leg to hip level, then lower it almost to the floor.
D. Complete 15 to 20 repetitions for a set.
E. Repeat on the other leg.
F. Eventual goal: two to three sets.

4. Side Lift
A. Assume a position on your side as shown.
B. Slowly raise the top leg through its full range of motion.
C. Slowly lower the leg to the floor, behind the bottom leg.
D. Complete 15 to 20 repetitions for a set.
E. Repeat on the other side.
F. Eventual goal: two to three sets.

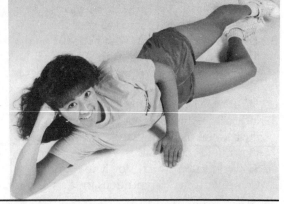

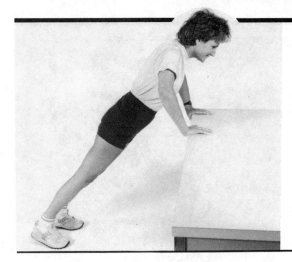

5. Push-ups (Modified)
A. Lean against a counter top, arms extended.
B. Keep your head, back and legs straight.
C. Lower your chest to the counter top, bending your elbows.
D. Extend the arms, breathing out. Don't lock elbows.
E. Complete 15 to 20 repetitions for a set.
F. Eventual goal: two to three sets.

6. Push-ups (Advanced)
A. Lie chest to floor, with your hands under your shoulders.
B. Keep your back and legs straight.
C. Extend your arms, breathe out, and don't lock elbows.
D. Return to the resting position.
E. Complete 15 to 20 repetitions for a set.
F. Eventual goal: two to three sets.

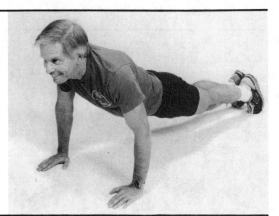

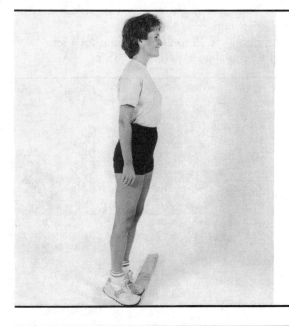

7. Calf Rise
A. Stand with the balls of the feet on a stable block of wood or step. Keep the heels lower than the toes.
B. Slowly raise the heels until you're up on your toes, keeping your arms at your sides.
C. Return slowly to the starting position.
D. Complete 15 to 20 repetitions for a set.
E. Eventual goal: two to three sets.

STRENGTH EXERCISES
Using Body Weight as Resistance

8. Wall Sit
A. Assume a sitting position with your back flat against a wall.
B. The thighs should be parallel to the floor. Hands are placed in your lap, on your kneecaps, or relaxed at your sides. **Don't hold your breath.**
C. Hold this position initially 20 seconds, gradually working up to a total of one minute for a set.
D. Eventual goal: two to three sets.

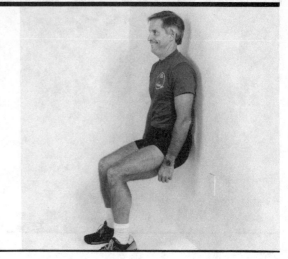

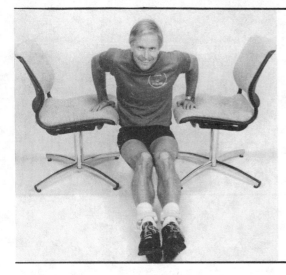

9. Parallel Dips
A. Position yourself between two sturdy chairs.
B. The body should be in a front lay-out position with one hand placed on each chair.
C. With the legs kept straight, the body is lowered and arms are bent until the elbows are at shoulder height.
D. Push up and extend the arms, keeping the body as straight as possible. Exhale as you come up.
E. Complete 15 to 20 repetitions for a set.
F. Eventual goal: two to three sets.

Dumbbell (Hand Weight) Exercises

1. Chest Press
A. Lie on your back on an exercise bench, with your feet flat on the floor.
B. Hold the dumbbells (hand weights) at your shoulders.
C. Press the weights toward the ceiling, exhaling as you lift.
D. Lower the weights with control and inhale.
E. Complete 15 to 20 repetitions for a set.
F. Eventual goal: two to three sets.

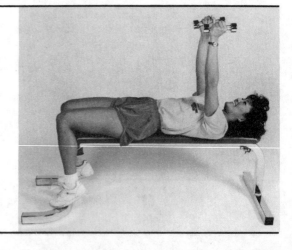

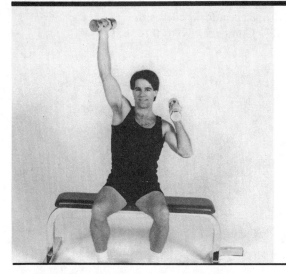

2. Shoulder Press
A. Sit on the bench with the dumbbells (hand weights) at your shoulders.
B. Alternating arms, lift each weight overhead to maximum extension. Exhale as you lift, keeping the back straight.
C. Lower the weights with control and inhale.
D. Complete 15 to 20 repetitions for a set.
F. Eventual goal: two to three sets.

3. Upright Rowing
A. Stand with your feet shoulder width apart.
B. Hold the dumbbells (hand weights) with your palms facing your body.
C. Keep your arms down at your sides, with the weights resting on top of your thighs.
D. Slowly raise both weights simultaneously, keeping the elbows above the hands, through the complete range of motion.
E. Raise the weights until they are even with your armpits. Breathe out when lifting.
F. Return to the starting position.
G. Complete 15 to 20 repetitions for a set.
H. Eventual goal: two to three sets.

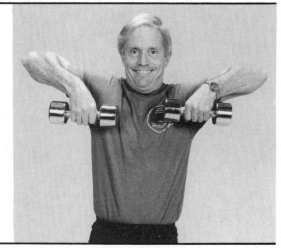

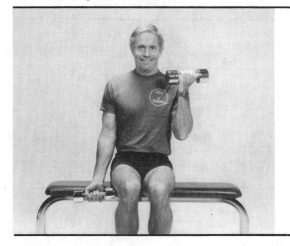

4. Bicep Curl
A. Sit on a bench or chair. Keep your back straight.
B. Hold a dumbbell (hand weight) in each hand, with your arms hanging.
C. Bend your right elbow, slowly raising the weight to your shoulder; exhale.
D. Slowly lower the weight to the starting position; inhale.
E. Repeat with the left arm.
F. Alternate lifting with the right and left arms.
G. Complete 15 to 20 repetitions for a set.
H. Eventual goal: two to three sets.

STRENGTH EXERCISES

Dumbbell (Hand Weight) Exercises

5. Tricep Extension

A. Sit on a bench or chair. Keep your back straight.

B. Grasp a dumbbell (hand weight) in your right hand. Place the weight behind your head, pointing the right elbow to the ceiling.

C. Stabilize your right arm with the left hand behind the right upper arm.

D. Slowly extend the right arm toward the ceiling. Exhale.

E. Slowly return to the starting position.

F. Complete 15 to 20 repetitions for a set using the right arm.

G. Repeat for the left arm.

H. Complete two to three sets.

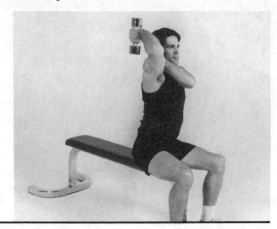

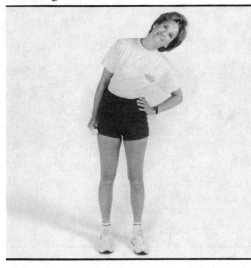

6. Side Bend

A. Stand with your feet shoulder width apart.

B. Grasp the dumbbell (hand weight) in your right hand, and place your left hand on your left hip.

C. Keeping the right arm straight, slowly bend to the left.

D. Feel the force pulling on your left side.

E. Return to the upright position.

F. Complete 15 to 20 repetitions for a set.

G. Eventual goal: two to three sets.

Ankle Weight Exercise

1. Double Leg Extension with Ankle Weights

A. Sit upright on a bench.

B. Hold the bench with your hands.

C. Slowly extend both legs until they are parallel to the floor.

D. Lower your legs with control, and inhale.

E. Complete 15 to 20 repetitions for a set.

F. Eventual goal: two to three sets.

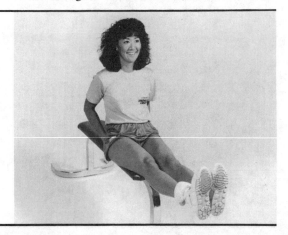

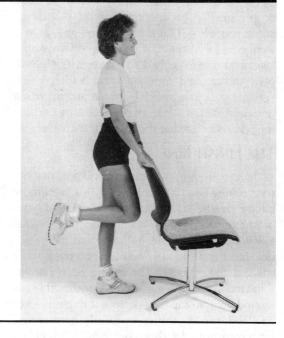

2. Standing Leg Curl

A. Stand upright, holding the top of a chair for support.

B. With an ankle weight on your right leg, slowly bring your heel to your buttocks.

C. Slowly lower the heel to the floor.

D. Complete 15 to 20 repetitions for a set.

E. Repeat on the left leg.

F. Eventual goal: two to three sets.

To use either weight machines or free weights safely and effectively, you need instruction. In fact, when you are using free weights heavy enough to cause strain, you also need a partner, called a spotter, to help you get the weight into position and work with it safely. Without a spotter there is too much danger that as you get fatigued, you'll lose control of the weights and hurt yourself or someone nearby.

Although weight machines don't "work the muscles" as well as free weights (body-builders don't think highly of them), your goal is not to compete as a Mr. or Ms. Universe. The machines are both safer and easier to use, and if you want to go beyond the strength exercises illustrated in this chapter, weight machines should be your first choice.

How To Handle Setbacks

Setbacks are bound to happen. During the first year, people average two to three interruptions in their exercise schedule, often because of minor injuries or illnesses unrelated to exercise. They are forced to slow down or stop altogether for a while.

During the second year, the setbacks tend to be fewer, and eventually they average about one a year. Studies with Olympic athletes suggest that you can actually miss exercise for seven to 14 days without seeing a major decline in conditioning. More than that and you'll be taking a big step backward.

When you resume your program, begin at a lower level—not at the beginning, but back a cou-

Activity vs. Exercise

There is real value to activity that is less strenuous than the recommended aerobic and strengthening exercises. This is true even if the activity is performed at a relatively low level and rather infrequently: Something is better than nothing. Gardening is good for you; so is walking up the stairs whenever you have a chance. However, if you want the full benefits of exercise, you need to develop a program that centers on vigorous activities, such as swimming and running.

ple of notches. If what you try seems too hard, drop your effort back another notch. To catch up, allow yourself the same amount of time as you were out; for instance, if you missed two weeks, take two weeks to get back to your previous level of performance. And common sense helps a lot: If you hurt your foot, switch from running to cycling or swimming for awhile. For specific problems, see the references listed at the end of this chapter.

THE FINISH LINE

As you get into shape, you will note that (1) your resting heart rate is lower, (2) it takes more intense exercise to raise the heart beat, and (3) your heart rate returns to the resting rate more quickly following exercise. This indicates that your muscles, heart and blood vessels are becoming more efficient and effective. The resting heart rate for someone who is fit but not a competitive athlete is around 60; for sedentary persons it might be over 75. Well-trained athletes frequently have resting heart rates around 40 beats per minute. John Havlicek of the Boston Celtics, who seemed never to stop running on the basketball court, is said to have a resting rate of 36. We can hope this isn't true for two reasons—it's so low that it's a little frightening, and it makes the rest of us seem so out of shape!

Exercise comes naturally. As cardiologist George Sheehan argues, people are animals, and you must first be a good animal before you can be a good worker or mother or anything else. Once you realize the importance of fitness, you need to leave yourself open to what exercise can do to make you happier and more productive. Then, if you stick with it long enough to enjoy the benefits of being fit, the situation will become self-reinforcing. You'll want to keep exercising to maintain those good feelings.

You don't need to buy fancy equipment, join a health club or hire a coach. You do need some common sense and a little perseverance. Once you experience the payoffs of exercise, it will be easy to find the time and the place. It's simply a matter of priorities. If you invest the effort to get started and become fit, you will never be satisfied to go back to being unfit.

Arthritis and Exercise

People with osteoarthritis or rheumatoid arthritis need a balanced approach to exercise. Pounding the joints with too much exercise is bad, but so is inactivity. Robert Ike, M.D., and his colleagues at the University of Michigan have shown that inactive arthritis patients who begin exercising on a stationary bicycle not only improve their endurance, they also decrease the severity of their arthritis. In fact, four out of five subjects studied had less pain and swelling after exercise. The Michigan group suggests that activities such as swimming, cycling, golf, dancing, gymnastics, fast walking and jogging may help to relieve arthritis symptoms.

And, contrary to popular belief, there is no evidence that any kind of exercise, even long-distance running, causes or contributes to any kind of arthritis.

ADDITIONAL RESOURCES

The New Aerobics, by Kenneth Cooper, M.D. New York: Bantam Books, 1983.

The Complete Book of Running, by James Fixx. New York: Random House, 1977.

The Complete Book of Exerwalking, by Gary Yanker. Chicago: Contemporary Books, 1983.

Gary Yanker's Walking Workouts, by Gary Yanker. New York: Warner Books, 1987.

Getting Physical: How to Stick with Your Exercise Program, by Art Turock. New York: Doubleday & Co., 1988.

Taking Care of Today and Tomorrow, by George Pfeiffer. Reston, VA: The Center for Corporate Health Promotion, 1988.

FOCUS LifeStyle Management Series on Fitness. The Center for Corporate Health Promotion, Reston, VA: 1988.

Dr. George Sheehan's Medical Advice for Runners, by George Sheehan, M.D. Mountain View, CA: Anderson World, 1978.

Running and Being: The Total Experience, by George Sheehan, M.D. New York: Warner Books, 1978.

This Running Life, by George Sheehan, M.D. New York: Simon & Schuster, 1981.

Dr. Sheehan on Fitness, by George Sheehan, M.D. New York: Simon & Schuster, 1983.

Take Care of Yourself, 4th edition, by Donald M. Vickery, M.D. and James F. Fries, M.D. The Center for Corporate Health Promotion, Reston, VA: 1990.

The Fitness Book, by Bud Getchell. Indianapolis: Benchmark Press, 1987.

Being Fit: A Personal Guide, by Bud Getchell and Wayne Anderson. New York: John Wiley and Sons, 1982.

Royal Canadian Air Force: Exercise Plans for Physical Fitness. New York: Pocket Books, 1972.

If you're interested in organized fitness programs or classes in particular exercise activities, contact these groups in your area:

- YMCA or YWCA
- Public school or community recreation department
- Parks department
- Aerobic-dance organizations
- Athletic clubs

FOOD FOR LIFE

WHAT'S YOUR DISH?

*H*ow much do you know about nutrition? Or better yet, how much do you *want* to know? While almost everyone is interested in food, people vary greatly in how much they want to know about food's connection to health. For this reason, this chapter presents you with jewels, rules and tools. The jewels, or gems of knowledge, lead to the rules—the nitty-gritty of healthy eating. Finally, tools for implementing the rules are provided. Use them as you need them.

In a nationwide survey conducted by the National Center for Health Statistics, 40 percent of the adults interviewed said they had not eaten a single piece of fruit in the past 24 hours. Approximately 20 percent had not eaten a vegetable. And more than 80 percent had not had any high-fiber cereals or whole-grain breads. Yet these very foods are the keys to a nutritious diet. They are high in nutrients and fiber, free of harmful fats and excess protein, and moderate in calories.

The not-so-great American diet has been famous for its bacon and eggs, cheeseburgers and fries, candy bars, cookies and hot fudge sundaes. But there are signs that a change is in the works. Sales of fresh produce and high-fiber cereals are up, while receipts for red meat, butter, eggs, whole milk and salt are down. And surveys by the U.S. Food and Drug Administration indicate that people are indeed responding to new information linking diet and health; more than six out of 10 Americans claimed they have made a "major" change in their eating patterns in the last two years.

Of course, good nutrition alone cannot guarantee good health; health and well-being are influenced by many factors, including heredity, environment, lifestyle and attitude. Nor will food work miracles. Vitamin C will not cure cancer, and vitamin E will not prevent aging. But eating wisely and well can help you feel and look your best. Moreover, evidence mounts daily to show that healthy eating can cut your chances of developing some devastating illnesses:

- **Heart disease.** A high level of cholesterol in the blood (see below) is one of the major risk factors for heart disease. The amount of saturated fat and cholesterol in your diet influences your blood cholesterol level, as do your exercise habits.

- **Cancer.** More than a third of all cancers may be related to the way we eat (see Chapter 19). A diet high in fat, with few fresh fruits and vegetables or whole-grain breads and cereals, has been linked to several types of cancer. Eating too much fat may increase the chances of cancers of the colon, breast, prostate and uterus. A diet high in fiber, in contrast, appears to protect against cancer of the colon. A diet containing nutrient-rich fruits and vegetables, especially dark green and deep yellow-orange vegetables and those in the cabbage family, may also fend off some cancers.

- **Stroke.** Most strokes are caused by atherosclerosis, the same condition that leads to coronary heart disease. And like heart disease, strokes are linked to high blood levels of cholesterol. A second type of stroke occurs when a blood vessel in the brain ruptures, perhaps in part because of high blood pressure.

- **High blood pressure.** About half the people with high blood pressure appear to be "sodium sensitive," that is, consuming sodium causes their blood pressure to go up. Most of the sodium that people eat comes from salt naturally in foods or added in processing, but much of it comes from table salt, too. So, for these people, salt restriction is a must. But because there's no way to tell in advance who is sodium sensitive and who is not, cutting down on salt is a good idea for everyone. Recently there has been evidence that sensitivity increases with age.

Table 7.1
Changing Diet to Reduce Risk of Diseases and Their Complications

Dietary Changes to Reduce the Risk of Diseases or their Complications Diet Change	Heart Disease	Cancer	Stroke	Diabetes	Gastrointestinal Diseases B	Osteoporosis	High Blood Pressure
Reduce Fats	✓	✓	✓	✓	✓		✓
Increase Starches, Fiber (Complex Carbohydrates) A	✓	✓		✓	✓		?
Reduce Sodium	✓		✓				✓
Limit Alcohol		✓	✓		✓		✓
Consume Adequate Calcium						✓	✓

A. Complex carbohydrates are provided by fruits, vegetables and whole-grain products.

B. Primarily gallbladder disease (fat and energy), diverticular disease (fiber), and cirrhosis (alcohol).

Source: *The Surgeon General's Report on Nutrition and Health, 1988.*

Consuming enough calcium may help to short-circuit the development of hypertension in those at risk and lower blood pressure in those already affected. Also, some evidence suggests that too little potassium may raise blood pressure; so potassium, which is plentiful in most fruits and vegetables, may also help to control this condition.

- **Osteoporosis.** The thinning of bones that often accompanies aging—and sets the stage for dangerous fractures—may in part reflect inadequate calcium intake (and, in part, lack of exercise). The usual intake of calcium by adult women is 450 to 550 milligrams per day, well below the 1,000 to 1,500 milligrams daily recommended for women after the menopause.

- **Gastrointestinal diseases.** A number of diseases fall into this category. They include gallbladder disease, which can be influenced by fat intake; liver disease, which results from too much alcohol; and several intestinal problems, which have been linked to fiber intake. A high-fiber diet prevents constipation and perhaps such related conditions as diverticulosis, in which the intestinal wall develops pouches and "irritable bowel."

THE RAW MATERIALS

Putting food in your mouth sets off an elaborate chemical reaction. Food, the most complex mixture the body encounters, is broken down into its primary building blocks. Then, the body extracts what it needs—vitamins, minerals, amino acids from proteins, essential fatty acids from vegetable oils and animal fats. It uses these materials to build tissues and produce vital chemicals, creating not only such hidden assets as supple arteries and rapidly firing nerve cells, but also such visible payoffs as clear skin, shiny hair and strong nails. In addition, the body draws out the energy it needs to keep its machinery running—calories from carbohydrates, proteins and fats.

Food contains five major classes of nutrients: proteins, fats, carbohydrates, vitamins and minerals.

Proteins

Proteins are organic compounds, present in plant and animal tissues. In the human body, they form part of every cell. Hundreds of different proteins help to make up muscle, bone, skin, blood and crucial body chemicals.

Protein is found in many foods of animal origin—meats, fish, poultry, dairy products and eggs—as well as in numerous vegetable sources. However, the body cannot use dietary protein as is; it must first be broken down in the digestive tract into its components, the amino acids. These

The High-Protein Diet

When a person restricts calories on a diet, the body's natural response is to break down muscle and save fat, as if faced with starvation. A dieter can best save muscle mass not by eating a high-protein diet (this has virtually no effect), but by exercising. Exercise causes protein-rich muscle to be spared and fat to be burned instead.

are then transported by the bloodstream to organs and tissues, where they can be fashioned into whatever new proteins are needed. Although the body can construct most amino acids from their basic elements, a few must be derived from food. These are known as essential amino acids.

The body cannot store protein; when a person eats more than the body needs, the excess is either excreted or stored as fat. As a result, protein must be part of each day's diet. If it is not, after a few days the body will begin to break down protein in nonessential tissues like muscles and use it to supply the organs vital for survival, such as the heart.

Proteins are used to build and repair tissues and carry out basic maintenance chores, but they do not normally add to the body's energy supplies. Thus, a person's need for protein depends on body size rather than activity level: A burly forester needs no more protein than an equally burly bureaucrat. The only exceptions might be athletes who work to build muscle or sustain repeated tissue injury. But even their extra needs are slight.

Many of us grew up hearing that it was healthy to eat lots of protein, but in fact the American diet is protein heavy. The average adult male needs less than 70 grams of protein a day—slightly more than two ounces. Thus, six to eight ounces of protein-rich foods will meet the daily needs of adults. When you realize that a single steak is often this large, you can see how easy it is to overdose. (The average American male eats 16 ounces of protein-rich food a day.)

A related problem arises from the fact that dietary protein comes packaged with other nutrients, such as carbohydrates and fat. Most Americans get the majority of their protein from animals sources, which can also contain saturated fat. Unfortunately, many of these sources contain more fat than protein. Hot dogs, for instance, have more than twice as much fat as protein; cheddar cheese contains about one-third more fat than protein; and the marbling that makes steaks tender consists of fat.

Many plants are a valuable, low-fat protein source. The richest lode of vegetable protein is found in *legumes*—peas and beans, including kidney, pinto, navy, lima, black and garbanzo beans, as well as soybeans, lentils and black-eyed peas. Nuts, seeds and peanuts are rich in protein, too, although they do contain some fat. Protein is also found in grains and cereals, and in such vegetables as potatoes, peas, broccoli and corn.

Most proteins from animal sources—eggs, dairy products and meat—are known as complete proteins, because they contain all of the essential amino acids, plus a variety of the nonessential ones. But you can get the amino acids you need from vegetable sources. While each may lack one or more amino acids, if you eat a wide variety of vegetables each day, you can get the full complement. You'll do even better if you add just a small amount of animal protein—a sprinkling of cheese, for instance, on a plate of pasta.

When choosing your protein sources, opt for these:
- Poultry without the skin.
- Fish.
- Lean cuts of meat.
- Low-fat dairy products.
- Cereals.
- Legumes and other vegetables.

Remember, you need only a few ounces a day.

Fats

Fats are a potent source of energy. They insulate the body against extremes of heat and cold, help in the transport of fat-soluble vitamins, are incorporated into essential body chemicals, and protect skin and hair against dryness.

Dietary fats are found in meats, poultry, dairy products, nuts and seeds. They can also be "invisible" in processed foods such as baked goods. Fats make foods tastier and help satisfy the appetite. However, they pack a mean caloric wallop: Where a gram of protein or carbohydrate provides about four calories, a gram of fat has nine. This makes it all too easy to down extra calories.

Dietary fats contain mixtures of the basic chemical units known as *fatty acids*. Depending on their makeup, fatty acids are classified as:

- Saturated. These occur in large amounts in fats of animal origin—meats and whole-milk dairy products. In addition, two vegetable oils—coconut oil and palm oil—are high in saturated fat. Saturated fats are solid at room temperature.
- Monounsaturated. These are most commonly found in olive oil and peanut oil.
- Polyunsaturated. These fats, which are usually liquid at room temperature, come primarily from plants, although some also are derived from fish.

The cholesterol connection. Fats in the diet are closely linked to levels of cholesterol in the blood. Cholesterol is a fat-like substance that forms an essential part of all body cells, nerve endings and certain hormones. It is also a central component of the atherosclerotic deposits that clog diseased blood vessels. (Cholesterol is also discussed in Chapter 18.)

About 80 percent of the body's cholesterol is manufactured in the liver from saturated fat and the rest is absorbed from foods of animal origin. Cholesterol forms part of all animal tissues, but it is never found in foods derived from plants.

It is the saturated fat that you eat, even more than the cholesterol, that can raise your blood level of cholesterol. Some studies suggest that dietary cholesterol has only a modest effect on blood cholesterol. Polyunsaturated and monounsaturated fats, in contrast, help to lower harmful cholesterol levels.

National dietary guidelines call for limiting cholesterol intake to 300 milligrams a day. For the

Table 7.2
Comparison of Dietary Fats

	Cholesterol (mg) Per Tablespoon	Saturated Fat	Monounsaturated Fat	Polyunsaturated Fat
Canola Oil	0	6%	58%	36%
Safflower Oil	0	9%	13%	78%
Sunflower Oil	0	11%	20%	69%
Corn Oil	0	13%	25%	62%
Olive Oil	0	14%	77%	9%
Soybean Oil	0	15%	24%	61%
Peanut Oil	0	18%	48%	34%
Cottonseed Oil	0	27%	19%	54%
Lard	12	41%	47%	12%
Palm Oil	0	51%	39%	10%
Beef Tallow	14	52%	44%	4%
Butterfat	33	66%	30%	4%
Coconut Oil	0	92%	6%	2%

■ Saturated Fat ▦ Monounsaturated Fat ☐ Polyunsaturated Fat

Source: U.S. Department of Agriculture, Science and Education Administration. *Agriculture Handbook No. 8-4*, June 1979.

most part, if you cut down on foods high in saturated fat you'll automatically limit foods that are high in cholesterol. There are a few exceptions: Egg yolks and organ meats are high in cholesterol, but fairly low in saturated fat. (An egg contains approximately 200 milligrams of cholesterol.) On the other hand, several plant oils, including coconut oil, palm oil and palm kernel oil, as well as the cocoa butter in chocolate, have no cholesterol, but they are very high in saturated fat. Other vegetable oils, such as soybean oil and cottonseed oil, can cause problems, too, if they undergo hydrogenation, a process that extends their shelf life but makes them more saturated.

Americans are eating less fat and fewer high-cholesterol foods than they did 25 years ago. This has contributed greatly to the drop in heart disease that has occurred during the last quarter century.

Still, daily fat intake far exceeds the single tablespoon of polyunsaturated fat that the body needs each day. The average American gets more than 40 percent of his or her calories from fat. Authorities, including the National Research Council, recommend that fats contribute no more than 30 percent of the calories in the diet. For a person whose daily intake totals 2,000 calories, this means limiting fat to no more than 600 of those calories, and saturated fat to 200. Virtually no American is in danger of eating too little fat, so the lower, the better. If you can get your fat intake down to 25 percent of total calories, or even 15 percent, so much the better.

The food choices you make can affect your health. Use this table to make wiser selections. (Remember that saturated fat is contained in foods of animal origin and in palm and coconut oils.)

It boils down to this: You can lower your

Table 7.3
How Much Fat and Cholesterol Do You Eat?

Food	Total Fat (grams)	Cholesterol (milligrams)
Beef liver, fried (3 ounces)	9	372
Egg, large, cooked:		
1 yolk	6	213
1 white	trace	0
Beef, roasted:		
Lean and fat (3 ounces)	16	80
Lean only (3 ounces)	6	77
Chicken, light and dark meat, roasted:		
With skin (3 ounces)	12	75
Without skin (3 ounces)	6	76
Halibut fillets, broiled, with		
margarine (3 ounces)	6	48
Lobster, steamed (3.5 ounces)	0.6	72
Shrimp, steamed (3.5 ounces)	0.3	195
Milk:		
Whole (1 cup)	8	33
2% fat (1 cup)	5	18
Skim	1	5
Vanilla ice cream (1/2 cup)	7	30
Vanilla ice milk (1/2 cup)	3	9
Potatoes:		
Au gratin (1/2 cup)	19	56
French fries, fried in		
vegetable oil (10)	8	0
Baked (1 medium)	trace	0
Danish pastry (1 piece)	12	49
Doughnut, yeast (1 doughnut)	13	21
Bagel, plain (1 bagel)	2	0
Waffle (1 waffle)	8	59
Oatmeal, cooked (1/2 cup)	1	0
Butter (1 tablespoon)	11	31
Margarine (1 tablespoon)	11	0
Mayonnaise (1 tablespoon)	11	8
Mayonnaise, imitation (1 tablespoon)	5	4
Cake, frosted, devil's food (1 slice)	11	50
Apple (1 medium)	trace	0

Source: *FOCUS on Cholesterol*. Reston, VA: The Center for Corporate Health Promotion, 1989.

Fish, Fish Oil and Cholesterol

The finding that Eskimos, who eat large amounts of fish, have low levels of heart disease sparked the idea that fish oil might protect against heart problems. The benefit is thought to come from components of fish oil known as omega-3 fatty acids. Several studies in which heart patients were given large doses of fish-oil supplements have found that omega-3 fatty acids seem to lower blood cholesterol levels and prevent blood from clotting. Also, they appear to lower blood pressure and provide some relief from arthritis. Unfortunately, the effect on these problems seems fairly small and probably decreases as time goes on.

On the minus side, fish-oil supplements may cause a number of side effects, such as diarrhea and, in diabetics, elevated blood sugar. Their effect on clotting could lead to severe bleeding in the event of injury. Much remains to be learned before high doses of fish oil can be widely recommended. In the meantime, you can safely add fish oil to your diet by eating fish two or three times a week, especially cold-water, fatty fish such as salmon, swordfish, mackerel, bluefish and fresh tuna. People who eat lots of all kinds of fish often have high HDL levels.

level of serum cholesterol, and also your risk of cancers of the colon, breast and prostate, by eating less fat, especially less saturated fat.

Carbohydrates

Carbohydrates are compounds made up of carbon, hydrogen and oxygen. They provide the body with its main source of energy. Carbohydrates are broken down into glucose, which is carried in the blood, and glycogen, which is stored in the liver and muscles.

Dietary carbohydrates come in two varieties, complex and simple. Complex carbohydrates are the starches in grain and grain-based foods, including cereals, breads and pasta; peas and beans; and "starchy" vegetables like potatoes and corn. The complex sugars contained in fruit and milk can also be placed in this group. Foods rich in complex carbohydrates tend to be high in vitamins and minerals as well as dietary fiber. Simple carbohydrates, sometimes called simple sugars, provide calories but little else. Some common sources are table sugar, honey and syrups. Gram for gram, starches and sugars supply about the same number of calories.

Many people shy away from starchy foods under the mistaken belief that they are fattening. In fact they contain fewer than half the calories of the same amount of fat. According to the 1989 recommendations of the National Research Council, carbohydrates should supply at least 55 percent of the calories in our diets.

The fiber imperative. Dietary fiber is the indigestible part of plant cells. It can be either soluble, meaning that it dissolves in hot water, or insoluble, in which case it doesn't. Most plant foods contain both kinds, but in different proportions.

By moving food and by-products through the intestines and out of the body, insoluble fiber helps prevent constipation and promotes a healthy digestive tract. Eating foods high in fiber has been found to reduce symptoms of diverticular disease and some types of "irritable bowel." It may also reduce the risk of colon cancer. Whole grains, beans and vegetables are especially rich in insoluble fiber; the most plentiful source is wheat bran. Some good high-fiber food choices are wholewheat bread, bran and corn muffins, bran cereals, shredded wheat, all fruits and vegetables, and popcorn. (Make popcorn unbuttered to avoid extra calories and saturated fat!)

Certain soluble fibers are known to lower serum cholesterol, although how they work is not clear. The leading theory is that they combine with bile to prevent the absorption of saturated fat from the intestine. Soluble fibers include oat bran, the outer covering of the oat kernel, and pectin, which is found in apples and other fruits. Soluble fiber is also found in legumes and vegetables. In one series of studies, men with high cholesterol levels were fed typical American diets supplemented with 100 grams of oat bran a day (the equivalent of about three servings of cooked oat-bran cereal or six oat-bran muffins), or 100 grams of dried beans. Overall, the men's cholesterol levels dropped by at least 19 percent.

Sugar: Calories and little else. In one or another of its many forms—sucrose, maltose, fructose, honey or corn syrup—sugar finds its way into most processed foods, including soups, peanut butter, ketchup and salad dressing. That's one reason the average American downs more than 120 pounds of sugar and sweeteners a year. Although sugar does not cause cellulite, depression or hyperactivity, its "empty calories" contribute to obesity and diabetes, heart disease and high blood pressure. Moreover, refined sugar is the major culprit in tooth decay.

Vitamins and Minerals

Vitamins are compounds derived from plants or animals that are needed for the hundreds of chemical reactions that go on non-stop in our bodies. However, because the human body cannot make vitamins, either at all or in large enough amounts, we must get them from the foods we eat.

Vitamins are classified as either fat soluble or water soluble. Because the fat-soluble vitamins—A, D, E and K—can be stored in body tissues, we do not need them every day. The water-soluble vitamins are the eight B vitamins—B_1 (thiamin), B_2 (riboflavin), B_3 (niacin), B_5 (pantothenic acid), B_6 (pyridoxine), B_{12} (cobalamin), folacin and biotin—plus vitamin C. With the exception of vitamin B_{12}, the water-soluble vitamins are not stored in the body and need to be part of the diet every day.

Minerals are inorganic substances, usually salts, that facilitate chemical reactions within cells. Of the more than two dozen that have been identified, several—calcium, phosphorus, magnesium, sodium, potassium and chloride—are known as

Artificial Sweetener

The trade-off between sugar and artificial sweetener is straightforward: 16 calories per teaspoon of sugar vs. the risk of the unknown. Aspartame (Nutra Sweet) is virtually the only sweetener used in the U.S. at present. It has virtually no *known* risks, at least at recommended levels of consumption. Are side effects not being recognized? Possibly, but not likely. The trade-off between sugar and aspartame only becomes important when large quantities are consumed. For example, the aspartame in a 12-ounce diet soda will save about 180 calories and probably not increase any risk very much. If you drink five such sodas per day, the savings of 900 calories is substantial—but any risk is increased also, and unfortunately, those 900 calories usually are made up for by eating other foods.

I must confess that I've always been amused by folks who insist on using an artificial sweetener in their coffee or tea and then use it to wash down high-calorie foods. They seem to feel that foregoing 16 calories of sugar makes up for the 400 calories in the dessert.

Again, unless huge amounts of artificial sweeetener are consumed (and this would be bad for you), the trade-off between sugar and aspartame is not a big deal. Take your choice.

macroelements, because they are needed in fairly large amounts. The rest, including iron, zinc, selenium and iodine, are known as trace elements.

How Much is Good For You?

Many conflicting claims are made about our needs for specific vitamins and minerals. One group of basic guidelines represents the consensus of a panel of experts from the National Academy of Sciences and is based on up-to-date scientific information. These are the U.S. Recommended Dietary

Vitamins and Cancer

Sweeping claims have been made for vitamin C's ability to cure cancer. However, careful studies, including a series at the Mayo Clinic, have failed to back up these claims.

On the other hand, vitamin C, as well as vitamins A and E, may play a role in cancer prevention. For example, researchers found that smokers who ate lots of vegetables, especially dark green and dark yellow-orange ones, were less likely to develop lung cancer than smokers who ate few vegetables. These foods contain high levels of beta-carotene, the dietary precursor of vitamin A. In another study, women smokers who ate diets rich in vegetables and fruits—and thus beta-carotene and vitamin C—were less likely to develop cancers of the mouth and throat. Several studies have shown a link between low rates of stomach cancer and diets rich in good sources of vitamin C. Finally, smokers with low blood levels of vitamin E are more likely to develop lung cancer than those with high levels.

Vitamins A, C and E are all antioxidants, substances that protect cells from highly reactive chemicals called free radicals. Many scientists believe that free radicals help cause cancer. Other antioxidants that have been linked to lower cancer risk are polyphenols, found in fruits, nuts and wheat bran, and lycopene, the compound that gives tomatoes, strawberries, cranberries and watermelon their red color.

If you want to get more of these antioxidants, it's probably better to seek them from food than through supplements. Eat heartily from vegetables such as carrots, spinach and other leafy greens; members of the cabbage family, including broccoli, brussels sprouts and cauliflower; cereals and breads containing wheat bran; and fruits, especially red ones. Nuts and peanut butter are rich in vitamin E and polyphenols; unfortunately, they're also high in fat. If you do decide to use supplements, 400 international units of vitamin E, 500 milligrams of vitamin C and 25,000 international units of beta-carotene should be plenty.

Large doses of vitamin C have also been promoted as a way to prevent colds or at least diminish their symptoms. Most tests of this claim have found little, if any, benefit. But if it makes you feel better, do it.

Allowances (RDAs). RDAs are not minimum requirements; they are set to meet the demands of people with the highest need, so they are more than enough for most people. For this reason this book does not focus on RDAs. Specific advice about foods and supplements is more useful.

Usually, vitamin or mineral supplements are not needed: You can meet your daily requirements by eating a balanced diet. This is especially true because so many American foods—including flour, cereals, juices, milk and margarine—are "fortified" with vitamins and minerals. Vitamin or mineral deficiency is unlikely to sneak up on you. In fact, you would have to eat a pretty lopsided diet for a long time before you suffered a disease from lack of a vitamin or mineral.

- In order for one presumably normal adult (a doctor) to develop signs of vitamin C deficiency, he had to eat nothing but milk and boiled potatoes for more than four months; one glass of orange juice would have botched the whole experiment.

- Human disease due to a diet deficient in vitamin E has never been reported, not even experimentally. Problems that *resemble* vitamin E deficiency in animals have been reported in children with serious intestinal diseases, but only very rarely.

- Pyridoxine (vitamin B_6) deficiency has been reported only rarely. It cannot be produced experimentally by excluding vitamin B_6 from the diet.

- Vitamin K is produced by bacteria in the large intestine, so adequate levels don't depend on diet.
- To produce disease from thiamine (vitamin B_1) deficiency, thiamine must be excluded from the diet for 50 to 200 days. To produce disease due to pantothenic acid (vitamin B_5) deficiency takes 12 weeks.
- Disease due to deficiency of such "vitamins" as biotin, choline and PABA has never been reported.

However, there are times when vitamin supplements may be needed: Women in their childbearing years may need extra iron; women who are pregnant or breastfeeding need more of many nutrients and may need supplements if their diets are inadequate (folacin is the most common supplement); breast-fed infants should receive a vitamin D supplement, while bottle-fed infants need extra iron.

Most vegetarians can meet all of their nutritional requirements by eating a wide variety of vegetables. However, persons who strictly avoid all foods of animal origin, including milk and eggs, should take a vitamin B_{12} supplement or be sure to eat plenty of tofu (a fermented bean product that contains vitamin B_{12}).

Contrary to popular belief, physical activity does not increase your need for vitamins or minerals, with a single important exception: You may need to increase your intake of potassium during intense, prolonged exercise in hot weather. (Orange juice and bananas are good and handy sources of potassium.) You do *not* need to eat salt during exercise.

While a lack of vitamins and minerals may lead to disease, overdosing can also be toxic. Large doses of vitamins A, D and B_6 are especially dangerous. High blood levels of iron have been associated with increased risk of colon cancer. Taking huge amounts of any nutrient has no known advantages—except profits for people who promote these overdoses.

The best way to obtain vitamins and minerals is to eat a variety of foods. If you are concerned

A Case for Vitamin Supplements?

As researchers learn more about the role of vitamins in health, recommendations about supplements may change. A recent Canadian study suggested that persons over 55 who took vitamin C supplements (at least 300 milligrams daily for the past five years) had a 70 percent lower risk of cataracts than those who did not. Persons who took a daily vitamin E capsule (400 international units) appeared to have about half the risk of those who did not.

Vitamins C and E are antioxidants, substances that protect cells against harmful chemicals called free radicals. They may protect against cancer as well. Most of the evidence for the benefits of antioxidants has come from studies in which people consumed *food* that contained them. The Canadian study is one of the few studies of supplement use. Supplements may prove to be useful, but at present the surest and safest way to obtain the benefits of antioxidants appears to be choosing the right foods.

about missing something and you want to take a daily supplement, fine. But unless they're prescribed to counter a specific problem, large doses of any nutrient should be avoided.

What about salt? Table salt contains the minerals sodium and chloride, both essential to nutrition. Salt—lots of it—shows up in processed foods, fast foods, canned vegetables, snacks, sandwich meats, sauces and pickles. Although the body can get along just fine with 0.2 gram of sodium per day, the average intake is 20 to 25 times that much—4 to 5 grams of sodium, or the equivalent of 2 1/2 to 3 teaspoons of table salt. Excess sodium, as we have seen, can lead to high blood pressure in persons who are sodium sensitive.

Table 7.4
Vitamins

Vitamin	Actions	Sources
A	Healthy skin and mucous membranes; needed for night vision, development of bones and teeth; possible anti-cancer effect	Found as *retinols* in liver, milk, butter and eggs, and as *carotenes* in dark green, leafy vegetables, yellow and orange vegetables and fruits
D	Permits proper use of calcium and phosphorus for healthy bones and teeth	Sunlight on skin, which converts body chemicals to vitamin D; milk fortified with vitamin D; egg yolk; tuna and salmon; liver
E	Helps form many body tissues, including muscles and red blood cells; protects vitamin A and fatty acids from breakdown	Vegetable oils; margarine; leafy green vegetables; whole-grain cereals and breads
K	Aids in making blood-clotting factors	Leafy green vegetables; cauliflower, peas and cabbage; meat
B_1 (thiamin)	Promotes energy release from carbohydrates; needed to make a vital nervous system substance	Starches enriched or made with whole grains; pork, liver and oysters
B_2 (riboflavin)	Helps maintain skin and mucous membranes; needed to extract energy from foods	Milk; eggs; whole grains; leafy green vegetables; liver and other meat

Food Additives

Food additives present some dilemmas. Some, such as food dyes, we could probably do without. They add nothing to nutrition, and at least some of them produce cancers in animals. (However, it is unlikely that they have anything to do with hyperactivity in children despite persistent claims to the contrary.)

Preservatives such as nitrites, in contrast, do make a contribution. Without them, foods such as sausages and luncheon meats would not be available. But they do cause bladder cancer in mice, and

Table 7.4
Vitamins, continued

Vitamin	Actions	Sources
B₃ (niacin)	Needed for body processes, including extraction of energy from food	Animal protein; green vegetables, peas, and beans; whole grains
B₅ (pantothenic acid)	Helps in food processing and synthesis of hormones and nervous system chemicals	Almost all plant and animal tissues
B₆ (pyridoxine and related compounds)	Vital for utilization of proteins in diet and for production of red blood cells	Fish, poultry, meat; whole grains, nuts; bananas, potatoes
B₁₂ (cobalamin)	Vital for production of red blood cells and genetic material; needed for nervous system function	Milk; eggs; animal tissue
Folacin (folic acid and related compounds)	Promotes production of hemoglobin (oxygen-carrying component of blood) and genetic material	Liver; leafy vegetables and fruit; dried beans and peas; milk
Biotin	Regulates fat and sugar processing	Liver and kidney; egg yolk; green vegetables
C (ascorbic acid)	Helps maintain bones, teeth and small blood vessels; promotes formation of the protein collagen; protects vitamins A and E from breakdown	Citrus fruits; tomatoes, melons, strawberries; potatoes and green vegetables

many of the foods in which they are used are high in fat. Avoiding them when possible seems a wise approach.

Just to keep things unsettled, we have the case of BHA and BHT antioxidants, added to cereals and other products to keep them fresh. There is evidence that these additives have contributed to the marked *decline* in stomach cancer that has occurred since the 1930s. Still, the evidence is inconclusive. Some animal studies suggest they prevent cancer while others indicate they could cause cancer.

Table 7.5
A Sampling of Minerals

Mineral	Action	Sources
Calcium	Builds bones and teeth; helps muscle contraction, blood clotting and enzyme activity	Milk and milk products; canned salmon and sardines; leafy green vegetables; citrus fruits; beans and peas
Phosphorus	Builds bones and teeth; helps release energy from food; helps form genetic material and many tissues	Milk and milk products; Meat, poultry, fish, and eggs; beans and peas
Magnesium	Helps build bones; manufactures proteins; produces energy from glycogen; conducts nerve impulses	Nuts, seeds and whole grains; leafy green vegetables
Potassium	Aids muscle contraction; regulates the balance of body chemistry; plays role in nerve impulses	Orange juice; bananas; apples; dried fruits; beans and peas; bran; avocados; potatoes; peanut butter; coffee, tea and cocoa
Sodium and Chloride	Regulate the balance of body fluids; activate an enzyme in saliva; part of stomach acid	Table salt and other naturally occurring salts
Iron	Helps form the system that supplies oxygen to cells	Liver, kidney, and red meat; leafy green vegetables; egg yolk; molasses; dried fruits; beans and peas; potatoes; enriched cereals
Zinc	Component of about 100 enzymes	Meat, liver, eggs and poultry; seafood; milk; whole grains
Iodine	Component of thyroid hormones; essential for reproduction	Seafood; iodized salt; sea salt
Copper	Helps form red blood cells and many enzymes; aids the work of the nervous system	Oysters; liver and kidney; dried beans; margarine
Selenium	Prevents breakdown of body chemicals	Seafood; meat and chicken; egg yolk; milk; cereals
Chromium	Helps form insulin for normal sugar utilization ·	Meat; cheese; dried beans; whole-grain breads and cereals; peanuts; brewer's yeast

Table 7.6
How the American Diet Stacks Up

Nutrient	Recommended Diet	Typical American Diet
Fiber[a]	20–30 g/day	11 g/day
Cholesterol[b]	300 mg/day	300–500 mg/day
Calcium[c]	800–1,000 mg/day	450 mg/day
Sodium[d]	3 g/day	4–5 g/day
Alcohol[e]	no more than 1 to 2 oz ethanol	

[a] A serving of 40 percent bran cereal provides 5 grams of fiber; a bowl of pea soup provides 4 grams.

[b] One egg contains approximately 200 milligrams of cholesterol.

[c] One cup of yogurt contains 415 milligrams of calcium; a cup of skim milk has 305 milligrams.

[d] One teaspoon equals approximately 2 grams (2,000 milligrams) of sodium. A bowl of corn flakes has 290 milligrams; a cup of skim milk has 120 milligrams.

[e] Half an ounce of ethanol is the equivalent of a 12-ounce can of beer, a 4-ounce glass of wine, or a cocktail made with 1 1/2 ounces of hard liquor.

Artificial sweeteners have been linked with cancer in laboratory experiments, but any risk clearly seems to be related to dosage. Using them occasionally seems to present little danger (see box on page 97). Diet foods can be useful when calories need to be restricted, but they are no substitute for exercise and reduced fat intake.

Nutrition and Performance

The body draws most of its energy from carbohydrates and fat. Carbohydrates, which are carried as glucose in the blood and stored as glycogen in the liver and muscles, are the most efficient and available source of energy. They supply energy to the brain, and they are needed for the processing of fat and protein.

At rest and at low levels of exercise, the body derives the energy it needs from fatty acids, the basic building blocks of fat. But when activity steps up, the body turns to glycogen, which can be quickly converted into glucose.

The amount of glycogen available in the muscles and the intensity of the exercise determine how long you can exercise. If there is enough glycogen, the muscles can do their work. But once the glycogen is used up, performance falters and muscles become tired and cramped. Marathon runners call this "hitting the wall."

To build up greater stores of glycogen in their muscles, many marathon runners and triathletes practice "carboloading." For several days before a competition, they fill up on pasta, bread and fruit. Although the technique is of little use to someone exercising less than several hours a day, choosing complex carbohydrates over fat, protein or sugar is always an advantage.

Nutrition and Aging

Many people gain weight more easily as they grow older, largely because they are less active. The best solution is simple: Exercise more (see Chapter 6). As always, eating less is important.

For other older people the problem is a shrinking appetite. This is more a problem of inactivity and depression than of food. It is part of a vicious cycle: Inactivity and depression lead to eating less; eating less leads to less energy, less activity and more depression. The way to break the cycle is to become more active. The rest will take care of itself.

Constipation is another common complaint of older people. Exercise, choosing high-fiber foods and drinking plenty of water and other fluids can help alleviate this problem.

Many older people, especially older women, suffer from osteoporosis, a gradual, abnormal loss of bone tissue that leaves them subject to broken bones, usually in the spine, hips and wrists. Experts recommend that premenopausal women and older women receiving estrogen, which also counters osteoporosis, consume 1,000 milligrams of calcium a day, and that other postmenopausal women take 1,500 milligrams a day. (This is hard to do when dieting!) In addition to dairy products, other good sources of calcium are leafy green vegetables, broccoli, sardines and canned salmon. Supplements make sense here. Also, weight-bearing exercise is necessary for normal calcium absorption.

PUTTING YOUR KNOWLEDGE TO WORK

This chapter began with a promise to offer "jewels, rules and tools." The jewels, or gems of knowledge, were to be followed by some basic principles of good nutrition (rules) and practical suggestions for improving poor eating habits (tools).

Now that you have sifted through the jewels, you should have a good understanding of how diet affects disease risk. You have read about the major classes of nutrients—proteins, fats and carbohydrates—as well as the role that vitamins and minerals play in maintaining health.

If your eating habits are like those of most Americans, you probably see a need to make them less harmful and more healthful. But it may seem that there are so many aspects of nutrition to remember, you may not know where to begin.

It's best to start by making those changes that yield the greatest health benefits—cutting down on fats, saturated fats in particular, and eating more of the complex carbohydrates found in bread, cereal, rice, beans, vegetables and fruits. Choosing a variety of foods is your best insurance of getting all of the vitamins and minerals your body needs.

To simplify healthful eating even more, I have combined these suggestions into a single recommendation, which I call the "Golden Rule":

Eat a varied diet that is low in fat and high in complex carbohydrates.

If you remember nothing else about healthy eating, memorize the golden rule and put it into practice whenever you can. You will find that other dietary concerns take care of themselves when you do. For example, by avoiding fat you will naturally consume more vegetables and fruits.

The Not-So-Great American Diet

Nutrient	Recommended Diet (% of total daily calorie intake)	Typical American Diet (% of total daily calorie intake)
Complex carbohydrates	40	20
Simple carbohydrates	15	25
Protein	15	15
Unsaturated fats	20	25
Saturated fats	10	15

Source: *Taking Care of Today and Tomorrow*. Reston, VA: The Center for Corporate Health Promotion, 1989.

Figure 7.1 presents some additional rules, or strategies, for implementing the Golden Rule. Each represents one thing you can do to improve your eating habits. Depending on the way you are eating now and your personal and family health history, you may want to pay special attention to particular rules. Along with each rule is a reference to one or more of the tools that follow. Make the tools that you need part of your personal LifePlan.

Figure 7.1
The Golden Rule

Eat a **varied diet** that is **low in fat** and **high in complex carbohydrates.**

A varied diet provides enough **vitamins, minerals** and **protein** for most people.

If you are in doubt, taking a daily **vitamin** and **mineral** supplement is better than worrying, but megadoses are not recommended. Some special groups may need supplements. See Do You Need a Supplement? (Tool #2).

Adequate levels of **calcium** in the diet can help to protect against osteoporosis and contribute to healthy blood pressure levels. See Do You Need a Supplement? (Tool #2) and Foods Rich in Calcium Tool #3).

Too much **sodium** and too little **potassium** contribute to hypertension. See Less Sodium, More Potassium (Tool #4).

Beta-carotene and other **antioxidants** appear to protect against some cancers. See Beta-Carotene and Other Antioxidants: Where to Find Them (Tool #5).

Substitute **low-fat** foods for high-fat choices. See How to Eat Less Fat (Tool #6), Guide to Healthful Restaurant Dining (Tool #10), Fast Food: Know What You're Ordering (Tool #11) and Recipes for Healthful Meals (Tool #12).

The fats you do consume should be **polyunsaturated** and **monounsaturated,** not saturated. See Fats: The Good vs. the Bad and the Ugly (Tool #7).

Most Americans consume more **protein** than they need. Animal studies suggest that low-calorie, low-protein diets mean longer lives. See Meal-Planning Guide (Tool #1), Guide to Healthful Restaurant Dining (Tool #10), Fast Food: Know What You're Ordering (Tool #11) and Recipes for Healthful Meals (Tool #12).

Choose **complex carbohydrates** that are rich in other nutrients and high in fiber. See Meal-Planning Guide (Tool #1), Guide to Healthful Restaurant Dining (Tool #10), Fast Food: Know What You're Ordering (Tool #11) and Recipes for Healthful Meals (Tool #12).

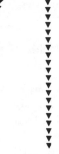

Soluble **fiber** promotes healthy cholesterol levels; insoluble fiber appears to protect against cancer of the colon and other disorders of the digestive tract. See Fiber: Soluble vs. Insoluble (Tool #8).

Avoid **simple carbohydrates,** or "simple sugars" which contribute calories to the diet but little nutrition. See Substitute Nutrition for Sugar's Empty Calories (Tool #9).

YOUR NUTRITION TOOLS
Tool #1: Meal-Planning Guide

Here are a week's worth of menus that emphasize complex carbohydrates while playing down protein and fat. They also stress variety and healthful food-preparation methods. You don't need to follow this menu plan exactly; rather, use it to get ideas as you start planning healthy meals of your own. Typical American "three square meals" are presented as well, so that you can compare the differences in terms of carbohydrates, protein and fat.

	Carbohydrates (g)	Protein (g)	Fat (g)
A TYPICAL AMERICAN DAILY DIET			
Breakfast			
Scrambled egg (1 large)	1.4	6.0	7.1
Pork sausage, 2 links	2.8	30.2	43.2
Croissant, Sara Lee	11.2	2.3	6.1
Margarine, 2 teaspoons	0	0	7.6
Orange juice, 4 oz.	14.4	0.8	0
Lunch			
Wendy's double cheeseburger	41.0	50.0	48.0
French fries	41.0	5.0	16.0
Chocolate shake	54.0	9.0	16.0
Dinner			
2 pork chops (7 oz. meat)	0	58.8	51.2
8 oz. macaroni and cheese	31.1	12.5	12.1
Broccoli, 1 cup	4.5	1.9	0.3
8 oz. whole milk	11.0	8.0	8.0
Daily Totals	212.4	184.5	215.6
A WEEK'S HEALTHFUL MENUS:			
SUNDAY			
Breakfast			
2 buckwheat pancakes	21.4	6.2	4.1
with 1 cup sliced strawberries	10.5	0.9	0.6
6 oz. grapefruit juice	14.5	1.0	0.2
Lunch			
1 cup vegetable soup	19.0	3.5	3.7
Ry Krisp, 2 triple crackers	10.0	1.3	0.2
1 oz. sliced Swiss cheese	1.0	8.1	7.8
2 oatmeal cookies	24.4	2.2	6.4
8 oz. skim milk	11.9	8.4	0.4
Dinner			
3.5 oz. baked chicken breast, skinless	0	30.9	4.5
Baked potato, medium	21.1	2.6	0.1
Margarine, 2 teaspoons	0	0	7.6
2/3 cup carrots, cooked	7.1	0.9	0.2
Tossed salad	2.5	1.2	0.2
Low-fat dressing	0.7	0	1.5
Homemade muffin	20.9	4.0	1.1
Daily Totals	165.0	71.2	38.6

Tool #1: Meal-Planning Guide, continued

	Carbohydrates (g)	Protein (g)	Fat (g)
MONDAY			
Breakfast			
Shredded wheat (1 biscuit)	18.8	2.6	0.3
Skim milk, 1/2 cup	6.0	4.2	0.2
Sliced peach	9.7	0.6	0.1
8 oz. orange juice	26.8	1.7	0.1
Lunch			
Sandwich:			
3.5 oz. sliced turkey breast, Louis Rich	0	21.0	3.0
2 slices whole-wheat bread	22.8	4.8	2.2
2 oz. lettuce	1.3	0.6	0.1
Low-fat mayonnaise, 1 tablespoon	0.4	0.2	5.5
Pear	25.1	0.7	0.7
8 oz. lemonade	23.9	0	0
Dinner			
French-bread pizza (homemade):			
2 slices bread	25.2	4.8	1.0
2/3 cup tomato sauce	7.3	1.3	0.3
1 oz. part-skim mozzarella cheese	0.8	6.9	4.5
2/3 cup Italian green beans	5.1	1.2	0.1
1 cup cantaloupe pieces	13.4	1.4	0.4
Daily Totals	186.6	52.0	18.5
TUESDAY			
Breakfast			
1 slice whole-wheat toast	10.9	2.3	6.1
1 tablespoon apple butter	9.1	0.1	0.2
1 cup low-fat yogurt, fruit flavored	31.3	11.2	2.8
1 orange	16.3	1.4	0.1
Lunch			
Microwave-baked potato, medium, topped with:	21.1	2.6	0.1
1/2 cup low-fat cottage cheese	6.2	14.0	2.3
1 cup Manhattan clam chowder	12.2	4.2	2.3
Dinner			
Stir-fry (pepper steak):			
3.5 oz. lean beef	0	30.0	9.5
1 green pepper	4.8	1.2	0.2
1/2 medium onion	4.4	0.8	0
4/5 cup cooked rice	36.3	3.0	0.2
Daily Totals	152.6	70.8	23.8
WEDNESDAY			
Breakfast			
3/4 cup oatmeal	18.9	4.5	1.8
Sliced banana	26.7	1.2	0.6
1/2 cup skim milk	6.0	4.2	0.2
8 oz. apple juice	27.6	0.3	0.3

Tool #1: Meal-Planning Guide, continued

	Carbohydrates (g)	Protein (g)	Fat (g)
Lunch			
Tuna salad sandwich	25.8	11.0	14.2
Carrot sticks	9.7	1.1	0.2
1/2 cup unsweetened applesauce	13.8	0.2	0.1
Dinner			
1 cup homemade minestrone soup	11.2	4.3	2.5
1 slice homemade bread	12.6	2.4	1.0
Tossed salad	2.5	1.5	0.2
Low-fat dressing	0.7	0	1.5
8 oz. skim milk	11.9	8.4	0.4
2 oatmeal cookies	24.4	2.2	6.4
Daily Totals	191.8	41.3	29.4

THURSDAY

	Carbohydrates (g)	Protein (g)	Fat (g)
Breakfast			
Bagel	30.9	6.0	1.4
1 tablespoon peanut butter	3.2	3.9	7.2
1/2 grapefruit	9.5	0.7	0.1
1/2 cup skim milk	6.0	4.2	0.2
Lunch			
1 cup minestrone soup (leftover from last night's dinner)	11.2	4.3	2.5
1 slice rye bread	12.0	2.1	0.9
Celery stalk	2.0	0.4	0.1
3/4 cup rice pudding	38.7	5.2	4.5
Dinner			
1 cup cooked spaghetti	44.0	7.3	0.7
2/3 cup tomato sauce	7.3	1.3	0.3
1 tablespoon grated cheese	0.2	2.1	1.5
Tossed salad	2.5	1.2	0.2
Low-fat dressing	0.7	0	1.5
1 slice Italian bread	11.3	1.8	0.2
Daily Totals	179.5	40.5	21.3

FRIDAY

	Carbohydrates (g)	Protein (g)	Fat (g)
Breakfast			
Bran muffin	16.7	3.0	5.1
1/2 cup low-fat cottage cheese	6.2	14.0	2.3
Sliced apple	21.1	0.3	0.5
Lunch			
Salad plate:			
3.5 oz. romaine lettuce	3.5	1.3	0.3
Medium tomato, sliced	7.0	1.6	0.3
Bean sprouts	6.6	3.8	0.2
1/2 cup cold, cooked shrimp	0.8	16.2	0.8
Low-calorie Italian dressing	0.7	0	1.5
2 bread sticks	9.0	1.4	0.4
1 cup skim milk	11.9	8.4	0.4

Tool #1: Meal-Planning Guide, continued

	Carbohydrates (g)	Protein (g)	Fat (g)
Dinner			
5 oz. Spanish rice	24.9	2.5	2.6
1/2 acorn squash, baked	21.8	3.0	0.2
Spinach salad	4.3	3.2	0.3
Low-fat dressing	0.7	0	1.5
Daily Totals	135.2	58.7	16.4
SATURDAY			
Breakfast			
English muffin, toasted	28.1	4.8	1.2
2 teaspoons margarine	0	0	7.6
Tangerine	9.4	0.5	0.2
1 cup skim milk	11.9	8.4	0.4
Lunch			
1/2 sandwich:			
2 oz. chicken breast	0	13.0	2.1
1 slice rye bread	12.0	2.1	0.9
1 cup low-fat vanilla yogurt	31.3	11.2	2.8
Alfalfa sprouts	5.5	5.1	0.6
8 oz. apple juice	27.6	0.3	0.3
Corn muffin	21.6	3.2	4.5
Dinner			
3.5 oz. broiled fish fillet	0	26.1	5.0
1/2 cup long-grain wild rice	24.7	2.8	4.1
Salad	2.5	1.2	0.2
Low-fat Dressing	0.7	0	1.5
1/2 cup steamed zucchini	3.3	1.1	0.1
Daily Totals	178.6	79.8	31.5

Tool #2: Do You Need a Supplement?

Group	Nutrient Possibly Needed	Form of Supplement Most Often Used
Women in their childbearing years	Iron	Iron supplements (Note: Too much iron can have toxic effects. Supplements should only be taken if a doctor determines that there is a deficiency.)
Pregnant and breastfeeding women	Iron, vitamins A, C, B_6, B_{12} and folacin	Multivitamin supplements
Breast-fed infants	Vitamin D	Multivitamin drops
Bottle-fed infants	Iron	Multivitamin drops with iron
Women past the menopause	Calcium	Calcium supplements (Note: Several kinds are on the market. Calcium carbonate (Tums, Oscal, Titrolac, etc.) is recommended; other forms may not be well absorbed by the body. Bone meal contains lead and can be toxic.
Persons who eat no food of animal origin	Vitamin B_{12}	Vitamin B_{12} supplements or tofu added to the diet

Tool #3: Foods Rich in Calcium

A serving of any of the following foods provides at least 10 percent of the U.S. Recommended Daily Allowance (USRDA) of calcium. The USRDA is 1,000 milligrams for adult men and women and 1,500 milligrams for postmenopausal women.

Food	Serving Size	Calcium (mg)
Plain, low-fat yogurt	8 ounces	415
Canned sardines, with bones	3 ounces	371
Part skim-milk ricotta cheese	1/2 cup	334
Skim milk	1 cup	302–316
Two-percent low-fat milk	1 cup	297–313
Swiss cheese	1 ounce	272
Soft-serve ice cream	1 cup	236
Non-fat dry milk	1/4 cup	209
Cheddar, muenster or part skim-milk mozzarella cheese	1 ounce	203–207
Raw oysters	4–6 medium	226
Slivered almonds	1/2 cup	179
Cooked, chopped collards	1/2 cup	178
Pasteurized processed American cheese	1 ounce	174
Canned salmon, with bones	3 ounces	167
Feta cheese	1 ounce	140
Cooked broccoli	3/4 cup	132
Tofu (2 1/2″ × 2 3/4″ × 1″)	1 piece	108

Source: U.S. Department of Agriculture. *Nutritive Value of Foods.* Home and Garden Bulletin Number 72.

Tool #4: Less Sodium, More Potassium

Salt Reduction: The Taste-First Method

- Use the "taste-first" method of salt reduction. The taste for salt is acquired. Heavy use of salt in preparing food raises the level at which food tastes salty enough to be satisfying. The taste-first method has been shown to reset this level downward. Try it out: You'll find that the amount of salt that you want becomes smaller and smaller.

    1. Prepare food without any salt.
    2. If the taste is not agreeable, add a little salt and taste again.
    3. If it's still not agreeable, add a little more and taste again.
    4. Repeat until salty enough to satisfy.

- Experiment with new ways to add flavor to food. Try fresh herbs, garlic, shallots, onion, lemon juice, black pepper and even hot peppers.
- Use a salt substitute that replaces sodium with potassium.

Tool #4: Less Sodium, More Potassium, continued

- Substitute foods low in sodium for high-sodium choices.

Instead of:	Choose:
Processed meats, such as bacon, cold cuts and ham	Fresh, lean cuts of meat
Canned vegetables	Fresh or frozen vegetables
Canned soups	Homemade soups with a low amount of added salt
Potato chips, pretzels, salted corn chips and popcorn	Unsalted chips, popcorn or breadsticks
Canned beans	Dried beans
Processed and American cheese	Swiss or Jarlsberg cheese
Pickles, sauerkraut and other vegetables marinated in brine	Fresh cucumbers, cabbage and other vegetables

- Learn to recognize the various forms of sodium listed on food labels. These include monosodium glutamate (MSG), brine, baking powder, baking soda, sodium citrate and saccharin. Use the chart below to add potassium-rich foods (especially low-fat, high-fiber fruits, vegetables and beans) to your diet.

Food	Potassium (mg.)	Food	Potassium (mg.)
Dairy Products		**Meat, Fish & Poultry (cooked, 4 oz.)**	
Yogurt, plain, low-fat (1 cup)	531	Rainbow trout	723
Milk, 1% fat (1 cup)	381	Halibut	657
Fruits and Juices		Pork, average, trimmed	416
Avocado (1/2 medium)	602	Beef, average, trimmed	401
Watermelon (1/16)	560	Flounder	392
Banana (1 medium)	451	Turkey, skinless	340
Cantaloupe (1/4 melon)	412	Chicken, skinless	277
Orange juice, frozen (6 oz.)	354	**Vegetables (cooked)**	
Raisins (1/4 cup)	308	Potato (1 large)	844
Grapefruit juice (6 oz.)	284	Squash, acorn (1/2 cup)	446
Orange (1 medium)	237	Spinach (1/2 cup)	419
Apple juice (6 oz.)	222	Sweet potato (1)	397
Pear (1)	208	Rutabaga (1/2 cup)	344
Beans (cooked, 1 cup)		Squash, butternut (1/2 cup)	290
Soybeans	886	Brussels sprouts (1/2 cup)	247
Lentils	731	Carrot, raw (1)	233
Red kidney beans	713	Zucchini (1/2 cup)	228
Split peas	710	Peas (1/2 cup)	217
White navy beans	669	Cauliflower (1/2 cup)	200
Black-eyed peas	476		

Source: *Nutrition Action Healthletter,* May 1989. Available from The Center for Science in the Public Interest, 1501 16th St., N.W., Washington, D.C. 20036, © 1989.

Tool #5: Beta-Carotene and Other Antioxidants:

Where to Find Them

Many fruits and vegetables are good sources of antioxidants such as beta-carotene, vitamins C and E, polyphenols and lycopene. Consider these:

- Carrots
- Cantaloupe
- Winter squash
- Oranges
- Green peas
- Spinach
- Swiss chard
- Kale
- Broccoli

- Turnip, mustard and collard greens
- Brussels sprouts
- Cauliflower
- Tomatoes
- Strawberries
- Cranberries
- Watermelon
- Wheat bran
- Nuts and peanut butter (but these are high in fat)

Tool #6: How to Eat Less Fat

- Avoid cooking foods in oil, shortening or grease. Boil, bake, broil or steam instead.
- Emphasize complex carbohydrates—pasta, rice, vegetables, grains and legumes—when planning meals.
- Use mayonnaise, sauces, salad dressing and cream sparingly.
- Coat frying pans with vegetable oil sprays (Pam) or use non-stick pans, which don't require oil or other fat.
- Substitute low-fat foods for high-fat choices.

Instead of:	Choose:
Bologna, salami or other luncheon meats	Sliced turkey or tuna packed in spring water
Doughnuts or pastry	Bagels
Sour cream	Yogurt or blended low-fat cottage cheese
Ground beef	Ground turkey
Fatty cuts of beef, lamb or pork	Lean red meat, poultry or fish
Whole milk	Low-fat or skim milk
Ice cream	Sherbet or Italian ice
Milkshakes	Fruit juice

Tool #7: Fats: The Good vs. The Bad and The Ugly

Reduce fat intake to no more than 30 percent of daily calories. Then, choose monounsaturated and polyunsaturated fats instead of saturated fats.

Monounsaturated Fats	Polyunsaturated Fats	Saturated Fats
Olive oil	Corn oil	Beef tallow
Peanut oil	Safflower oil	Poultry fat
The fats in peanut butter, cashews and avocados	Soybean oil	Lard
	Sunflower oil	Butter
	Cottonseed oil	Milk Fat
	Mayonnaise	Cheese
	Most margarines	Palm oil
		Coconut oil

Tool #8: Fiber: Soluble vs. Insoluble

Food	Total Fiber (%)	Insoluble Fiber (%)	Soluble Fiber (%)
Wheat bran	42.2	38.9	3.3
Oat bran	27.8	13.8	14.0
Rolled oats	13.9	6.2	7.7
Corn flakes	12.2	5.0	7.2
Pinto beans	10.5	6.0	4.5
Kidney beans	10.2	5.5	4.7
Lima beans	9.7	6.4	3.3
Corn	3.3	1.5	1.8
Sweet potato	2.5	1.4	1.1
Apple	2.0	1.1	0.9
Asparagus	1.6	1.1	0.5

Oat Bran Cholesterol-Lowering Guide

In this chart, the far right column tells you about how many cookies, muffins or bowls of cereal you'd have to eat every day to lower your cholesterol by around 3 percent. If you've got to eat 10 servings, for example, multiply the calories per serving by 10 to find the true calorie cost of your oats.

Product	Serving	Oat Bran (g)	Calories	Servings to Get 3% Drop
Cereal [a]				
Quaker Oat Bran	1/3 cup, dry	28.0	90	1
Quaker Oatmeal (all flavors) [b]	1/3 cup, dry	9.0	100	1
Erewhon Instant Oatmeal	2/3 cup	28.0	100	1 1/3
w/Added Oat Bran	2/3 cup	15.0	125	1 1/3
Total Oatmeal w/Oat Bran	2/3 cup	10.0	100 [b]	1 1/3
General Mills Oatmeal Swirlers	2/3 cup	7.0	160	1 1/3
Erewhon Oat Bran w/Toasted Wheat Germ	2/3 cup	22.0	115	1 2/3
Breadshop Triple Bran	1/3 cup	21.0	100	1 2/3
Nabisco 100% Bran w/Oat Bran	1/2 cup	20.0	80	1 2/3
Barbara's Crunchy Oat Bran	1/4 cup	20.0	120	1 2/3
Health Valley Oat Bran Hot Cereal	1/4 cup	20.0	100	2
Kolln Oat Bran Crunch	1/3 cup	20.0	120	2
Health Valley Oat Bran O's	3/4 cup	15.0	90	2
Health Valley Oat Bran Flakes	1/2 cup	15.0	100	2
Kellogg Common Sense Oat Bran	2/3 cup	13.0	100	3
Kolln Fruit N Oat Bran Crunch	1/3 cup	11.1	110	3
Nabisco Wholesome 'N Hearty Oat Bran	2/3 cup	14.0	90	3
New Morning Ultimate Oat Bran	2/3 cup	14.0	110	3
Arrowhead Mills Oat Bran Flakes	2/3 cup	12.0	110	3
Kellogg Cracklin' Oat Bran	1/2 cup	9.0	110	4 [c]
New Morning Oatios with Oat Bran	1 cup	8.4	110	4
Kolln Crispy Oats Cereal	1/3 cup	8.3	110	4
General Mills Cheerios	1 1/4 cup	8.0	110	4
Ralston Oat Bran Options	1 cup	10.0	130	4
Post Oat Flakes	2/3 cup	5.0	110	7
Quaker Oat Squares	1/2 cup	5.0	100	7
New Morning Fruit-e-O's	1 cup	4.0	113	9
Breadshop Branana	1/3 cup	4.0	110	9
Breadshop Crunchy Oat Bran	1/3 cup	4.0	110	9
Kellogg's Bran Mueslix	1/2 cup	4.0	140	9
General Mills Oatmeal Raisin Crisp	1/2 cup	3.0	110	12
Ralston Bran Chex	2/3 cup	2.0	90	23
Post Honey Bunches of Oats	2/3 cup	1.0	114	35

Oat Bran Cholesterol-Lowering Guide, continued

Product	Serving	Oat Bran (g)	Calories	Servings to Get 3% Drop
Cookies, Breads, Muffins, Doughnuts				
Joseph's Oat Bran Pita	1 (1.4 oz.)	20.0	80	1 2/3
Arrowhead Mills Apple Spice Oat Bran Muffin Mix	1 (1/8 pkg.)	29.0	120	1 2/3
Health Valley Oat Bran Fruit Muffins	1 (2 oz.)	16.9–17.2	140–170	2
Health Valley Jumbo Fruit Bars	1 (1.5 oz.)	12.5	150	3
Dunkin' Donuts Plain Oat Bran Muffin	1 (3.6 oz.)	12.0	350	3
Sara Lee Oat Bran Muffin	1 (2.5 oz.)	11.0	220	3
Dunkin' Donuts Blueberry Oat Bran Muffin	1 (3.5 oz.)	10.0	270	4
Oatmeal Goodness English Muffin	1 (2 oz.)	7.0	140	5
Safeway Oat Bran Donuts	1 (1.7 oz.)	5.0	180	7
Health Valley Fruit Jumbos Oat Bran Cookies	2 (1.1 oz.)	4.6	140	8
Hostess Oat Bran Muffin	1 (1.5 oz.)	5.0	170	8
Dunkin' Donuts Oat Bran Doughnut	1 (2.6 oz.)	4.0	320	8
Dunkin' Donuts Glazed Oat Bran Cruller	1 (3.1 oz.)	4.0	350	8
Health Valley Fruit & Nut Oat Bran Cookies	2 (0.8 oz.)	4.0	88	9
Health Valley Oat Bran Graham Crackers	6 (1 oz.)	3.6	86	10
Lender's Oat Bran Bagels	1 (2.5 oz.)	3.0	170	11
Duncan Hines Oat Bran Muffin	1 (1/12 pkg.)	3.0	100	12
Duncan Hines Blueberry Oat Bran Muffin	1 (1/12 pkg.)	3.0	110	12
Arrowhead Mills Wheat-Free Oat Bran Muffin Mix	1 (1/12 pkg.)	12.0	100	13
Health Valley Oat Bran Animal Cookies	7 (1 oz.)	2.6	90	13
Continental Oatmeal Goodness Bread	1 slice (1.3 oz.)	2.3	90	15
Snack Foods				
Robert's American Gourmet Pretzels w/Oat Bran	4 (1 oz.)	6.0	110	6
Season's Oat Bran Puffs	20 (1 oz.)	6.0	150	6
Ralston Oat Bran Krisp crackers	2 (1/2 oz.)	5.0	60	7
Robert's American Gourmet Potato Chips w/Oat Bran	12 (1 oz.)	4.0	140	9
Keystone Oatzels	2 (1 oz.)	1.0	111	35
Pritikin Rice Cakes	1 (1/3 oz.)	1.0	35	50
Other				
Arrowhead Mills Pancake Mix	4 (4″ ea.)	28.0	200	1 1/3
Health Valley Oat Bran Fettucini Dinner	1 (9 oz.)	21.0	320	1 2/3
Edward & Sons Oat Bran Pasta	2 oz., dry	14.0	180	3
Kellogg's Common Sense Oat Bran Waffles	1 (1.4 oz.)	2.0	110	18
For Comparison				
Beans, lentils, split peas	1/2 cup, cooked	—	105–135	1

[a] All serving sizes for cereals are one ounce, dry.

[b] Packets of instant oatmeal contain dried fruit and flavorings in addition to 1/3 cup oatmeal.

[c] Contains coconut oil, which may cancel out the drop in cholesterol from the oat bran.

Sources: *Nutrition Action Health Letter*, December 1988, July/August 1989. Available from The Center for Science in the Public Interest, 1501 16th St., N.W., Washington, D.C. 20036, © 1989.

Tool #9: Substitute Nutrition for Sugar's Empty Calories

Instead of:	Choose:
Candy	Nuts or unbuttered popcorn
Cake, doughnuts or pastry	A whole-grain muffin or crusty roll
Cookies	Rice cake
Soft drinks	Fruit juice mixed with seltzer or club soda
Fruit pies	Fresh fruit
Ice cream	Fruit topped with plain, low-fat yogurt
Sweetened breakfast cereals	Shredded wheat, oatmeal or Wheatena

Some additional strategies:
- Don't buy sweets or have them in the house.
- Add less sugar than is called for when preparing recipes.

Tool #10: Guide to Healthful Restaurant Dining

Here are some ways to eat healthfully away from home.
- **Keep your appetite in check.** Starving yourself all day to enjoy dinner in a restaurant usually leads to overeating. Eat a healthful breakfast and lunch, and have a small nutritious snack, such as some carrot sticks or fruit, before leaving home.
- **Be careful with alcohol.** Not only does alcohol add calories, it can stimulate your appetite—so use caution. Sparkling water or fruit juice is a better choice than wine, beer or liquor.
- **Order a la carte.** Why order food that you don't really want just because it is served with a meal? Avoid temptation by ordering only those items that you really want to eat.
- **Ask questions.** Find out how dishes are prepared. As you would at home, choose food that is baked or broiled, rather than fried. If a dish comes with a sauce, ask that it be served on the side.
- **Use a light hand with toppings.** Butter, salad dressing and other sauces tend to be high in fat and calories. Add them sparingly, or not at all.
- **Put down your fork when you've had enough.** Restaurant portions are often larger than the ones you serve at home. If you hate to waste what you can't finish, ask to have it wrapped in a "doggie bag."
- **Beware of dessert!** Tempting desserts can be a careful diner's downfall. If you want something tasty to top off your meal, order fresh fruit or another healthful offering, or nibble on a fresh roll saved from dinner. You might also share a sweet treat with a dining companion.

Tool #11: Fast Food: Know What You're Ordering

Restaurant and Food	Total Calories	Sugar (tsp.)	Fat (tsp.)	Sodium (mg)	Gloom Rating*
Arby's					
Apple Turnover	303	3.4	4.2	178	25
Bac'n Cheddar Deluxe	526		8.3	1672	54
Beef 'N Cheddar	455		6.0	955	38
Chicken Breast Sandwich	509		6.6	1082	39
Deluxe Potato	657		8.4	685	49
French Fries	215		2.2	114	14
Hot Ham 'N Cheese Sandwich	292		3.1	1350	29
Junior Roast Beef Sandwich	218		1.9	345	15
Milk Shake (avg.)	383	10.5	2.5	295	20
Potato Cakes (2)	201		2.9	397	21
Regular Roast Beef Sandwich	353		3.4	588	25
Super Roast Beef Sandwich	501		5.0	798	32
Burger King					
Apple Pie	305	3.4	2.7	412	21
Bacon Double Cheeseburger	510		7.0	728	46
Breakfast Croissan'wich w/Bacon	355		5.5	762	38
Cheeseburger	317		3.4	651	26
Chicken Specialty Sandwich	688		9.1	1423	56
Chicken Tenders, 6 pc.	204		2.3	636	17
Double Beef Whopper	863		12.0	948	71
Double Beef Whopper w/Cheese	946		13.6	1232	83
French Fries, Regular	227		3.0	160	22
French Toast Sticks	499		6.6	498	38
Ham and Cheese Specialty Sandwich	471		5.2	1534	42
Hamburger	275		2.7	509	20
Milk Shake (avg.)	321	8.8	2.5	204	19
Onion Rings	274		3.6	665	16
Scrambled Egg Platter w/out Meat	468		6.8	808	49
Whaler Sandwich	488		6.1	592	36
Whaler Sandwich w/Cheese	530		6.8	734	41
Whopper	628		8.2	880	49
Whopper Jr.	322		3.9	486	25
Whopper Jr. w/Cheese	364		4.5	628	30
Whpper w/Cheese	711		9.8	1164	61
Church's					
Catfish, 1 pc.	67		0.9	151	6
Chicken Breast, Fried	278		3.9	560	24
Chicken Leg, Fried	147		2.0	286	12
Chicken Thigh, Fried	305		4.9	448	28
Chicken Wing, Fried	303		4.5	583	27
Corn on the Cob, w/Butter Oil	237		2.1	20	11
French Fries	138		1.3	126	8
Nuggets, Regular, 6 pc.	330		4.2	750	28
Nuggets, Spicy, 6 pc.	312		4.0	546	24

Tool #11: Fast Food: Know What You're Ordering, continued

Restaurant and Food	Total Calories	Sugar (tsp.)	Fat (tsp.)	Sodium (mg)	Gloom Rating*
Domino's Pizza					
Cheese, 12," 5-oz. slice	305		1.7	404	15
Cheese, 16," 6-oz. slice	377		2.3	484	19
Deluxe, 12," 7-oz. slice	414		4.2	756	31
Deluxe, 16," 8 1/4-oz. slice	498		4.6	954	36
Double Cheese/Pepperoni, 12," 6 2/3-oz. slice	466		4.4	728	33
Double Cheese/Pepperoni, 16," 8-oz. slice	545		5.8	1042	44
Ham, 12," 5 1/2-oz. slice	331		2.1	593	19
Ham, 16," 6 3/5-oz. slice	417		2.5	810	24
Pepperoni, 12," 5 3/5-oz. slice	374		3.2	652	25
Pepperoni, 16," 6 2/3-oz. slice	460		4.0	826	31
Sausage/Mushroom, 12," 6-oz. sl.	355		2.9	573	23
Sausage/Mushroom, 16," 7-oz. sl.	430		3.6	553	26
Veggie, 12," 7 3/4-oz. slice	414		3.4	773	28
Veggie, 16," 9 1/4-oz. slice	499		4.2	1037	36
Hardee's					
Bacon & Egg Biscuit	410		5.8	1175	43
Bacon Cheeseburger	556		7.5	2042	54
Big Country Breakfast w/Bacon	761		11.4	1238	74
Big Country Breakfast w/Sausage	849		15.9	1820	100
Big Deluxe Hamburger	503		6.6	868	38
Big Roast Beef Sandwich	440		4.9	1434	38
Biscuit w/Egg	336		4.3	575	29
Canadian Sunrise Biscuit	482		6.8	1121	47
Cheeseburger	327		3.4	745	24
Chef Salad	309		3.0	788	24
Chicken Fillet Sandwich	413		3.5	1258	29
Chicken Stix, 6 pc.	234		2.2	887	20
Cinnamon 'N Raisin Biscuit	276		3.7	346	22
Fisherman's Fillet Sandwich	510		5.7	861	38
French Fries, regular	197		2.2	78	11
Garden Salad	246		2.4	207	14
Ham & Egg Biscuit	379		4.7	1166	37
Hamburger	244		2.1	548	17
Hash Rounds	232		3.1	558	22
Hot Dog	285		3.2	796	25
Hot Ham 'N Cheese Sandwich	316		2.2	1833	29
Milk Shake	390	10.7	2.4	241	20
Mushroom 'N Swiss Hamburger	509		5.3	1051	37
Roast Beef Sandwich	312		2.8	966	24
Sausage & Egg Biscuit	503		7.9	885	49
Sausage Biscuit	426		6.4	831	39

Tool #11: Fast Food: Know What You're Ordering, continued

Restaurant and Food	Total Calories	Sugar (tsp.)	Fat (tsp.)	Sodium (mg)	Gloom Rating*
Jack in the Box					
Apple Turnover	410	4.6	5.5	350	41
Bacon Cheeseburger	705		8.9	1127	56
Breakfast Jack	307		3.0	871	26
Canadian Crescent	452		7.0	851	45
Cheeseburger	325		3.9	746	30
Chicken Supreme	575		8.2	1525	59
Club Pita w/out Sauce	277		1.8	931	20
French Fries, regular	221		2.7	164	18
Ham & Swiss Burger	754		11.1	1217	74
Hamburger	288		3.0	556	22
Jumbo Jack	584		7.7	733	46
Jumbo Jack w/Cheese	677		9.1	1090	57
Milk Shake (avg.)	323	8.9	1.5	247	17
Moby Jack	444		5.7	820	37
Mushroom Burger	470		5.5	910	40
Onion Rings	382		5.2	407	37
Pasta & Seafood Salad	394		5.0	1570	34
Sausage Crescent	584		9.8	1012	62
Scrambled Egg Platter	662		9.1	1188	64
Supreme Crescent	547		9.1	1053	58
Supreme Nachos	787		10.2	2194	71
Swiss & Bacon Burger	678		10.7	1458	73
Taco	191		2.5	406	18
Kentucky Fried Chicken					
Baked Beans	105		0.3	387	5
Buttermilk Biscuit	269		3.1	521	20
Cole Slaw	103		1.3	171	7
Extra Crispy Center Breast	353		4.8	842	32
Extra Crispy Drumstick	173		2.5	346	17
Extra Crispy Side Breast	354		5.4	797	35
Extra Crispy Thigh	371		6.0	766	38
Extra Crispy Wing	218		3.5	437	23
Kentucky Fries	268		2.9	81	14
Kentucky Nuggets, 6 pc.	276		3.9	840	28
Mashed Potatoes w/Gravy	62		0.3	297	5
Original Recipe Center Breast	257		3.1	532	21
Original Recipe Drumstick	147		2.0	269	14
Original Recipe Side Breast	276		3.9	654	27
Original Recipe Thigh	278		4.4	517	28
Original Recipe Wing	181		2.8	387	19
Potato Salad	141		2.1	396	14

Tool #11: Fast Food: Know What You're Ordering, continued

Restaurant and Food	Total Calories	Sugar (tsp.)	Fat (tsp.)	Sodium (mg)	Gloom Rating*
Long John Silver's					
Battered Shrimp Dinner, 6 pc.	740		8.4	1110	50
Cajun Shrimp Platter	900		10.0	1800	62
Catfish Fillet Dinner	900		10.2	1070	57
Chef's Combo Salad	280		2.5	1230	20
Chicken Plank Dinner, 3 pc.	830		8.7	1340	43
Chicken Plank Dinner, Child, 2 pc.	510		5.5	730	33
Clam Dinner	980		10.2	1200	58
Crispy Breaded Fish Sandwich	600		6.4	1220	40
Fish & Fryes, 2 pc.	660		6.8	1120	43
Fish & Fryes, Children's, 1 pc.	440		4.5	590	28
Fish Dinner, 3 pc.	960		10.0	1890	64
Fryes, 1 order	220		2.3	60	14
Hawaiian Chicken Salad	420		5.7	570	28
Hushpuppies, 1 pc.	70		0.5	25	3
Ocean Chef Salad	250		2.0	1340	20
Seafood Platter	970		10.5	1540	65
Seafood Salad w/out Dressing	270		1.6	660	14
Shrimp, Fish & Chicken Dinner	840		9.1	1450	56
McDonald's					
Apple Pie	262	2.9	3.4	240	21
Big Mac	562		7.4	950	45
Biscuit w/Bacon, Egg, Cheese	449		6.2	1230	46
Biscuit w/Biscuit spread	260		2.9	730	21
Biscuit w/Sausage	440		6.6	1080	46
Biscuit w/Sausage and Egg	529		8.0	1250	57
Blue Cheese Dressing (2.5 oz.)	345		7.8	750	45
Cheeseburger	308		3.1	750	24
Chef Salad	231		3.1	490	21
Chicken McNuggets, 6 pc.	288		3.7	520	24
Chicken Salad Oriental	141		0.8	230	7
Chocolaty Chip Cookies	325	6.7	3.5	280	23
Cinnamon Raisin Danish	445		4.8	430	29
Egg McMuffin	293		2.7	740	25
English Muffin w/Butter	169		1.0	270	9
Filet-O-Fish	442		5.9	1030	38
French Dressing (2 oz.)	232		4.7	720	29
Fries, Regular	220		2.6	110	15
Garden Salad	112		1.5	160	11
Hamburger	257		2.2	460	17
Hash Brown Potatoes	131		1.7	330	14
Hot Fudge/Caramel Sundae (avg.)	328	9.4	2.1	160	19
Hotcakes w/Butter, Syrup	413	10.0	2.1	640	24
Lite Vinaigrette Dressing (2 oz.)	60		0.5	240	4
McDLT	674		9.6	1170	56
McDonaldland Cookies	288	5.6	2.1	300	15
Milk Shake (avg.)	375	10.3	2.3	193	21

Tool #11: Fast Food: Know What You're Ordering, continued

Restaurant and Food	Total Calories	Sugar (tsp.)	Fat (tsp.)	Sodium (mg)	Gloom Rating*
McDonald's, continued					
Pork Sausage	180		3.7	350	24
Quarter Pounder	414		4.7	660	32
Quarter Pounder w/Cheese	517		6.6	1150	45
Ranch Dressing (2.5 oz.)	332		7.8	520	43
Sausage McMuffin	372		5.0	830	34
Sausage McMuffin w/Egg	451		6.2	980	44
Scrambled Eggs	157		2.5	290	21
Shrimp Salad	104		0.6	480	10
Side Salad	57		0.8	85	6
Soft Serve w/Cone	144	4.2	1.0	70	9
Strawberry Sundae	283	8.1	1.7	85	16
Thousand Island Dressing (2 oz.)	390		8.5	500	45
Roy Rogers					
Apple Danish	249	1.4	2.6	255	17
Bacon Cheeseburger	581		8.9	1536	58
Biscuit	231		2.8	575	20
Breakfast Crescent Sandwich	401		6.2	867	42
Breakfast Crescent w/Meat (avg.)	479		7.6	1172	52
Cheeseburger	563		8.5	1404	55
Chicken Breast, Fried	412		5.4	609	34
Chicken Leg, Fried	140		1.8	190	12
Chicken Thigh, Fried	296		4.4	406	28
Chicken Wing, Fried	192		2.9	285	19
Egg & Biscuit Platter	394		6.0	734	41
Egg & Biscuit Platter w/Bacon or Ham	439		6.6	1057	47
Egg & Biscuit Platter w/Sausage	550		9.3	1059	60
French Fries	268		3.1	165	19
Hamburger	456		6.4	495	37
Hot Fudge/Caramel Sundae (avg.)	315	9.1	2.4	190	19
Milk Shake (avg.)	326	9.0	2.4	278	20
Pancake Platter w/Bacon or Ham	500	7.5	4.0	1165	38
Pancake Platter w/Sausage	608	7.5	6.7	1167	51
Pancake Platter w/Syrup, Butter	452	7.5	3.5	842	31
RR Bar Burger	611		9.0	1826	61
Roast Beef Sandwich w/Cheese, large	467		4.8	1953	42
Roast Beef Sandwich w/Cheese, regular	424		4.4	1694	38
Roast Beef Sandwich, large	360		2.7	1044	24
Roast Beef Sandwich, regular	317		2.3	785	20
Strawberry Shortcake	447	6.5	4.4	674	32
Strawberry Sundae	216	6.2	1.6	99	12

Tool #11: Fast Food: Know What You're Ordering, continued

Restaurant and Food	Total Calories	Sugar (tsp.)	Fat (tsp.)	Sodium (mg)	Gloom Rating*
Taco Bell					
Bean Burrito	360		2.5	922	24
Beef Burrito	402		3.9	994	28
Beefy Tostada	238		4.2	706	31
Bellbeefer	312		3.0	855	25
Burrito Supreme	422		4.3	952	33
Burrito Supreme Platter	774		8.4	1920	65
Cinnamon Crispas	266	n/a	3.6	122	21
Combo Burrito	380		3.2	958	28
Double Beef Burrito Supreme	464		5.2	1054	39
Enchirito	381		4.6	1260	38
Nachos	356		4.4	423	33
Nachos Bellgrande	719		9.3	1312	68
Pintos & Cheese	194		2.2	733	20
Pizzazz Pizza	714		10.9	1364	80
Seafood Salad	921		16.0	1577	103
Seafood Salad w/out Dressing	648		9.4	917	69
Soft Taco	228		2.7	516	20
Taco	184		2.5	273	18
Taco Bellgrande	351		4.9	470	34
Taco Light	411		6.6	575	46
Taco Salad	949		14.1	1741	100
Taco Salad w/Ranch Dressing	1204		20.6	2047	132
Tostada	243		2.5	670	21
Wendy's					
Bacon & Cheese Potato	570		6.8	1180	43
Bacon Cheeseburger, White Bun	455		5.7	843	36
Baked Potato, Plain	250		0.5	60	2
Chicken Sandwich, Multi-Grain Bun	340		3.0	525	22
Chili, 8 oz.	240		1.8	990	18
Double Hamburger, White Bun	560		6.8	465	39
French Fries, Regular	310		3.4	105	19
Frosty Dairy Dessert, 12 oz.	400	10.0	3.2	220	24
Garden Salad (takeout)	102		1.1	110	5
Hamburger, Kid's Meal	200		2.0	225	14
Hamburger, Multi-Grain Bun	350		3.9	320	23
Hamburger, White Bun	350		3.6	360	23
Sour Cream & Chives Potato	460		5.5	230	28
Taco Salad	430		4.3	1260	32

Tool #11: Fast Food: Know What You're Ordering, continued

Restaurant and Food	Total Calories	Sugar (tsp.)	Fat (tsp.)	Sodium (mg)	Gloom Rating*
Beverages					
Coca-Cola Classic (12 fl. oz.)	144	9.0	0.0	14	5
Coffee, Black (8 fl. oz.)	0		0.0	3	0
Diet Coke (12 fl. oz.)	1	0.1	0.0	16	0
Diet Pepsi (12 fl. oz.)	1	0.1	0.0	23	0
Milk 2%, Low fat (8 fl. oz.)	120		5.0	122	8
Milk, Whole (8 fl. oz.)	150		8.0	120	13
Orange Juice (8 fl. oz.)	110		1.0	2	1
Pepsi Cola (12 fl. oz.)	160	9.9	0.0	18	5
7-Up (12 fl. oz.)	144	8.8	0.0	32	5
Sprite (12 fl. oz.)	142	8.7	0.0	46	5
Tea, Hot or Iced (8 fl. oz.)	0		0.0	1	0

*In general, the higher the GLOOM rating, the more unhealthful the food. This number reflects a food's overall fat, sodium, sugar and calorie content. A food's high vitamin, mineral and protein content will improve (lower) the GLOOM score. Try to limit yourself to 50–100 GLOOM points per day.

n/a, Not available.

Source: Michael F. Jacobsen and Sarah Fritschner. *The Fast Food Guide*. New York: Workman Publishing, 1986.

Tool #12: Recipes for Healthful Meals

Spinach Salad with Mexican Salsa Dressing

4 to 6 cups spinach leaves, washed and drained
1 cup bean sprouts
Several mushrooms and scallions, sliced

Dressing:
1/2 cup plain, low-fat yogurt
1/2 cup Mexican salsa

Place the vegetables in a large salad bowl. Combine the yogurt and salsa to make the dressing. Pour the dressing over the vegetables; toss well.

Lentils, Rice and Barley

1 cup lentils
1 bay leaf
1 cup rice
1/2 cup barley

1 medium onion, sliced
2 tablespoons margarine
2 tablespoons flour
3/4 cup plain, low-fat yogurt

Cook the lentils with the bay leaf in 2 1/2 cups water until tender (about 35 minutes). At the same time, cook the rice and barley, each separately, according to package directions.

In a skillet, saute the onion in margarine; add the flour, and brown it well. Stir the onion and browned flour into the lentils.

Combine the cooked rice and barley in a bowl. Stir in the yogurt. Serve the lentils in a separate bowl. (Remove the bay leaf.) Diners can spoon the rice and barley onto their plates, then top them with lentils. Anyone who misses the taste of salt may add a little soy sauce at this time.

This recipe serves three or four adults as a main course.

Chickpea and Pasta Soup

4 servings (about 6 cups)
1 tablespoon unsalted butter or margarine
1 medium onion, minced
1/2 teaspoon dried thyme
1 16-oz. can tomatoes, including juice, chopped
2 garlic cloves, minced (about 2 teaspoons)
2 cups beef broth (canned, cubes or homemade), or more

2 cups cooked chickpeas (garbanzo beans), drained and rinsed if canned
1/2 cup small pasta (shells, elbows, etc.), cooked al dente
Freshly ground black pepper to taste
1/4 cup grated Parmesan cheese

In a large saucepan, melt the butter or margarine, and cook the onion with the thyme, stirring, for 5 minutes. Add the tomatoes, their juice and the garlic, and simmer the mixture, stirring occasionally, for 15 minutes. Add the broth and chickpeas, and simmer the soup, stirring occasionally, for another 15 minutes. Add the pasta and pepper, and cook the soup until the pasta is warm. Thin the soup with additional stock or water, if necessary. Serve the soup with a tablespoon of Parmesan sprinkled in each bowl.

Source: *Jane Brody's Good Food Book*. New York: W. W. Norton & Company, 1985.

Tool #12: Recipes for Healthful Meals, continued

Vegetable-Bean Salad with Rice or Pasta

4 main-dish servings

Preparation tip: The salad can be prepared several hours to one day in advance.

Salad
1 cup raw long-grain rice, white or brown, cooked without butter, or 3 cups cooked orzo
1 15-oz. can kidney beans, drained and rinsed
1 large stalk broccoli, flowerets cut, stems sliced, and steamed for 5 minutes or blanched for 2 minutes
1/2 pound snow peas or sugar snap peas
1/2 pound mushrooms, sliced thin (about 2 1/2 cups)
1 green or red sweet pepper (or both), cut in strips about 1/4 inch wide
4 to 6 scallions, sliced thin

Dressing
1/4 cup olive oil
2 tablespoons lemon juice
3 tablespoons vinegar
2 large cloves garlic, crushed
1 teaspoon dry mustard
3/4 teaspoon tarragon, crumbled
1/2 teaspoon salt, if desired
1/2 teaspoon freshly ground black pepper, or to taste

Garnish
Greens for serving
1 pint cherry tomatoes, halved (optional)

In a large bowl, combine all the salad ingredients. In a jar, combine all the dressing ingredients. Cover the jar, shake it well, and pour the dressing over the rice and vegetable mixture. Toss the salad to mix it thoroughly. Refrigerate the salad until serving time. On a large platter, serve the salad on a bed of greens surrounded by a necklace of cherry tomato halves, if desired.

Source: *Jane Brody's Good Food Book*. New York: W. W. Norton & Company, 1985.

Chilied Chicken Fricassee

6 servings

Preparation tip: It can be prepared ahead and frozen. It can also be made with turkey breasts.

1/4 cup yellow corn meal
1/2 teaspoon salt, if desired
1/4 teaspoon American Heart Association herb mix or other no-salt seasoning
1/4 teaspoon freshly ground black pepper
1 1/4 pounds boneless chicken breast, skin removed and flesh cut into 1 1/2 inch cubes
4 teaspoons vegetable oil, divided
1 large onion, coarsely chopped (1 cup)
1 large green pepper, diced (3/4 cup)

1 teaspoon minced garlic
2 to 3 teaspoons chili powder, or to taste
1/2 teaspoon ground cumin
1 cup no-salt chicken broth
1 28-oz. can tomatoes (without salt, if available), with juice, coarsely chopped
1 cup cooked corn kernels
1 cup green peas (frozen or, if fresh, boiled for 3 minutes)
1 cup cooked pink beans (optional)

Combine the corn meal, salt, herb mix and pepper in a shallow bowl or paper bag. Add the chicken pieces in batches, tossing them to coat them thoroughly with the corn meal mixture.

Heat 3 teaspoons of the oil in a 4- to 5-quart Dutch oven or comparable heavy pot, preferably with a nonstick surface. Lightly brown the chicken chunks on all sides, remove them from the pot, place them in a bowl and set the bowl aside.

Add the remaining teaspoon of oil to the pot, reduce the heat to moderately low, and add the onion, green pepper, garlic, chili powder and cumin. Cook the mixture for about 5 minutes, stirring it often, until the onions are translucent.

Add the broth and the tomatoes with their juice to the pot, and bring the mixture to a boil. Reduce the heat to low, cover the pot and simmer the mixture for 20 minutes.

Add the reserved chicken, cover the pot and simmer the fricassee for another 25 minutes.

Add the corn, peas and beans, if desired, and simmer the fricassee 5 minutes longer.

Source: *Jane Brody's Good Food Book*. New York: W. W. Norton & Company, 1985.

Tool #12: Recipes for Healthful Meals, continued

40-Clove Garlic Chicken

8 servings

8 chicken legs and thighs, skinned and separated
2 tablespoons oil
1 large onion, coarsely chopped (1 cup)
4 ribs celery, sliced into 1/4-inch pieces (1 1/2 to 2 cups)
2 tablespoons minced fresh parsley or 2 teaspoons dried
   parsley flakes

1 teaspoon dried tarragon
1/2 cup dry vermouth
1/2 teaspoon salt, if desired
1/4 teaspoon freshly ground black pepper
Dash nutmeg
40 cloves garlic, separated but not peeled

Brush the chicken pieces on all sides with the oil.

In a large casserole or heavy Dutch oven (5 to 6 quarts), combine the onion, celery, parsley and tarragon. Lay the chicken pieces over the vegetables and herbs, and pour the vermouth over the chicken. Sprinkle the chicken with salt, pepper and nutmeg. Distribute the unpeeled garlic cloves throughout the casserole, tucking them under the chicken pieces. Cover the casserole tightly (you might fit a piece of foil around the top under the lid).

Bake the chicken in a preheated 325 degrees Fahrenheit oven for 1 1/2 hours. Do not uncover the casserole until after this time has elapsed.

Serve the chicken with the garlic, advising the diners to squeeze the flesh from its papery coat. The garlic is especially tasty when eaten on crusty bread.

Source: *Jane Brody's Good Food Book*. New York: W. W. Norton & Company, 1985.

Pizza Sandwiches

12 pizza sandwiches

Sauce

2 tablespoons oil
1/2 cup chopped onion
2 1/2 tablespoons chopped celery
2 1/2 tablespoons chopped green pepper
1 cup canned tomatoes

6 tablespoons tomato paste
1 teaspoon oregano
1/8 teaspoon sweet basil
Freshly ground black pepper
1/4 teaspoon rosemary (optional)

Saute onion, celery and pepper in vegetable oil until tender and translucent. Add tomatoes, tomato paste and seasonings. Cook over low heat on stove top for approximately 30 minutes, stirring occasionally.

Yield: approximately 1 1/2 cups sauce

Sandwich

1 1/2 cups pizza sauce
1 1/2 cups low-fat cottage cheese

6 English muffins, toasted
4 tablespoons Parmesan cheese, grated

Mix 2 tablespoons cottage cheese with 2 tablespoons sauce. Spread mixture on half of a toasted English muffin. Sprinkle 1 teaspoon Parmesan cheese over top. Broil in oven for approximately 5 minutes or until Parmesan cheese just starts to turn golden.

Nutritional Analysis Per Serving

Calories: 130
Protein: 7.1 g
Total Fat (est.): 3.7 g
Saturated Fat: .79 g
Polyunsaturated Fat: 1.36 g
Monounsaturated Fat: 1.55 g

Cholesterol: 3 mg
Carbohydrates: 17.1 g
Calcium: 94.85 mg
Potassium: 325 mg
Sodium: 359 mg

Source: *American Heart Association Cookbook*, 4th edition, pg. 234

Tool #12: Recipes for Healthful Meals, continued

Sauteed Collard Greens

3 to 4 servings

1 pound fresh collard greens, washed, stems removed,
cut into shreds
2 quarts boiling water, salted if desired

2 teaspoons butter or margarine
1 teaspoon minced garlic
2 tablespoons broth or water

Plunge the shredded greens into the boiling water for 3 minutes. Drain them immediately. In a skillet, heat the butter or margarine, and cook the garlic, stirring it, for 30 seconds. Then add the blanched greens and the broth or water, tossing the ingredients well. Cover the pan, and cook the greens over low heat for 15 minutes, stirring them occasionally.

Source: *Jane Brody's Good Food Book*. New York: W. W. Norton & Company, 1985.

Half-the-Beef Tacos

4 to 6 servings

Preparation tip: You can buy ready-made taco sauce in a jar or can. Taco shells are also readily available in supermarkets, or you can make your own by toasting or frying corn or flour tortillas according to package directions.

Filling

1/2 pound lean ground beef
1/2 pound new potatoes
2 teaspoons vegetable oil
1 medium onion, finely chopped (1/2 cup)
2 teaspoons minced garlic (2 large cloves)
1/2 teaspoon ground cumin
3 tablespoons taco sauce (mild or hot)

12 taco shells,
sprinkled with water,
wrapped in foil and
heated in the oven

Toppings

1 cup shredded cheese (e.g., Cheddar or Monterey Jack) (about 4 oz.)
1/4 to 1/3 cup finely chopped onion, to taste
1 1/2 cups finely diced tomato
1 1/2 cups finely shredded lettuce
1/3 cup taco sauce

In a nonstick or cast-iron skillet, brown the meat over medium heat, crumbling it with a spatula. Pour off all the accumulated fat, and transfer the beef to a plate lined with a paper towel. Set the beef aside. When the skillet is cool enough to handle, wipe it with a paper towel, or wash and dry it.

Peel and coarsely shred the potatoes.

Heat the oil in the skillet, and add the potatoes, spreading them out and pressing them into a cake. Fry them over medium-high heat until the cake is lightly browned on one side. Then, divide the cake in half with the spatula, and flip the halves over to brown the other side. When browned, break up the potato cake with the spatula.

Add the onion, garlic and cumin, and saute the mixture for about 3 minutes. Stir in the reserved cooked beef and 3 tablespoons of taco sauce. Cook the mixture, stirring to combine it thoroughly, 2 minutes longer to heat it through.

To serve, distribute the meat-and-potato mixture among the taco shells. Provide diners with separate bowls of the cheese, onion, tomato, lettuce and taco sauce to add to their tacos according to taste.

Source: *Jane Brody's Good Food Book*. New York: W. W. Norton & Company, 1985.

Tool #12: Recipes for Healthful Meals, continued

Jane's Tabbouli
(Bulgur Salad)
6 to 8 servings

Preparation tip: Bulgur can be found in supermarkets (check near the rice or hot cereals) as well as in natural food and specialty stores. Both the salad ingredients and the dressing can be prepared ahead separately and mixed together about an hour before serving.

Salad
1 cup bulgur (cracked fine or medium)
2 cups boiling water
2 tomatoes, finely diced
1 bunch scallions (about 6), with tops, finely chopped
1 cup finely chopped fresh parsley, or more, to taste
3 tablespoons chopped fresh mint leaves or 2 teaspoons dried mint

Dressing
1/4 cup lemon juice
2 tablespoons olive or salad oil
1/2 teaspoon salt, if desired
1/4 teaspoon (or more) freshly ground black pepper
1/4 teaspoon oregano (ground or crumbled leaves)
1/4 teaspoon ground cumin
Dash allspice (optional)
Dash coriander (optional)

In a medium bowl, soak the bulgur in the boiling water for 1 hour. Drain the bulgur well, pressing out the excess water through a fine strainer or cloth.

Add the tomatoes, scallions, parsley and mint to the bulgur. Combine the ingredients well.

Mix all the dressing ingredients in a small bowl. About 1 hour or less before serving, add the dressing to the bulgur mixture, and toss the salad to coat the ingredients thoroughly.

Source: *Jane Brody's Good Food Book*. New York: W. W. Norton & Company, 1985.

Steamed Chicken with Spinach Pesto
6 servings

8 oz. uncooked macaroni or other small pasta
1 1/2 pounds skinned and boneless chicken, cut in 1-inch cubes

2 cups sliced carrots
Spinach pesto sauce (see below)

Prepare pasta according to package directions. Drain and transfer to a serving bowl. Meanwhile, place chicken and carrots in a steamer. Steam until fully cooked, about 7–10 minutes, stirring twice.

Combine chicken, carrots and pasta. Toss with pesto sauce. Serve warm or at room temperature.

Spinach Pesto Sauce

10 oz. fresh or frozen spinach
1/4 cup chopped walnuts
1/4 cup grated Parmesan cheese
2 tablespoons chopped fresh parsley

1 tablespoon bread crumbs
2 tablespoons olive or vegetable oil
1 teaspoon salt
1 clove garlic, peeled and crushed

Steam spinach just until tender. When cool enough to handle, press out all excess liquid.

In a food processor or blender, puree spinach, walnuts, cheese, parsley, bread crumbs, oil, salt and garlic until ingredients are thoroughly blended.

Nutritional Analysis Per Serving

Calories: 384
Protein: 35 g
Total Fat (est.): 12.8 g
Saturated Fat: 2.56 g
Polyunsaturated Fat: 2.93 g
Monounsaturated Fat: 7.31 g

Cholesterol: 78 mg
Carbohydrates: 31.5 g
Calcium: 136.8 mg
Potassium: 678 mg
Sodium: 558 mg

Source: "LIGHTEN UP" Quantity Recipe Cards, Copyright 1982, American Heart Association. Reprinted with permission.

Tool #12: Recipes for Healthful Meals, continued

Beef Kabobs

8 servings

1 cup red wine
3/8 cup sherry
1/8 cup soy sauce
1 teaspoon sesame hot oil
1/2 teaspoon freshly ground ginger
1 cup pineapple juice
1 teaspoon thyme
1 teaspoon rosemary
1/4 cup worcestershire sauce
1 onion, finely chopped

1/2 teaspoon pepper
1 1/2 pounds sirloin, cut into cubes
3 tomatoes, cut into eighths, if large; or use whole cherry tomatoes
3 onions, cut in 1-inch wedges, or small whole boiling onions
12 whole mushrooms
1 small eggplant, peeled and chopped in 1-inch pieces
1 green pepper, cut in large cubes
12 small whole potatoes, cooked fresh, or canned

Make a marinade by mixing the first 11 ingredients together. Pour over the meat. Let stand 2 hours at room temperature or overnight in the refrigerator.

Alternate the beef on skewers with the vegetables. Broil 3 inches from the heat for about 15 minutes, or grill over charcoal turning frequently and basting with the marinade.

Nutritional Analysis Per Serving

Calories: 163
Protein: 16.1 g
Total Fat (est.): 3.5 g
Saturated Fat: 1.52 g
Polyunsaturated Fat: .09 g
Monounsaturated Fat: 1.89 g

Cholesterol: 37 mg
Carbohydrates: 16 g
Calcium: 29.61 mg
Potassium: 580 mg
Sodium: 90 mg

Source: *American Heart Association Cookbook*, 4th edition, New York: David McKay Company, 1984, pg. 59.

Scalloped Potatoes

6 servings

4 cups thinly sliced, peeled raw potatoes
1 onion, peeled and sliced thinly
1 tablespoon chopped parsley, if desired
3 tablespoons flour

1 tablespoon curry powder
Freshly ground black pepper
3 tablespoons margarine
1 1/2 cups skim milk

In a lightly oiled casserole, place a layer of potatoes. Sprinkle with flour and curry powder; then, place a layer of onions. Sprinkling each layer with flour and curry powder, alternate potatoes and onions until all are used. Season with pepper.

Heat the milk and margarine together and pour over the potatoes. Cover casserole and bake at 350 degrees Fahrenheit for one hour, then remove cover and bake another 1/2 hour to brown.

Nutritional Analysis Per Serving

Calories: 161
Protein: 4.9 g
Total Fat (est.): 6.0 g
Saturated Fat: 1.16 g
Polyunsaturated Fat: 1.76 g
Monounsaturated Fat: 3.08 g

Cholesterol: 1 mg
Carbohydrates: 22.9 g
Calcium: 95.4 mg
Potassium: 450 mg
Sodium: 101 mg

Source: *American Heart Association Cookbook*, 4th edition, New York: David McKay Company, 1984, pg. 334.

Food for a Healthy Life

I called this chapter "Food for Life" to draw attention to the close tie between diet and survival. Certainly, without food, people could not live. But choosing the right kind of food can enable people to live *well*. It raises the chances of survival to a healthy old age and helps make the years in-between full and productive.

Did you find it strange that a chapter on "diet" made little mention of "weight loss"? The next chapter, "Fat Control," explains why losing fat, not weight, can be important and describes ways to go about it.

Additional Resources

The American Heart Association Cookbook. New York: David McKay Company, 1984.

The California Diet and Exercise Program, by Dr. Peter Wood. Mountain View, CA: Anderson World Books, 1982.

The Fit or Fat Target Diet, by Covert Bailey. Boston: Houghton Mifflin Company, 1984.

Jane Brody's Good Food Book. New York: W. W. Norton & Company, 1985.

Jane Brody's Nutrition Book. New York: W. W. Norton & Company, 1981.

The Fast Food Guide, by Michael F. Jacobsen and Sarah Fritschner. New York: Workman Publishing, 1986. Available from the Center for Science in the Public Interest, 1501 16th Street, N.W., Washington, DC 20036.

Eater's Choice. A Food Lover's Guide to Lower Cholesterol, by Ron and Nancy Goor. Boston: Houghton Mifflin Company, 1987.

Don't Eat Your Heart Out, by Joseph C. Piscatella. Takoma, WA: Institute for Fitness and Health, 1987.

Choices for a Healthy Heart, by Joseph C. Piscatella. Takoma, WA: Institute for Fitness and Health, 1987.

FAT CONTROL

FAT IS WHERE IT'S AT

When you look at Arnold Schwartzenegger, you're likely to think "massive," but you won't think "fat." Fatness is more than a matter of pounds. After all, muscular people with little fat may be overweight when compared to average or "desirable" weights. Being fat—actually, being *overfat*—means having a body that carries too much fatty tissue.

I use the term "fat control" rather than "weight control" not to be unkind, but simply to stress that the real issue is not weight but fat. It is common to use weight as a way of gauging fat, because fat itself is not easy to measure. But our goal—yours and mine—is to focus on a lifestyle that defends against being overfat and produces a healthy, attractive body.

The key to a trim, good-looking body—and this may surprise you—is not strict dieting, but rather exercise combined with improved eating habits. Although we live in a sea of diet aids —books, magazines, videos, programs, strategies, companies, foods, drinks, suits and pills—a starvation diet without exercise can be worse than no diet at all. It can set you up for an unhappy shift in the proportions of fat and muscle in your body. With less muscle, it becomes ever harder to keep off additional fat, even when you're eating the same amount of food.

HOW FAT ARE YOU?

The best place to start is in front of your mirror. Fat, like beauty, is in the eye of the beholder—so long as the beholder is fairly honest. How do you look? Is your waistline thick? Does your tummy bulge? Have your ribs disappeared? Either you have a fair amount of fat on you or you don't, and your mirror will be the first to tell you.

Scientists have devised some more precise ways to measure the body's fat content. In the most accurate technique, the person is weighed while completely underwater. This indicates body density and makes it possible to calculate the proportion of fat, which floats. (If two men of the same height and weight were weighed underwater, but one was fat and one lean, the fat man would appear to weigh much less.)

The second-best way to determine body fat is to measure skin thickness with calipers. This method measures a pinch of skin and the fatty layer beneath it on six parts of the body: the waist, chest, shoulder blade, abdomen, thigh and upper arm. These measurements are added up and checked against tables showing proportions of body fat.

Neither of these techniques is very practical to use every day or even every month. A much more accessible tool is the tape measure, used with the charts included in the LifeScore questionnaire (see Chapter 1).

For men, a body fat between 12 percent and 17 percent is desirable, and less than 12 percent is excellent. More than 25 percent is considered obese; between 20 percent and 25 percent is borderline obesity.

The desirable range of body fat for women is between 19 percent and 24 percent. More than 30 percent is considered obese; between 25 percent and 30 percent is borderline obesity.

How Do You "Get" Fat?

Fatness has nothing to do with medicines, wholesome food, cellulite or baby fat. You "get fat" by regularly taking in more calories than your body burns. The excess is stored as fatty tissue, to be drawn on in times of increased activity. Engorged fat cells grow large; in extremely obese people, the number of fat cells also increases. Each pound of body fat contains about 3,500 calories worth of energy.

The basic principle of fat control is straightforward: You lose fat by burning more calories than you take in. If you eat less than you burn, fat decreases. If you eat more than you burn, fat increases. It is simply a law of physics.

However, not everyone burns off, or metabolizes, calories at the same rate. Heredity seems to influence a person's metabolic rate. What's more,

Yes, But What Is Your Real Weight?

Data from the second National Health and Nutrition Examination Survey show that when men and women report their weight, they don't often tell the truth. But they err in opposite directions.

Men tend to report that they weigh more than they actually do, on average about a pound. The youngest men surveyed (age 20 to 24) reported that they weighed about 1.35 pounds more than they actually did. The reports became more accurate with age, so that in the 55-to-64 age group, men reported weighing only 0.4 pound more than they actually did. Then, for reasons unknown, the error jumped back up to 1.38 pounds in the 65-to-74 age group.

Women, in contrast, reported that they weighed about 2.3 pounds less than they actually did. Women age 35 to 44 were least accurate, reporting that they weighed 2.6 pounds less, on average, than they actually did.

both heredity and calorie intake during the first year of life seem to affect the number of fat cells in a person's body. Researchers in England studied babies born to normal-weight and overfat mothers. They found that as early as three months of age, babies born to the overfat mothers were burning off about 20 percent fewer calories than those born to the normal-weight women. These babies added fat cells and weight until they were about a year old, when their metabolic rates caught up with those of the babies born to the normal-weight mothers. Unfortunately, they were already fat, even though they had "normal" metabolic rates.

This and other research implies that the body may have a "set point" for its metabolic rate, which it seeks to maintain by storing fat. It is as if the body wants to be sure that it has plenty of fat to burn before it will burn it at a normal rate. Unfortunately, it appears that obese people may have set

Fat and the Boob Tube

William Dietz, M.D., Ph.D., studied the relationship between obesity and television watching in children. As you might have guessed, he found that the more time a child spent watching television, the more likely it was that he or she would be obese.

Over the course of a year, the average child watches 23 to 25 hours of TV a week. That's about as much time as the child spends at school.

points that call for high levels of body fat. The good news is that the set point may be altered by exercise and healthful eating patterns.

The number of fat cells appears to be set for life by the time a baby is one year old. The body accommodates growing stores of fat by letting the existing fat cells grow larger. Fat cells may be very large or very small, depending on how much fat is being stored. Thus, you can go from being fat to being lean and vice versa, even though your number of fat cells doesn't change.

In the United States, fat typically creeps up slowly and steadily with age, with many people adding about a pound a year. This isn't hard. You can do it by eating just 10 calories more each day than you expend. Moreover, as a person becomes less active with age, half a pound of lean tissue —mostly muscle and bone—shifts to fat every year. As Jack Wilmore, author of *Sensible Fitness*, points out, at the rate of 1.5 pounds per year, the average 25-year-old American can look forward to piling on 45 pounds of fat by age 55.

Luckily, the shift works both ways, and you don't have to change very much to reverse the trend. If you establish a deficit of 500 calories a day (by skipping three or four soft drinks, for example), in seven days you will lose a pound. Giving up a couple of soft drinks won't cause you to waste away to nothing, however. As you lose weight, it takes fewer calories to accomplish any given task. Just as it takes more energy to lift 200 pounds than 150 pounds, it takes more energy to heft your 200-pound body up the stairs than to move your 150-pound version. If your activities remain exactly the same, the deficit caused by foregoing the soft drinks will get smaller and smaller, until finally you come into balance again and your weight becomes steady.

THE DANGERS OF FAT VS. THE VIRTUES OF LEAN

Being overfat is a major problem in this country. An estimated 34 million Americans between the ages of 20 and 75 are far above the "desirable" weight for people of their height and frame. Many millions more are overfat to a lesser degree.

Being fat has a lot going against it. It is inconvenient: Excess pounds make it hard to find clothes that fit, get up out of chairs, squeeze into airplane seats, bend over or cross your legs. It is demoralizing and unhealthy. People who are overfat risk a variety of diseases, and they don't live as long as other people. And the heavier they are, the greater the toll, as Table 8.1 (at right) demonstrates.

Excess fat damages the body in many ways. It stresses your bones, joints and muscles, including your heart. It distorts your body's metabolism and raises blood pressure. It contributes to many serious disorders. Moreover, the location of fatty tissue has proven to be important. Fat cells lodged

What Is a Calorie?

The ever-present calorie is actually a measure of heat. It is the amount of heat required to raise the temperature of one kilogram of water one degree centigrade. Because it takes energy to produce heat, the term "calories" is used to express the amount of energy generated as a person burns fuel, or the energy content of food. In a typical day, a man who weighs 170 pounds uses 2,890 calories. In order to keep his weight constant, he must take in 2,890 calories in what he eats and drinks.

around the waist—the typical pot belly—appear to be less active metabolically than those in the thighs and buttocks, and they are more likely to increase the risk of heart disease.

The overfat person is at a higher risk of the following health problems:

- **Heart disease.** Heart disease afflicts more overweight than normal-weight people. Data from the National Health and Nutrition Examination Surveys, which are obtained from a representative sample of U.S. residents, show that being overweight is strongly associated with two of the main risks for cardiovascular disease —high blood pressure and high blood cholesterol—especially in younger persons. The links are even stronger when scientists consider not total weight, but only body fat. What's more, data from the famous Framingham (Massachusetts) study have shown that obesity itself is a risk factor for coronary heart disease.

- **Elevated blood levels of cholesterol.** Twenty- to forty-five year-olds who are overfat are twice as likely as trimmer people their age to have elevated blood levels of cholesterol. Also, losing fat can raise levels of the "good" cholesterol, high-density lipoprotein (HDL-C). In a new study from Stanford University, obese men who lost weight through either exercise or diet experienced not only a significant increase in levels of HDL-C, but also a marked improvement in their risk of heart disease.

- **High blood pressure.** Having high blood pressure is almost three times more common among the overfat. And among persons between 20 and 45, hypertension is five times more common. Gaining fat greatly increases your chances of developing high blood pressure; losing fat—even 10 percent of body weight—often lowers blood pressure and makes drug treatment unnecessary. (During the siege of Leningrad in World War II, when food was scarce, low blood pressure was common and heart disease declined.

Table 8.1
Fat Kills: 1979 Build Study

Percentage of Average Weight	Risk of Death (100% equals the average risk for all individuals)
65–75%*	105%*
75–95%	93%
95–105%	95%
105–115%	110%
115–125%	127%
125–135%	134%
135–145%	141%
145–155%	211%
155–165%	227%

*The chances of dying are above average—105 percent—for people who weigh the least (65 percent to 75 percent of average weight) because this group includes some persons who are very thin due to illness, which may not yet have been diagnosed. It's not that thin people get sick, but that sick people often get thin.

When the siege was lifted and food again became available, blood pressures rose and so did the incidence of heart disease.)

- **Cancer.** A major study by the American Cancer Society, involving more than 1 million men and women, found that obese men, smokers as well as non-smokers, were more likely to die of cancer of the colon, rectum or prostate. Obese women had higher death rates due to cancer of the gallbladder, breast, cervix, womb or ovaries.

- **Diabetes.** Four-fifths of all cases of non-insulin-dependent diabetes mellitus (NIDDM), sometimes called adult-onset diabetes, occur in persons who are overfat. Diabetes is almost three times more common in overfat than non-overfat persons, and as fat goes up, so does risk. The chances of developing NIDDM are 15 times higher in people with the highest waist–hip ratio (those whose fat is concentrated around the waist and on the upper body) than in those with the lowest, even when their overall weight is the same.

The mainstay of diabetes treatment is fat loss through exercise and diet. As weight goes down, levels of blood sugar (glucose) quickly move toward normal. New studies show that for many obese people, even small weight losses—often only 10 percent of body weight—can correct a tendency toward diabetes.

- **Osteoarthritis.** Carrying around excess pounds not only stresses the joints, it discourages exercising, which can strengthen bones and muscles and keep tendons and ligaments supple.
- **Chronic obstructive lung disease.** Extra fat impairs lung function by crowding the chest and abdominal cavities and makes extra demands on the heart and lungs.
- **Gout.** Usually it is not clear why some of us suffer the uric acid buildup that causes joints—especially the joint in the big toe—to become hot, swollen and painful. But it's often possible to decrease uric acid and the risk of gout by losing fat and avoiding alcohol.

IF YOU LOSE, YOU WIN

There are lots of pluses to losing fat. You'll look better, feel better, have more energy and be more productive. You'll enjoy a greater sense of control, and you'll reduce your risk of fat-related disease. The Framingham study showed that by losing weight you can lower blood pressure, blood sugar and uric acid and raise levels of HDL-C.

As we have seen, you become overfat when your calorie intake exceeds your calorie output, and you lose fat by reversing the process. You can produce a calorie deficit by eating less or burning more. But the combination of more exercise and a little less munching seems to be the best and most natural way to achieve this result.

Table 8.2 shows how many calories you need to eat each day to maintain a given weight. Locate the number that matches your present weight. To determine how many calories you should take in each day if you want to lose one pound a week, subtract 500 calories from the daily

allotment. To lose two pounds a week, subtract 1,000 calories from your current daily intake. (Note: Altogether, you must consume 3,500 fewer calories in one week to lose a pound of fat.)

DIET IS A FOUR-LETTER WORD

"Going on a diet" has come to mean enduring an unpleasant period of food deprivation. The dieter is sustained through his or her suffering by visions of one day enjoying real food again. First you starve, then you celebrate not starving—by eating.

The trouble is that when you sharply reduce the amount you eat but don't increase the amount you exercise, all the wrong things happen. As your body tries to compensate for what it perceives as starvation, your metabolism drops and you burn calories more slowly. This makes it harder to lose fat; your body is waiting for the time when it can increase its fat and raise its metabolic rate to its set point again.

Of course you lose weight anyway, but at first it's mostly water weight. This is another of the body's responses to perceived starvation; as stored carbohydrates are broken down and excreted, they take lots of water with them. (This is also what causes the frequent urination of diabetics.) It's water loss like this that leads to the fleeting popularity of quick-loss miracle diets. Eventually you'll have to drink liquids that will replace the water losses, and the apparent weight loss will be erased. Losing fat takes time.

A major problem with dieting is that it depletes both lean body mass and fat. This is the body's way of saving fat, the most efficient form of stored energy, to see you through the period of starvation. Not only does muscle loss sap your strength and endurance, if it's severe enough it can endanger your life: The deaths associated with very-low-calorie diets have been triggered by damage to the heart, which is, after all, a muscle. And unfortunately, high-protein diets do *not* preserve muscle. But exercise does.

When you go off your diet (and you will —dieters live for the moment they can get back to

Table 8.2
How Many Calories Do You Need?

Present Weight	Present Daily Intake (PDI: Calories to maintain present body weight)*	Daily Calorie Intake to Lose 1 Lb/Wk (500 calories/day less than PDI)	Daily Calorie Intake to Lose 2 Lbs/Wk (1000 calories/day less than PDI)
295	5,015	4,515	4,015
290	4,930	4,430	3,930
285	4,845	4,345	3,845
280	4,760	4,260	3,760
275	4,675	4,175	3,675
270	4,590	4,090	3,590
265	4,505	4,005	3,505
260	4,420	3,920	3,420
255	4,335	3,835	3,335
250	4,250	3,750	3,250
245	4,165	3,665	3,165
240	4,080	3,580	3,080
235	3,995	3,495	2,995
230	3,910	3,410	2,910
225	3,825	3,325	2,825
220	3,740	3,240	2,740
215	3,655	3,155	2,655
210	3,570	3,070	2,570
205	3,485	2,985	2,485
200	3,400	2,900	2,400
195	3,315	2,815	2,315
190	3,230	2,730	2,230
185	3,145	2,645	2,145
180	3,060	2,560	2,060
175	2,975	2,475	1,975
170	2,890	2,390	1,890
165	2,805	2,305	1,805
160	2,720	2,220	1,720
155	2,635	2,135	1,635
150	2,550	2,050	1,550
145	2,465	1,965	1,465
140	2,380	1,880	1,380
135	2,295	1,795	1,295
130	2,210	1,710	1,210
125	2,125	1,625	1,125

* Your weight x 17 = Approximate number of calories to maintain present weight of active person.

Using the Exercise High to Lose Fat

Your body's metabolic rate not only increases while you exercise, it stays high even after you stop. Based on a study at the University of Victoria, British Columbia, the figure below shows that the longer you exercise, the more calories you burn after you stop. The study showed that after a 30-minute bike ride, subjects' metabolic rates stayed high for about 130 minutes, causing them to burn an extra 6.8 liters of oxygen. But when the riding time was doubled to 60 minutes, the high metabolic rate continued for 455 minutes, rather than the expected 260 minutes. Oxygen consumption was a very surprising 36 liters instead of the expected 13.4 liters. This suggests that the best exercise pattern for losing

fat is one that increases the length rather than the frequency of exercise sessions. This after-exercise "high" is substantial: If you exercise vigorously for 60 minutes, not only will you burn more calories while you exercise, you will keep on burning more calories for 7-1/2 hours afterward.

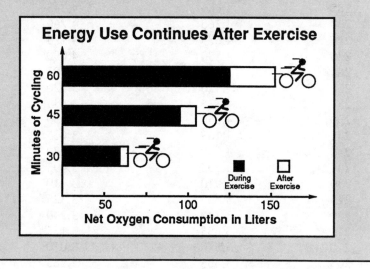

"normal" eating), your body will be at a lower metabolic rate. This means it will be easier to regain weight, which will consist of more fat and less muscle than you lost. And it gets worse: Because muscle burns calories more efficiently than fat does, having less muscle means that it will be easier than ever to gain weight, even if you eat no more than you used to. After you've dieted off 20 pounds and then regained them, eating just what you ate before the diet will cause you to gain even more.

The final blow is that you become less able to lose fat. Studies have shown that "yo-yo dieting" —losing weight, regaining it, losing and regaining it again—ends up increasing body fatness and makes it more difficult to lose fat, probably by resetting the set point upward. This means that the body requires more fat to reach its normal meta-

bolic rate. Ultimately the yo-yo dieter, with progressively more fat and less muscle, may be unable to lose fat even on a very low-calorie diet.

FIGHTING FAT THROUGH EXERCISE

Exercise, in contrast to dieting, fights fat in several ways. First, and most obviously, it burns calories.

Second, exercise steps up the body's metabolism. You burn calories more quickly as your body strives to meet the greater demand for energy. During aerobic exercise, the metabolic rate increases by 10 percent to 15 percent. And your metabolic rate stays up even after you have finished exercising (see box). This "post-exercise burn" alone can easily consume a half-pound or more of fat each week.

Table 8.3
Burning Up Calories

This chart shows how many calories a 150-pound man can burn in 20 minutes through a variety of activities.

Activity	Calories Burned in 20 Minutes
Walking (2 1/2 mph)	70
Bicycling (5 1/2 mph)	70
Gardening	73
Walking (3 3/4 mph)	100
Swimming (1/4 mph)	100
Disco dancing	100
Wood chopping or sawing	133
Aerobic dancing	133
Tennis	140
Skiing (10 mph)	200
Bicycling (13 mph)	220
Running (10 mph)	300

Source: FOCUS on Weight. Reston, VA: The Center for Corporate Health Promotion, 1986.

Third, exercise increases your muscle mass. And muscle mass can be important. Having more muscle makes it much easier to burn up calories, because muscle burns calories more efficiently than other types of body tissue. And fat, the best source of energy, is the first to go. That's what you're after, a reduction in *fat*.

Exercise may also decrease your appetite. Researchers have found that obese people in particular cut back on food intake when they begin an exercise program.

THE PERFECT COUPLE

It's ideal to combine exercise with a good diet. Studies comparing diet alone with diet plus exercise have found that while both methods may cause people to lose about the same amount of weight, persons who only diet lose a great deal of muscle mass. In contrast, those who also exercise increase muscle mass. In one study, non-exercising dieters lost 18 pounds, including seven pounds of muscle, whereas exercising dieters lost 19 pounds total—but they gained four pounds of muscle and lost 23 pounds of fat. So even when their weight loss was identical, the difference in how people looked and felt was enormous.

NOT ALL CALORIES ARE CREATED EQUAL

It appears that a calorie from fat that you eat poses more threat than a calorie of carbohydrate —one from bread, cereal, pasta, fruit or vegetables. (Fats, proteins, carbohydrates and the many other components of healthful eating are discussed at length in Chapter 7.) Fat is readily stored in the body, whereas storing carbohydrates takes more processing. This processing uses up about 25 percent of the carbohydrate calories, but only 2.5 percent of the calories in fat. So, if you use 100 calories worth of a high-fat salad dressing, 97.5 of the calories can be stored as body fat. But when you eat an apple that contains 100 carbohydrate calories, 25 are used up right away, and only 75 can be stored as fat. Thus, simply switching from a high-fat diet to one high in carbohydrates can result in a net calorie loss, even if you eat the same number of calories. Moreover, you don't need to eat many fatty foods to reach your calorie quota: An ounce of fat packs more than twice the calories of an ounce of protein or carbohydrate. Thus, an ounce of fat can generate three times as much fat as an ounce of carbohydrate or protein.

Two recent reports have linked obesity not with total calories, but with the proportion of calories that come from fat. People who ate more fat were fatter, whatever their calorie intake. The nation's high-fat diet, researchers believe, may help to explain why so many Americans are overfat. The best way to cut calories is to cut down on high-fat foods: whole milk, butter, ice cream, oils, fatty meats, fried foods, cookies, cakes, etc. (see Chapter 7, Food for Life).

THE ROAD TO FAT CONTROL

If you are among the millions of Americans who are overfat, you should slim down, but don't "go on a diet." As we've seen, most diets are destined to fail, and many make it harder to lose weight in the long run. Rather, you should exercise, make some food substitutions and, if necessary, change harmful eating patterns.

Exercising

To gain the most from the new eating patterns you plan to establish, you'll want to become more active both formally and informally. Your formal exercise program should consist of at least 20 minutes of aerobic activity three times a week. Chapter 6 offers lots of help on making exercise part of your life.

Make Some Food Substitutions

Most people find it much easier to substitute one food for another than to eliminate food altogether. The most important substitution for all of us, whether or not we are trying to lose fat, is replacing high-fat foods with low-fat ones. Chapter 7 suggests such substitutions. Some changes will almost always lead to eating lower-calorie

foods as well. It is also possible to look at substitutions simply as replacing high-calorie with low-calorie foods. Refer to Table 8.4 for a table of such substitutions.

Change Harmful Eating Patterns

Exercise and food substitutions are the basics of fat control. But sometimes our eating patterns themselves cause a problem. These patterns allow us to impulsively eat or to consume large amounts of food unconsciously. Understanding and improving eating patterns can be important for many people. If exercise seems to be having little effect, or if food substitutions seem hard to make, try to get a handle on your eating habits. These suggestions may help:

- **Find out what, when, where and why you eat.** Most of us never give much thought to our eating habits. Often we can't even remember what we've eaten. Keeping a food diary for two weeks can be a real eye-opener.

Food Diary

	Time	Food	Amount	Location	Reason
S					
M					
T					
W					
T					
F					
S					
S					
M					
T					
W					
T					
F					
S					

- **Analyze why you eat.** People eat for many different reasons, but not usually to ease hunger pangs. Most people eat out of habit, or in response to cues from the environment—the sight or smell of food, scheduled breaks, formal meal times or food-associated settings (a kitchen or restaurant). What's more, feelings have a great deal to do with eating. Many, if not most, overfat people have learned to eat because they are anxious or bored. Importantly, eating in response to these cues brings real rewards, which can be represented as follows:

Cue	Reaction	Reward
Hungry	→ Eating	→ Satisfied
Nervous	→ Eating	→ More relaxed
Angry	→ Eating	→ Composed
Bored	→ Eating	→ Occupied

Studying your food diary will show you which cues are important to you.

- **Change your eating cues.** Decide what you can do to develop better eating habits, and then map a strategy for change. This strategy is not a diet in the usual sense. No foods are off limits. You will not have to restrict yourself to low-calorie choices. In fact, you will not even have to count calories.

It helps some people to eat in only one place at home. You may be packing away lots of calories without realizing it, under the guise of "snacking." During the first month, try to avoid going out to dinner.

You should also avoid doing anything else while eating. You won't believe how many "munchies" people consume unconsciously in front of the TV or while reading a book. If you are going to eat, sit down and enjoy it.

Finally, keep food out of sight. It's hard to resist taking a bite when food is visible and within easy reach. And don't put serving dishes on the table.

- **Create small changes in your eating habits.** After keeping a food diary for a few weeks, you will have a much clearer picture of your eating habits. You will then be in a better position to control them. This is the time to change those habits that affect your food intake.

Great changes are not needed. You have months, even years, to reduce your weight. Eliminating "unconscious" snacking may itself trigger weight loss. Still, if weight loss seems very slow, try these seven ploys:

1. Eat only when you are hungry.
2. Try not to eat between meals.
3. Reduce serving sizes by about a quarter.
4. Serve with a teaspoon instead of a tablespoon.
5. Never eat standing up.
6. Stretch your meal by eating slowly and putting your fork down between bites. You'll enjoy your food more and give the "hunger center" in your brain enough time to be satisfied. (It takes about 20 minutes.)
7. Brush your teeth right after meals; you'll be less likely to go back for more.

- **Choose reasonable goals.** One to three pounds of fat a week is all that you should try to lose. More than that can upset your metabolism, and it's almost always only water weight, anyway.

Each week, on the same day and at the same time, recalculate your percentage of body fat. As you lose fat, your waist or hip measurement will decrease. Your weight will depend upon the balance between fat loss and muscle gain. Until you reach the advanced levels of exercise (including strength exercises), fat loss will usually outweigh muscle gain—but don't let the chart's limitations discourage you. Often, change can be seen and felt before it is confirmed by the chart. After all, most likely you are only looking for a change of a few percentage points in your body fat composition. If you are on a good program, stick with it. It can be several weeks before the chart confirms what you already know.

- **Reward yourself.** Recognizing your own success is important. Every time your body fat drops a percentage point, give yourself a reward. It should be something that you can give yourself promptly, that will really please you and that you can't eat!

  Your reward can be anything from magazines to new clothes. But a small amount of money—a dollar or two—often works well. The important thing is to act promptly and make the reward something you really like or need.

- **This is forever.** To rephrase the famous quote, "Fat control is a thing of beauty and of joy, but only if it is forever." You must develop habits that you can live with for the rest of your life. If you think of losing fat as a short-term activity and plan to get back to living "normally," forget it. If your goal is to lose 10 pounds a week of anything—fat, water, muscle, even hair—you cannot succeed. But if you make permanent changes in exercise and eating habits, the benefits of fat control will be permanent also.

LOOKING FOR SUCCESS

Remember, the basic rules are simple:

1. **Exercise.** This is the most important rule of all.
2. **Make good choices.** Substitute low-fat foods for high-fat foods (see Chapter 7). Also, substitute low-calorie foods for high-calorie foods.
3. **Gain control of your eating habits.**

Table 8.4
Food Substitutions

For This		Substitute This		
Beverages	**Calories**		**Calories**	**Calories Saved**
Milk (whole), 8 oz.	165	Milk (buttermilk, skim), 8 oz.	80	85
Prune juice, 8 oz.	170	Tomato juice, 8 oz.	50	120
Soft drinks, 8 oz.	105	Diet soft drinks, 8 oz.	1*	104
Coffee (with cream and 2 tsp. sugar)	110	Coffee (black with artificial sweetener)	0	110
Cocoa (all milk), 8 oz.	235	Cocoa (milk and water), 8 oz.	140	95
Chocolate malted-milk shake, 8 oz.	500	Lemonade (sweetened), 8 oz.	100	400
Beer (1 bottle), 12 oz.	175	Liquor (1 1/2 oz.), with soda or water, 8 oz.	120	55

Table 8.4
Food Substitutions, continued

For This		Substitute This		
Breakfast Foods	**Calories**		**Calories**	**Calories Saved**
Rice flakes, 1 cup	110	Puffed rice, 1 cup	50	60
Eggs (scrambled), 2	220	Eggs (boiled or poached), 2	160	60
Butter and Cheese				
Butter on toast	170	Apple butter on toast	90	80
Cheese (blue, cheddar, cream or Swiss),1 oz.	105	Cheese (cottage, uncreamed), 1 oz.	25	80
Desserts				
Angel food cake, 2" piece	110	Cantaloupe, 1/2	40	70
Cheesecake, 2" piece	200	Watermelon, 1/2" slice (10" diameter)	60	140
Chocolate cake with icing, 2" piece	425	Sponge cake, 2" piece	120	305
Fruitcake, 2" piece	115	Grapes, 1 cup	65	50
Pound cake, 1 oz. piece	140	Plums, 2	50	90
Pudding (flavored), 1/2 cup	140	Pudding (dietetic, made with non-fat milk), 1/2 cup	60	80
Cupcake, white icing, 1	230	Plain cupcake, 1	115	115
Cookies, assorted (3" diameter), 1	120	Vanilla wafer (dietetic), 1	25	95
Ice cream, 4 oz.	150	Yogurt (flavored), 4 oz.	60	90

Table 8.4
Food Substitutions, continued

For This		Substitute This		
Fish and Fowl	**Calories**		**Calories**	**Calories Saved**
Tuna (canned), 3 oz.	165	Crabmeat (canned), 3 oz.	80	85
Oysters (fried), 6	400	Oysters (shell w/sauce), 6	100	300
Ocean perch (fried), 4 oz.	260	Bass, 4 oz.	105	155
Fish sticks, 5 sticks or 4 oz.	200	Swordfish, (broiled), 3 oz.	140	60
Lobster meat, 4 oz., with 2 tbsp. butter	300	Lobster meat, 4 oz., with lemon	95	205
Duck (roasted), 3 oz.	310	Chicken (roasted), 3 oz.	160	150
Meats				
Loin roast, 3 oz.	290	Pot roast (round), 3 oz.	160	130
Rump roast, 3 oz.	290	Rib roast, 3 oz.	200	90
Swiss steak, 3 1/2 oz.	300	Liver (fried), 2 1/2 oz.	210	90
Hamburger (average fat, broiled), 3 oz.	240	Hamburger (lean, broiled), 3 oz.	145	95
Porterhouse steak, 3 oz.	250	Club steak, 3 oz.	160	90
Rib lamb chop (medium fat), 3 oz.	300	Lamb leg roast, (lean only), 3 oz.	160	140
Pork chop (medium fat), 3 oz.	340	Veal chop (medium fat), 3 oz.	185	155
Pork roast, 3 oz.	310	Veal roast, 3 oz.	230	80
Pork sausage, 3 oz.	405	Ham (boiled, lean), 3 oz.	200	205

Table 8.4
Food Substitutions, continued

For This		Substitute This		
Pie (1/7 piece of a 9″ pie)	**Calories**		**Calories**	**Calories Saved**
Apple, 1 piece	345	Tangerine (fresh), 1	40	305
Blueberry, 1 piece	290	Blueberries (frozen, unsweetened), 1/2 cup	45	245
Cherry, 1 piece	355	Cherries (whole), 1/2 cup	40	315
Custard, 1 piece	280	Banana, small, 1	85	195
Lemon meringue, 1 piece	305	Lemon-flavored gelatin, 1/2 cup	70	235
Peach, 1 piece	280	Peach (whole), 1	35	245
Rhubarb, 1 piece	265	Grapefruit, 1/2	55	210
Potatoes				
Fried, 1 cup	480	Baked (2 1/2″ diameter)	100	380
Mashed, 1 cup	245	Boiled (2 1/2″ diameter)	100	145
Salads				
Chef salad with oil dressing, 1 tbsp.	180	Chef salad with dietetic dressing, 1 tbsp.	40	140
Chef salad with mayonnaise, 1 tbsp.	125	Chef salad with dietetic dressing, 1 tbsp.	40	85
Chef salad with Roquefort, blue cheese, Russian, or French dressing, 1 tbsp.	105	Chef salad with dietetic dressing, 1 tbsp.	40	65

Table 8.4
Food Substitutions, continued

For This		Substitute This		
Sandwiches	**Calories**		**Calories**	**Calories Saved**
Club	375	Bacon and tomato (open)	200	175
Peanut butter and jelly	275	Egg salad (open)	165	110
Turkey with gravy, 3 tbsp.	520	Hamburger, lean, (open), 3 oz.	200	320
Snacks				
Fudge, 1 oz.	115	Vanilla wafers, (dietetic), 2	50	65
Peanuts (salted), 1 oz.	170	Apple, 1	100	70
Peanuts (roasted), 1 cup, shelled	1375	Grapes, 1 cup	65	1310
Potato chips, 10 medium	115	Pretzels, 10 small sticks	35	80
Chocolate, 1-oz. bar	145	Toasted marshmallows, 3	75	70

ADDITIONAL RESOURCES
Books

The California Diet and Exercise Program, by Dr. Peter Wood. Mountain View, CA: Anderson World Books, Inc., 1983.

The Fat-to-Muscle Diet, by Victoria Zak, Cris Carlin, M.S., R.D., and Peter Vash, M.D., M.P.H. New York: G. P. Putnam's Sons, 1986.

The Fit or Fat Target Diet, by Covert Bailey. Boston: Houghton Mifflin Company, 1984.

Mind Over Weight, by William Macleod. Englewood Cliffs, NJ: Prentice-Hall, 1983.

Sensible Fitness, by Jack H. Wilmore, Ph.D. Champaign, IL: Leisure Press, 1986.

A Minibook About Healthful Eating is available from NutriWork, a division of The Network. The company also offers Food for the Health of It (book/teacher's guide). NutriWork, 290 South Main Street, Andover, MA 01810. (508) 470-1080.

Audiovisuals

A catalog of materials for purchase or lease is available from Milner-Fenwick, Inc., 2125 Greenspring Drive, Timonium, MD 21093. The toll-free number is (800) 638-8652.

Table 8.4
Food Substitutions, continued

For This		Substitute This		
Soups (1 cup)	**Calories**		**Calories**	**Calories Saved**
Creamed	210	Chicken noodle	110	100
Bean	190	Beef noodle	110	80
Minestrone	105	Beef bouillon	10	95
Vegetables (1 cup)				
Baked beans	320	Green beans	30	90
Lima beans	160	Asparagus	30	130
Corn (canned)	185	Cauliflower	30	155
Peas (canned)	145	Peas (fresh)	115	30
Winter squash	75	Summer squash	30	45
Succotash	260	Spinach	40	220

* See individual bottle label for possible variations.

Source: Pharmaceutical Division, Pennwalt Corporation. Used by permission.

PRI (Professional Research, Inc.) also has some good materials. It is located at 930 Pitner Avenue, Evanston, IL 60202. (800) 421-2363.

Associations

The American Diabetes Association (ADA) offers some good, inexpensive materials, including food-exchange brochures and two cookbooks, *The ADA Cookbook* and *Recipes for Health*. Contact your local ADA chapter for ordering information and prices.

The American Heart Association (AHA) publishes *The American Heart Association Cookbook* and numerous brochures. Call or write your local chapter or the AHA National Center, 7320 Greenville Avenue, Dallas, TX 75231. (214) 373-6300.

Government

Source Book for Health Education Materials and Community Resources (Publication #017-023-00144-2) is available for $5.50 from the Superintendent of Documents, U.S. Government Printing Office, Washington, DC 20402. (202) 783-3238.

A publications list can be obtained from the President's Council on Physical Fitness and Sports, 450 Fifth Street, N.W., Suite 7103, Washington, DC 20001. (202) 272-3430.

SMOKING:
The Black Cloud

In January 1989, William Bennett became the country's most famous quitter. Nominated by President George Bush to be Director of the Office of Drug Control Policy, Bennett vowed to quit smoking before he took office. He had tried before without success. But this time, prodded by the publicity of his pledge, he worked hard to make it stick. In the quiet of a rustic West Virginia retreat, the future "drug czar" spent six days exercising, hiking and meditating in an attempt to kick his two-pack-a-day habit.

Bennett's effort put him in the company of more than 40 million Americans who have given up cigarettes since the landmark report to the Surgeon General in 1964. But 46 million—more than a quarter of the adult population—continue to smoke, at grave peril to themselves and to those around them.

According to the Surgeon General's 1989 report, smoking contributes to close to 400,000 deaths each year, primarily from cancer, heart disease and lung disease. Consider these facts:

- **Smokers are twice as likely as non-smokers to have a heart attack and two to four times more likely to die suddenly.** Heart disease is the country's leading killer, and smoking actually causes more deaths through heart disease than through lung cancer. This year more than 1.5 million Americans will suffer heart attacks, and more than a million will die.
- **Smoking triggers stroke deaths.** The Surgeon General's 1989 report was the first to confirm smoking as a cause of strokes. It is estimated that more than 25,000 lethal strokes each year are linked to smoking.
- **Men who smoke have 22 times the chance of dying from lung cancer as men who don't smoke.** A smoker who's exposed to asbestos runs a risk of getting lung cancer about 60 times that of a non-smoker; alcohol and certain drugs also in-

tensify smoking's adverse effects. And lung cancer has now passed breast cancer as the number-one cancer killer of women. Smoking also increases the risk of cancers of the larynx (voice box), lip, mouth, pancreas, bladder and cervix.

- **Emphysema is a sure thing.** Cigarette smoke directly damages lung tissue. Every smoker develops emphysema to some degree, depending on how much he or she has smoked. If smokers live long enough, their emphysema gets to the point where just getting up to go to the bathroom leaves them winded and exhausted. If you find this hard to imagine, try breathing through a straw. Use one that is narrow enough to make you work to breathe while sitting down. Then get up, and try to move around and do something—still breathing through the straw. This is called suffocation.

- **Smoking is harmful to your baby's health.** Smoking during pregnancy can kill an otherwise healthy fetus. Mothers who smoke increase their risk of miscarriage, stillbirth or infant death during the neona-

Table 9.1
Smoking's Contribution to Disease

Smoking cigarettes, cigars and pipes is responsible for an appalling number of deaths.

Disease	Percentage of Deaths Due to Smoking
All cancers	30%
Lung cancer	87%
Coronary heart disease	21%
Coronary heart disease (in people under the age of 65)	40%
Stroke	18%
Chronic obstructive lung disease (emphysema)	82%

Source: Surgeon General's Report, *Reducing the Health Consequences of Smoking: 25 Years of Progress*, 1989.

tal period. They are 55 percent more likely to give birth to babies who are deformed. The smoker's baby is more likely to be small at birth and to lag in physical, mental and behavioral development. Furthermore, infants and young children exposed to cigarette smoke are prone to acute respiratory illnesses, such as bronchitis or pneumonia, and often need to be hospitalized. Or they may develop chronic symptoms, such as coughing or wheezing.

- **Smoking is harmful to your neighbor's health.** So-called "involuntary smoking" —breathing in the smoke from someone else's cigarette—can cause disease, including lung cancer, in healthy non-smokers. National Cancer Institute scientists who analyzed more than a dozen published studies found that the risk of lung cancer is increased 30 percent for non-smokers married to smokers, and 70 percent for the spouses of heavy smokers. Separating

The Country That Smokes Together

You say that you don't smoke? Not so fast. Virtually every non-smoker engages in passive smoking, be it at home, at work, in restaurants or in airplanes. Current estimates are that almost 50,000 Americans die each year from cancer and heart attacks caused by inhaling *other people's smoke*.

You get a really heavy dose when you fly. A National Cancer Institute study shows that someone on a four-hour flight inhales so much smoke that nicotine remains in the body for up to three days after flying, even though the person sat in the non-smoking section.

Test Yourself: Why Do You Smoke?

Here are some statements that describe what people get out of smoking cigarettes. How often do you feel this way when smoking? Circle one number for each statement. **Important: Respond to every statement.**

	Always	Frequently	Occasionally	Seldom	Never
A. I smoke cigarettes to keep myself from slowing down.	5	4	3	2	1
B. Handling a cigarette is part of the enjoyment of smoking it.	5	4	3	2	1
C. Smoking cigarettes is pleasant and relaxing.	5	4	3	2	1
D. I light up a cigarette when I feel angry about something.	5	4	3	2	1
E. When I have run out of cigarettes I find it almost unbearable until I can get them.	5	4	3	2	1
F. I smoke cigarettes automatically without even being aware of it.	5	4	3	2	1
G. I smoke cigarettes for stimulation, or to perk myself up.	5	4	3	2	1
H. Part of the enjoyment of smoking a cigarette comes from the steps I take to light up.	5	4	3	2	1
I. I find cigarettes pleasurable.	5	4	3	2	1
J. When I feel uncomfortable or upset about something, I light up a cigarette.	5	4	3	2	1
K. I am very much aware of the fact when I am not smoking a cigarette.	5	4	3	2	1
L. I light up a cigarette without realizing I still have one burning in the ashtray.	5	4	3	2	1
M. I smoke cigarettes to give me a "lift."	5	4	3	2	1
N. When I smoke a cigarette, part of the enjoyment is watching the smoke as I exhale it.	5	4	3	2	1
O. I want a cigarette most when I am comfortable and relaxed.	5	4	3	2	1
P. When I feel "blue" or want to take my mind off cares and worries, I smoke cigarettes.	5	4	3	2	1
Q. I get a real gnawing hunger for a cigarette when I haven't smoked for a while.	5	4	3	2	1
R. I've found a cigarette in my mouth and didn't remember putting it there.	5	4	3	2	1

1. Enter the numbers you have circled in the spaces below, putting the number you have circled for Question A over line A, for Question B over line B, etc.
2. Add up the three scores on each line to get your totals. For example, the sum of your scores over lines A, G, and M gives you your score on Stimulation—lines B, H and N give the score on Handling, etc. Scores can vary from 3 to 15. Any score of 11 or above is **high**; any score of 7 or below is **low**.

_____ + _____ + _____ = _____ Stimulation				
A	G	M		
_____ + _____ + _____ = _____ Handling				
B	H	N		
_____ + _____ + _____ = _____ Pleasurable Relaxation				
C	I	O		
_____ + _____ + _____ = _____ Crutch: Tension Reduction				
D	J	P		
_____ + _____ + _____ = _____ Craving: Psychological Addiction				
E	K	Q		
_____ + _____ + _____ = _____ Habit				
F	L	R		

Adapted from material provided by the National Clearing House for Smoking and Health, Bureau of Health Education, Centers for Disease Control, U.S. Department of Health, Education and Welfare, Atlanta, Georgia.

Reprinted from *American Health: Fitness of Body and Mind,* 1983, American Health Partners.

This test is designed to provide you with a score on each of six factors that describe many people's smoking. Your smoking may be well characterized by only one of these factors, or by a combination of factors.

A score of 11 or above on any factor indicates that this factor is an important source of satisfaction for you. The higher your score (15 is the highest), the more important a particular factor is in your smoking and the more useful the discussion of that factor can be in your attempt to quit.

Stimulation

If you score high or fairly high on this factor, it means that you are one of those smokers who are stimulated by the cigarette—you feel that it helps wake you up, organizes your energies and keeps you going. If you try to give up smoking, you may want a safe substitute (a brisk walk or moderate exercise, for example) whenever you feel the urge to smoke.

Handling

Handling things can be satisfying, but there are many ways to keep your hands busy without lighting up or playing with a cigarette. Why not toy with a pen or pencil? Or try doodling. Or play with a coin, a piece of jewelry or some other harmless object.

Accentuation of Pleasure—Pleasurable Relaxation

It is not always easy to find out whether you use the cigarette to feel good, whether you get real, honest pleasure out of smoking (Factor 3), or whether you smoke to keep from feeling bad (Factor 4). About two-thirds of smokers score high or fairly high on accentuation of pleasure, and about half also score as high or higher on reduction of negative feelings.

Those who do get real pleasure out of smoking often find that an honest consideration of the harmful effects of their habit is enough to help them quit.

Reduction of Negative Feelings or "Crutch"

Many smokers use the cigarette as a kind of crutch in moments of stress or discomfort, and on occasion it may work; the cigarette is sometimes used as a tranquilizer. But heavy smokers, those who try to handle severe personal problems by smoking many times a day, are apt to discover that cigarettes do not help them deal with problems effectively.

"Craving" or Psychological Addiction

Quitting smoking is difficult for those who score high on this factor. For them, the craving for the next cigarette begins to build up the moment they put one out.

Giving up cigarettes may be so difficult and cause so much discomfort that once they do quit, they will find it easy to resist the temptation to go back to smoking because they know that some day they will have to go through the same agony again.

Habit

These smokers no longer get much satisfaction from cigarettes. They light them frequently without even realizing they are doing so. They may find it easy to quit and stay off if they can break the habit patterns they have built up. Cutting down gradually may be quite effective if there is a change in the way the cigarettes are smoked and the conditions under which they are smoked. The key to success is becoming aware of each cigarette you smoke. This can be done by asking yourself, "Do I really want this cigarette?" You may be surprised at how many you do not want.

smokers from non-smokers within the same airspace may reduce the danger, but it does not eliminate it, according to the Surgeon General.

- **Smoking and oral contraceptives are a deadly combination.** The death rate for smokers on the pill is about six times that for non-smokers, according to studies by the Population Council. This is far greater than if the risk of smoking were simply added to the risk of oral contraceptives. The combination of smoking and birth control pills is especially dangerous with regard to heart disease: Women who smoke and take birth control pills are up to 39 times more likely to have a heart attack and up to 22 times more likely to have a stroke than women who neither smoke nor use birth control pills.

- **Smoking accelerates the menopause.** While studying the relationship between heart attacks and the menopause, investigators were surprised to discover that smokers experience the menopause at much younger ages than non-smokers do. Smoking also raises blood levels of cadmium, a mineral that contributes to osteoporosis in animals.

- **Other forms of tobacco also cause cancer.** Both snuff and chewing tobacco have been linked to cancers of the mouth and throat and to other health problems, including gum disease, tooth loss and high blood pressure. Pipe and cigar smokers are at increased risk for cancers of the mouth and lips. Moreover, a British study found that cigar smokers who continue to smoke following a heart attack have higher death rates than those who quit. Cigarette smokers who switch to pipes and cigars may be even worse off, because they tend to inhale, and pipe and cigar smoke is high in tar.

- **The country pays a high price for smoking.** It costs the American public about $65 billion a year to cover cigarette-related health care costs and loss of worker pro-

Equality Isn't Always Good

Has it seemed to you that as many women are smoking as men? If so, your observation is correct. The decline in smoking has been much slower among women than among men. More high-school girls than high-school boys smoke, and they're starting earlier every year. Smoking is actually increasing among older women. If current trends continue, more women than men will be smoking by 1994.

ductivity. The tobacco industry spends $2.5 billion on advertising and promotion —about $10 for every man, woman and child. To buy cigarettes, Americans pay out at least $35 billion.

KNOWING WHEN TO QUIT

No doubt you knew at least some of these facts. Surveys indicate that smokers and non-smokers alike know that smoking destroys health. Such knowledge is important in keeping non-smokers from beginning and in getting smokers to think about stopping and make an effort to stop. Eighty percent to 90 percent of smokers say they would like to quit, and more than half have made serious efforts to do so.

When you quit, you can get back much of what you have lost through smoking. (Not the money; that's gone forever.) Naturally, the longer you wait, the more advanced the damage. Yet your body has a remarkable ability to come back if you will give it a chance. The risk of heart disease declines rapidly in ex-smokers; within one week they have much less risk of having a heart attack, and within two years their risk is almost the same as that of people who have never smoked. For people who have emphysema and/or chronic bronchitis, quitting won't restore lost function, but it will prevent further deterioration.

Figure 9.1 shows the results of one study of the risk of lung cancer after quitting the noxious

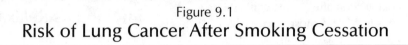

Figure 9.1
Risk of Lung Cancer After Smoking Cessation

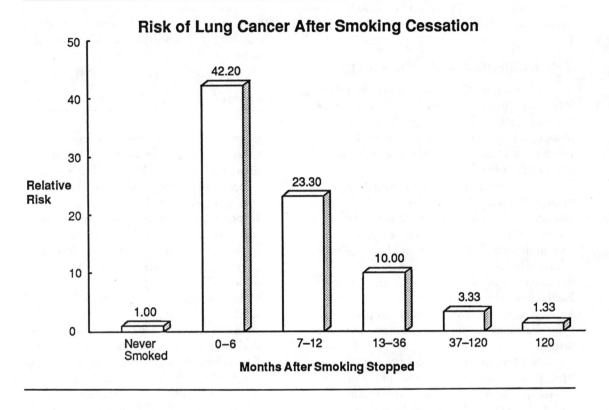

weed. Note that smokers who have just quit have very high risks of cancer. It is not uncommon for doctors to see heavy smokers soon after they have stopped and to diagnose lung cancer at that time. Undoubtedly many of these people have developed symptoms that scared them into quitting—the proverbial "closing the barn door after the horse gets out."

The moral is clear: If you wait until you have symptoms, you have waited far too long. Fewer than 5 percent of people with lung cancer live for five years, and most are dead within one year. Relying on chest X-rays to pick it up "early"? By the time lung cancer changes can be seen on an X-ray, the disease is too advanced to be helped.

SMOKING AS AN ADDICTION

Smoking is not just a nasty habit, something that keeps hands and mouth occupied and lets you look poised when you don't known what to do or say. If you are a smoker, you are addicted. Experts, including the Surgeon General, have found that nicotine is every bit as addictive as heroin, alcohol or cocaine, and probably more so. And withdrawal is painful—a major reason why so many people stay hooked.

Because they are addicted, smokers persist even though they know they are harming themselves and others—including their own children, born or unborn. Even more extreme are the patients recovering from heart surgery or cancer: Half resume smoking soon after, some while they are still in the hospital. And most doctors have heard horror stories such as the one about the emphysema patient who rigs up tubing to keep a lit cigarette at a safe distance from his or her oxygen tank.

THE INGREDIENTS OF ADDICTION

Cigarette smoke contains more than 4,000 ingredients, including many that are toxic or able to produce mutations or cancer. These include ammonia, benzene and carbon monoxide. The component that causes addiction, however, is the potent drug nicotine.

Each puff on a cigarette delivers a dose of nicotine that is rapidly absorbed through the lungs and into the bloodstream. Within seconds it is racing to the brain, where it acts on special receptors on the outside of brain cells. This triggers the release of hormones and other chemicals that affect numerous physical and psychological changes. Furthermore, brain cells respond to nicotine by forming additional receptors; this may partially explain the addictive effects of nicotine (and other drugs).

Nicotine stimulates and relaxes at the same time. It speeds up the heart, raises blood pressure, relaxes muscles, cuts circulation to the hands and feet, and suppresses the appetite for carbohydrates. (Carbon monoxide, for its part, reduces the amount of oxygen available to the heart and other tissues.) Whenever a smoker lights up and inhales, the immediate result is a feeling of energy, mental sharpness and control over life—in short, a bit of euphoria. And each puff strengthens the effect.

THE LURE OF SMOKING

As Tom Ferguson, M.D., points out in *The No-Nag, No-Guilt, Do-It-Your-Own-Way Guide to Quitting Smoking*, nicotine provides the smoker with a number of short-term rewards:

- **Mood control.** By regulating various brain hormones, nicotine "tunes" the smoker's mood up or down.
- **Keener attention and performance.** Nic-

Smoking as Relaxation

Smokers often feel that lighting up and taking a drag calms them down. And they're right. But it's not because nicotine has a sedative effect. It's because they are addicted and were entering withdrawal; the cigarette stops this by giving them the drug they crave, nicotine.

otine influences adrenalin and dopamine, two chemicals responsible for attention.
- **Sustained alertness.** With the help of nicotine, smokers can concentrate better on boring, repetitive tasks.
- **Improved long-term memory and learning.** Nicotine enhances long-term memory by helping smokers consolidate learned material—though day-to-day events are more likely to be forgotten.
- **Control of anger and anxiety.** Perhaps by subduing the brain structures that control emotions, nicotine allows the smoker to deal more calmly with annoyances.
- **Pain relief.** Nicotine serves as an analgesic, numbing the smoker's awareness of pain.
- **A sense of control.** By "self-dosing" with additional puffs throughout the day—typically 200 to 300 times—the smoker can maintain the blood levels of nicotine needed to regulate moods and alertness.

These effects, and addiction, are what make it so hard to quit. Smoking-cessation techniques must address what Ferguson calls "the smoker's dilemma"—the need to risk smoking's long-term health hazards for its short-term psychological benefits.

WEIGHT CONTROL

One of the most common reasons for not wanting to quit is fear of gaining weight. Indeed, some evidence suggests that the drugs in cigarette smoke increase metabolism and burn more calories. Some weight gain is common—about half of those who quit experience it—but it can be prevented. Regular exercise and proper nutrition are vital to any smoking-cessation program (see "Getting into Condition," below); they are vital if you find your weight creeping up. Should you put on a few pounds, take comfort in the fact that most ex-smokers revert to their former weight over time. Don't try to fool yourself into thinking that the health benefits of being a few pounds lighter outweigh the risks of smoking. That is a deadly deception. Finally, don't rely on smoking to keep you thin. The fact is, more smokers than non-smokers are overweight.

PUTTING CIGARETTES OUT (OF YOUR LIFE)

Many techniques have been developed to help people stop smoking. Most seem to "work" permanently for about 20 percent of the people who try them. The good news is that it is not the same 20 percent for each method and a method that did not work on one occasion may on another. If one approach doesn't help, try another. If an approach helped but you resumed smoking, you can still try it again. The most important thing is not the method but making a try at stopping. In fact, 95 percent of the people who quit do so on their own, without classes, acupuncture, aversive therapy or hypnosis.

A PLAN FOR SUCCESS

Quitting is the easy part; lots of people do it. Sticking to your decision, however, is another matter. The trick to long-term success is to find harmless ways to gain the mental and physical benefits you used to get from using nicotine. The following five-step smoking-cessation program includes proven techniques for success. You may not want to use all of them, but be wary of choosing only the easiest—you may be choosing failure.

Step One: Getting into Condition

In many smoking-cessation programs, eating healthfully and learning to relax come as after-thoughts. But these vital skills can form the groundwork for a successful transition, because they provide benefits similar to those gained from nicotine use. For example:

- Regular exercise reduces stress and tension.
- Relaxation exercises can help control moods, concentration and attention.
- Proper diet and exercise can offset weight gain, a common excuse for not wanting to quit.

Someone who is disciplined in these areas demonstrates the self-mastery that is needed for remaining smoke free.

When you have made the decision to quit, prepare for your life as a non-smoker by getting in shape. *Thirty to 45 days before you plan to quit*:

- Begin regular physical activity—*formal* aerobic exercise—at least three days a week (see Chapter 6).
- Observe your eating habits and make any needed adjustments (see Chapter 7).
- Learn to relax at will through self-control exercises (see Chapter 11).

Step Two: Setting a Quit Date

For most people, trying to ease out of the habit by gradually smoking less doesn't work well; instead it seems just to prolong the symptoms of withdrawal. Switching to brands low in tar and nicotine doesn't help either; many people compensate by smoking more cigarettes, inhaling more deeply or smoking the cigarette down to the butt.

A modified "cold-turkey" approach seems best. First cut down for a few weeks, to let your body adjust to a cutback in nicotine. Then stop.

Set a date for stopping completely—about 30 days ahead—and don't let anything interfere with it.

To motivate yourself, list all the reasons you want to quit:

- **You stink.** So do your clothes, car, office and home. To the extent that you expose them to your smoke, so do your spouse and kids. (If they smoke, tell them that they stink all by themselves.)
- **You are not looking good.** Dermatologists report that smokers develop more wrinkles, and sooner, than people who don't smoke.

- **You are tough to love.** Kissing a smoker may not be exactly like kissing a dirty ashtray, but it comes close.
- **You have a feeble sense of taste or smell.** Smoking impairs these senses. You don't know what you're missing.
- **You're squandering the vacation money.** A two-pack-a-day habit can cost more than $1,000 a year.
- **You are a fire hazard.** According to the National Fire Protection Association, smoking is the major cause of fatal residential fires.
- **You are setting yourself up for major illness.**

Step Three: Preparing to Quit

To find out when and why you smoke, use a smoking diary, a "Pack Wrap" or both. Then practice techniques for coping with the desire to smoke, and begin to smoke less.

The Pack Wrap is designed to give you a simple measure of how much you're smoking. Make a photocopy and wrap it around your pack of cigarettes. Each day, tally the number of cigarettes you smoke in the morning, afternoon and evening. As you gradually cut down, you'll see the number drop.

A diary lets you keep track of every cigarette you smoke and why you smoke it. On a sheet of lined paper, draw five columns with these headings: **Time, Need, Place or Activity, With Whom**, and **Mood or Reasons**. Then, whenever you light up, make a note of the factors at work. In the column marked **Need**, use numbers to rate the cigarettes, from 5, for those you felt you absolutely had to have, down to 1, for those you could easily have done without. At the end of the day, review the entries for any patterns. Perhaps you smoke most with certain people, after meals, at parties or when you're anxious.

The LifePlan Pack Wrap
Photocopy for additional wraps

	Morning	Afternoon	Evening	Total
S				
M				
T				
W				
T				
F				
S				

Sample of a Filled-Out Smoking Diary

Time	Need*	Place/Activity	With Whom	Mood/Reason
6:30 am	5	Kitchen/coffee	Self	Sleepy
7:15 am	4	Kitchen/after shower	Self	?
7:45 am	3	Car/driving	Self	Something to do with hands
8:30 am	4	Office/proofreading	Self	Frustrated
Noon	5	Restaurant/lunch	Co-Worker	Anxious

*In the column marked "Need," use numbers to rate the cigarettes, from 5, for those you felt you absolutely had to have, down to 1, for those you could easily have done without.

There are lots of little tricks you can use to cut down. Try some of these:

- Postpone lighting your first cigarette by 15 minutes the first day and 15 minutes more each day thereafter.

- Don't light up as soon as you crave a cigarette. Distract yourself: Start a conversation, or find something else to do, even if it's only drinking a glass of water.

- When you get the urge to smoke, take a mental trip: Close your eyes, breathe deeply and imagine yourself in your favorite spot.

- Set aside "non-smoking hours," and then gradually extend them.

- After a meal, leave the table promptly: Take a walk—or brush your teeth.

- When you have a strong urge to smoke, exercise. Exercise will both relax and distract you until the urge has passed.

- Practice a self-control relaxation exercise daily, such as the progressive relaxation exercise on page 176. And while you are in that part of the book, why not read all of Chapter 11, Mind ↔ Body, in order to give yourself the best chance for a healthy mind and body.

- Switch to a brand you hate.

- Try not to smoke two packs of the same brand in a row.

- Buy cigarettes by the pack, not by the carton. Finish one pack before buying another.

- Make your cigarettes harder to get. Wrap them in paper, lock them in a drawer—or roll them yourself.

- Try smoking with the hand you don't normally use.

- Smoke only half of each cigarette.

- Stop carrying matches or lighters.

- Chart your progress. Seeing is believing. Your daily records will encourage you as you count down toward cold-turkey day.

- Sit in non-smoking areas in restaurants, airplanes, etc.

- View smoking cessation as a positive move rather than a sacrifice. Tell yourself that you are becoming a non-smoker. Picture yourself enjoying the good feelings and benefits of not smoking.

- Tell others you are quitting. They'll support you and encourage you to succeed.

- Make a bet with someone that you'll quit on your target date.

- Form a "quit team" with people who will help you quit or who are also quitting.

- Ask your spouse, a friend or co-worker to quit with you.

- Don't empty ashtrays. Stale cigarettes are a turnoff. For about a week save your butts in a glass jar.

- Drink more fluids than usual, and get plenty of rest.

- Aim at not smoking for one hour at a time.
- Avoid parties or other situations (bars, etc.) where people are sure to smoke.
- Use substitutes—sugarless mints, gum and so forth—to replace the oral activity provided by smoking.

Something new that helps some people break away from nicotine addiction is a nicotine-containing gum. Used in combination with a smoking-cessation program, it appears to improve success rates. A hard, waxy and bitter substance, the "gum" is available only by prescription, and it must be used correctly—chewing deliberately and intermittently for 20 to 30 minutes. If it is to work, the nicotine should not be swallowed. It must be absorbed through the lining of the mouth.

The gum is used only after a person has stopped smoking. Because it delivers a lower dose of nicotine than a cigarette, more slowly and more regularly, it provides less pleasure than a cigarette. The idea is to pop a piece in your mouth whenever you feel the need for a cigarette, so as to fend off withdrawal symptoms (cravings, irritability, anxiety, trouble concentrating, restlessness, headache, drowsiness and digestive disturbances). It is to be used for the first couple of months, until you're safely weaned off the weed.

Step Four: On the Day You Quit

The keys to success are to focus on what you are doing rather than what you are not doing, and to build pleasure into the day. For example:

- Reward yourself. Buy something you've had your eye on or do something special to celebrate. Keep rewarding yourself with little things—a paperback or a movie.
- Keep practicing the "big three": regular exercise, proper nutrition and relaxation exercises.
- Make sure all your cigarettes are gone. Hiding them is cheating.
- Keep busy. Go to the movies, exercise, take long walks or go biking.
- Spend as much time as possible in "No-Smoking" areas.
- Avoid stressful situations if you can't apply stress-management techniques.
- Have your teeth cleaned at the dentist's office.
- Give yourself a break. Withdrawal is a fact of life, and you can expect to be a little cranky for the first 48 hours. Don't be hard on yourself, but do let others know what you're up to. That way, they can support you (and they will), rather than get on your case.

Step Five: After You've Stopped

Being unprepared when the urge strikes can lead to panic smoking—you find yourself smoking because you don't know what else to do. The following suggestions should help you remain a non-smoker:

- Take one day at a time.
- Keep up the "big three"—regular exercise, proper nutrition and daily relaxation exercises.
- If you link certain foods or drinks with smoking (consult your diary), try to avoid them, at least for now. After a while, you'll be able to ease back to them.
- Avoid situations in which people are sure to smoke (bars, etc.). Try to be with non-smokers.
- If you feel your will weakening, take a few deep breaths, light a match, and then slowly blow it out. Crush it in an ashtray as you would a cigarette.
- Most important, keep rewarding yourself for succeeding. Each day of not smoking takes effort, and you deserve a pat on the back.
- If you have trouble keeping your hands busy, fiddle with a paper clip, worry beads or a pencil. Do whatever you love to do, except smoking cigarettes.
- When the desire to smoke is strong, brush your teeth, wash your hands or take a shower.
- If you miss having something in your mouth, use a fake cigarette or keep toothpicks handy.

- Keep a stock of sugarless gum or mints, apples, celery, or carrots to munch on.
- Drink lots of water and juice. Some ex-smokers swear by orange or tomato juice.
- Make a calendar for the first 90 days. Cross off each smoke-free day and record the money saved by not smoking.
- Beware of the notion that just one cigarette won't hurt. On the other hand, if you give in and have one, don't think of yourself as a failure or a permanent smoker. Stop again immediately. You will succeed.

If you want to stop smoking and think you can, the chances are very good that you will succeed. If your spirit is willing but you fear that the flesh is too weak, take heart. Over 40 *million* Americans have quit. It does not require superhuman will power, but you must persist. If one method doesn't work, try another. You don't have to do it on your own; smoking-cessation programs and treatments do help many people. But don't look for any method to do it *for* you—at best it will *help* you to stop.

ADDITIONAL RESOURCES

There are lots of organizations that would love to help you quit smoking. Here are just a few:

- Contact your local chapter of the American Cancer Society, American Lung Association, and/or American Heart Association. They have all developed materials and programs to encourage quitting and keep you on the right path.
- Your local or state health department can put you in touch with programs and support groups in your community.
- Call the National Cancer Institute's toll-free number, (800) 4-CANCER, for a variety of publications, including a booklet called "Clearing the Air," a questionnaire called "Why Do You Smoke?" and the self-help "Quit Kit."
- A booklet called "No More Butts," as well as publications on smoking and pregnancy and the effects of family smoking on infants and children, is available from the Centers for Disease Control's Office on Smoking and Health, 5600 Fishers Lane, Parklawn Building, Room 1-16, Rockville, MD 20857.
- For more information on relaxation techniques, see the resources listed at the end of Chapter 11, Mind ↔ Body.
- Check out *The No-Nag, No-Guilt, Do-It-Your-Own-Way Guide to Quitting Smoking* by Tom Ferguson, M.D., New York: Ballantine Books, 1987.

PUTTING ALCOHOL IN ITS PLACE

Champagne at weddings, beer at ball games, fine wines with candle-lit dinners. Alcohol is very much a part of the current American scene. It is also the country's number-one drug of abuse.

In moderation, alcohol relaxes and sedates. It can convey a sense of power and create euphoria. It spurs merry-making in social settings and has meaning in religious ceremonies. Alcohol may even exert some health benefits: Some studies have linked a drink or so a day to a lower risk of heart attack.

But like all drugs, alcohol is a poison, and "intoxication" is more than a figure of speech. In large amounts alcohol ravages the body, blurs judgment, shreds the memory and destroys coordination. Alcohol abuse leads to 97,500 deaths in this country each year, some directly, through physical damage to the body, others indirectly, through accidents, violent crimes and suicide.

THE HIGH COST OF ALCOHOL ABUSE

In a given year Americans drink an estimated 2.65 gallons per capita of pure alcohol. That amounts to about 50 gallons of beer, 20 gallons of wine, or more than 4 gallons of whiskey, gin or vodka per person. But one-third of the population doesn't drink at all, and another third takes less than three drinks a week. Thus 95 percent of all drinking is done by the remaining third of the population. Heavy drinkers—people who consume more than 14 drinks per week—constitute 10 percent of the drinking population and account for half the alcohol consumed in the United States.

An estimated 10 million Americans are alcoholics, people unable to control their drinking. Another 7 million must cope with problems created by drinking while driving, drinking illegally or drinking just to get drunk.

Moreover, the shock waves of alcohol abuse spread far beyond the drinker. It is estimated that every alcoholic has a direct and harmful impact on the lives of four other people—mostly family members, friends and co-workers. A 1987 Gallup poll found that about one-fourth of all American homes have been touched by alcohol-centered problems. Excessive use of alcohol is a factor in about half of all divorces, and it lies behind many cases of spouse abuse and child abuse.

As if that were not bad enough, the stains of alcohol abuse spread across generations. The children of alcoholics are four times more likely to become alcoholics themselves than are the children of non-alcoholics. And heavy drinking by pregnant women can produce babies who are mentally retarded and/or physically deformed. Lighter drinking may create lesser abnormalities, such as poor coordination and hyperactivity.

The cost of alcohol abuse to the nation is estimated at more than $175 billion a year, $110 billion of which is due to lost employment and productivity. Between 5 percent and 10 percent of all employees—and as many as one-tenth of all executives—have a drinking problem. On average, the problem drinker costs his or her company from $4,800 to $7,500 a year.

ALCOHOL IN THE BODY

Once swallowed, alcohol is rapidly absorbed from the stomach and intestines into the bloodstream, which ferries it throughout the body. Because alcohol can travel anywhere water does, it can freely cross all membranes and enter all cells. Within moments, a sip can be found in all the tissues of the body.

Alcohol is broken down in the liver, and its byproducts are excreted through the lungs (creating a telltale breath odor) and urine. The body burns alcohol at the rate of about one drink an hour. (Contrary to folklore, the process cannot be speeded up by tricks such as drinking coffee or breathing pure oxygen.)

Taking more than one drink an hour causes alcohol to build up. The amount of alcohol in the blood (the blood alcohol concentration, or BAC) is used to gauge sobriety. In most states, drivers are considered legally drunk (and thus guilty of "driving while intoxicated," or DWI) when their BAC exceeds 0.10 percent. This is too high. Significant

What's in a "Drink"?

Beer, wine and hard liquor, such as whiskey, gin or vodka, all contain ethyl alcohol, a natural product of fermentation that is a colorless, inflammable liquid. Beer contains about 5 percent alcohol (light beer contains about 3 percent); table wine, about 12 percent; and whiskey, about 40 percent. (The strength of hard liquor is often stated as "proof," which doubles the percentage: 80 proof is equal to 40 percent.)

These differences in alcohol content are offset by the way drinks are served. There is about a half an ounce of alcohol in:

- A 12-ounce can of beer
- A 5-ounce glass of wine
- A cocktail with 1 1/2 ounces (a "jigger") of spirits.

Each drink contains about 100 calories, but few nutrients. (Of course, fancy drinks with added ingredients, as well as oversized drinks, add to the calorie toll.)

problems with both mental and physical functions begin at much lower BAC levels—0.05 or less.

IT GOES TO YOUR HEAD

"The wine urges me on, the bewitching wine, which sets even a wise man to singing and to laughing gently and rouses him up to dance and brings forth words which were better unspoken."

The Odyssey

Although alcohol is a sedative and slows down brain activity, for many people it seems to act at first as a stimulant. This is because it affects the parts of the brain that control learned behavior patterns, including self-control. Many people find that drinking relaxes their inner restraints and makes them more cordial. For other people, however, drinking uncovers depression or unleashes aggressiveness.

Here's a sobering thought: Any euphoria

Table 10.1
How Much Can You Drink?

For One Hour of Drinking

Number of Drinks	Approximate Blood Alcohol Concentration (Percentage of Alcohol in the Bloodstream) of person weighing (pounds):							
	100	120	140	160	180	200	220	240
1	.03	.03	.02	.02	.02	.01	.01	—
2	.06	.05	.04	.04	.03	.03	.03	.02
3	.10	.08	.07	.06	.05	.05	.04	.04
4	.13	.10	.09	.08	.07	.06	.06	.05
5	.16	.13	.11	.10	.09	.08	.07	.07
6	.19	.16	.13	.12	.11	.10	.09	.08
7	.23	.19	.16	.14	.13	.11	.10	.09
8	.26	.22	.18	.16	.14	.13	.12	.11

For Two Hours of Drinking

Number of Drinks	Approximate Blood Alcohol Concentration (Percentage of Alcohol in the Bloodstream) of person weighing (pounds):							
	100	120	140	160	180	200	220	240
1	.01	.01	—	—	—	—	—	—
2	.04	.03	.02	.01	.01	.01	—	—
3	.18	.06	.04	.03	.03	.02	.02	.01
4	.11	.09	.07	.06	.05	.04	.03	.03
5	.15	.12	.10	.08	.07	.06	.05	.04
6	.18	.14	.12	.10	.09	.08	.07	.06
7	.22	.18	.15	.12	.11	.09	.08	.07
8	.25	.20	.17	.15	.13	.11	.10	.09

Source: An Invitation to Health, 4th Edition, by Dianne Hales. Redwood City, CA: Benjamin/Cummings Publishing Co., 1989.

that you feel from drinking may be due in part to your brain being deprived of oxygen. "Drunk" feelings are experienced in other situations in which there is a lack of oxygen. For example, pilots whose oxygen systems fail are often euphoric even in the face of disaster.

As more alcohol enters the system, it impairs memory, muscle coordination and balance. As it reaches deeper into the brain, it can hamper judgment and dull the senses. A person with a BAC between 0.15 and 0.30 percent can pass out (and can even die by inhaling vomit). At extreme levels, alcohol can cause death by slowing heart function and breathing.

An overdose of alcohol leads to the pangs of a hangover. The headache, nausea, heartburn, abdominal pain, lack of coordination, slowed reflexes and other problems—including guilt—that most of us have suffered at some time attest to the alcohol's toxic effects. The fact that we recover does not mean there is no real damage, but rather that the body has considerable power to heal itself.

SAME DRINK, DIFFERENT DRINKER

How is it that one person quaffs a martini with little effect, yet another person is left reeling? How does a single glass of beer, on two occasions, affect the same person very differently? Part of the answer lies in individual makeup: Some people are genetically equipped to metabolize alcohol more quickly than others. Size is another factor: One drink will have less effect on the blood level of alcohol in a large person than in a smaller person, simply because the alcohol flows through a larger circulatory system.

Also, having food in your stomach can slow the absorption of alcohol. Diluting drinks with water or juice also slows alcohol absorption—but mixing alcohol with carbonated beverages actually increases the rate of uptake. And your reaction to drinking depends on how you are feeling: Someone who is upset, stressed or tired can become intoxicated more readily. If you expect to get drunk, you are likely to do so more quickly.

POSSIBLE HEALTH BENEFITS

In small amounts, alcohol may improve circulation, reduce blood fats and help to calm you down. Several studies suggest that moderate alcohol consumption, defined as no more than two drinks per day, increases the "good" cholesterol, high-density lipoprotein (HDL-C); this may ex-

Table 10.2
How Your BAC Affects You

.02%	Moderate drinkers feel some effect.
.04%	Most people begin to feel relaxed. This is after about two drinks.
.06%	Judgment begins to be impaired. There is less concern with environment. It becomes difficult to make rational decisions about your capabilities, such as driving or operating machinery.
.08%	The drinker becomes talkative, noisy and moody. Muscle coordination and driving skills are definitely impaired. In Idaho and Utah, you're legally drunk.
.10%	Reaction time and control have clearly declined. In all but six of the 50 states, you're legally drunk.
.12%	Serious loss of judgment and coordination occurs. The person is clumsy and may vomit.
.15%	The drinker staggers and speech is slurred. You're legally drunk in Maryland, Mississippi, New Jersey and Wisconsin.
.30%	The person may lose consciousness.
.40%	Loss of consciousness occurs at this level, and possibly death.
.45%	You are dead.

Source: Girdano and Dusek, *Drug Education*, 1980.

plain why moderate drinkers seem to have less risk of heart disease. Other studies indicate that moderate drinkers live longer than both heavy drinkers and teetotalers. But two studies found evidence that even moderate drinking could cause brain damage. Putting this all together suggests that drinking in moderation can be neither condemned nor encouraged.

THE SLIDE FROM SOCIAL TO LETHAL

About nine out of 10 people who drink have little problem controlling their drinking: They can take it or leave it. In *The Lost Weekend*, Charles Jackson wrote that alcoholics, too, can take it or leave it—so they take it.

Alcoholism is characterized by a growing inability to control one's drinking. Over a period of years the person goes from enjoying a drink to needing one. He or she develops a greater tolerance for liquor, grows concerned about maintaining a ready supply and becomes unable to stop drinking once he or she starts.

Alcohol wreaks havoc throughout the body. The damage is reversible in the early stages, but over time it becomes permanent and untreatable. Alcohol is especially hard on the liver, where it is

True or False: How to Keep From Getting Drunk

Question: Which of the following will keep you from getting drunk?

1. Don't mix different kinds of drinks.
2. Just drink beer.
3. Run or exercise to work off the alcohol.
4. Drink coffee.
5. Take vitamins.
6. Use other drugs.
7. Eat before and during drinking.
8. Drink in moderation—that is, not more than 1–2 drinks per hour.

Answer: Only 7 and 8 will work. If you drink on an empty stomach, the alcohol goes directly into the bloodstream and brain; eating slows its down. Since drunkenness depends on how much you weigh and how much you drink in how short of time, moderation is the most certain way of staying sober.

But note number 2: Stronger drinks make you drunk quicker because more will be absorbed. Thus, it is better if you order beer, table wines, or highballs (liquor with water) than cocktails or liquor (straight or on the rocks), or even fortified wines such as sherry or port.

Control Your Drinking

1. Dilute alcoholic beverages with water or soda, or consume low-alcohol-content drinks, such as light beer and white wine.
2. Eat something before and while you drink.
3. Never gulp your drinks. Pace yourself and set limits on your drinking, especially when planning to drive.
4. Don't be pressured into drinking if you don't want to drink. Learn to say no.
5. Know what you are drinking and how strong it is.
6. Don't mix alcohol with any drugs, including over-the-counter medications.

Alcohol can serve a social purpose, but too much or inappropriate drinking can easily destroy any positive effects. Knowledge of yourself and how alcohol affects you is the key to control.

broken down. Overwhelmed, liver cells become inflamed and die, leaving useless scar tissue in their wake; the result is the disorder known as cirrhosis, which claims about 28,000 lives a year. Alcohol also damages the brain and spinal cord; brain scans of advanced alcoholics reveal that their brains have literally withered away.

Alcohol can cause heartburn, diarrhea, insomnia and impotence. Large doses may raise blood pressure. Alcoholics are at increased risk for cancers of the throat, mouth, breast, stomach, pancreas and liver. They are more likely to be malnourished, and to suffer profound mental problems. The slow death of an alcoholic is never pretty, marked as it is by bloody vomiting, staggering, a bloated abdomen and dementia.

Fast deaths due to alcohol will turn your stomach as well. The smashed bodies of drunk drivers and their victims are all-too-common sights on our highways. The National Highway Traffic Safety Administration has determined that more than half of the drivers causing fatal accidents are

drunk. The more violent the crash, the more likely it is that the driver has been drinking. Moreover, thousands of pedestrian deaths as well as drownings, falls and other fatal accidents are alcohol-related. *As a rule, half the deaths from all accidents involve alcohol.*

Why people become alcoholics is not settled, but a growing number of studies point to a genetic link. Children of alcoholics are three to four times more likely to become alcoholics themselves than are the children of non-alcoholics—even when they have been raised by non-alcoholic foster parents. Sons and daughters of alcoholics show marked physical responses when tested after drinking. And identical twins tend to develop comparable drinking patterns even when raised apart.

HOW MUCH IS TOO MUCH?

If a little alcohol may be OK and a lot is truly bad, how much is too much? In my opinion, if someone averages more than two cocktails or beers per day, he or she has crossed the line and alcohol is a problem. Such a person may not be an alcoholic in the usual sense, but alcohol is harming his or her chances for a long and healthy life. Most likely it is hurting the chances of friends and family as well. Before you tell yourself that such a habit is still on the safe side, think about this: To my knowledge, there has never been a documented case of someone *over*estimating the amount of alcohol consumed. Traditionally, physicians are taught to *double* whatever patients tell them about alcohol use as a way of coming up with a more realistic estimate of alcohol intake. So if someone thinks he or she may be borderline and might have a problem, it's probably true.

Although some studies define an average of two drinks per day as moderate, I think this is a lot, and I am uncomfortable saying it has benefits or is even all right. Averaging one drink per day or less seems wiser.

HOW TO STOP THE DOWNWARD SPIRAL

Alcoholism is not hopeless. There are about a million recovered alcoholics in this country, and between half and three-quarters of the people who attempt rehabilitation will succeed; their success depends on their personal characteristics, early treatment, the skill of their counselors, access to the right medical and outpatient services, and the strong support of family, friends and co-workers. Among some highly motivated groups, the success rate is much higher. For example, more than 90 percent of physicians and airline pilots who go into highly structured, monitored programs stay in recovery.

However, someone with a drinking problem seldom changes this harmful behavior alone. Although the "cure" must come from within, the decisive nudge often comes from without. The drinker needs input, feedback and support from a friend, co-worker or spouse. If, like most Americans, you know someone who drinks too much, you can provide this help.

BARRIERS TO HELPING

There are many reasons why people hesitate to discuss drinking with a person who has a drinking problem. They may be afraid of butting in, of sparking an argument or of getting too involved. They may also be unsure whether the alcoholic is driven by physical, emotional or moral problems.

People wonder whether to view the abuser as a sick person who deserves sympathy and treatment or as a no-good bum who needs to have the law laid down. Thinking of the alcoholic as sick may be a disservice, because treatment involves neither drugs nor surgery, and a cure cannot be bought. However, condemning the person and not providing help will only make the problem worse.

It is best to think of the alcohol abuser as someone with a problem that is harming *your* ability to get along, work together or enjoy each other's company. This means that you are responsible for helping the alcoholic own up to his or her behavior toward you with the hope that your former good relationship will be restored.

By exploring some of the common barriers to helping, you may overcome your reluctance to step in.

Who Has a Problem?

One method for gauging the seriousness of a drinking problem is known as the CAGE questionnaire. It was created to help physicians decide if their patients had drinking problems. CAGE stands for Cutting down, Annoyed by criticism, Guilty feelings and Eye-openers.

CAGE Questions

Yes   No

☐   ☐   1. Has the person ever mentioned the need to *cut down* on drinking?

☐   ☐   2. If anyone has criticized the person for drinking, was he or she *annoyed*?

☐   ☐   3. Has the person ever expressed *guilt* feelings about drinking?

☐   ☐   4. Does the person ever take an "*eye-opener*" first thing in the morning?

_____ **TOTAL YES**

_____ **TOTAL NO**

Answering "yes" to even one question may signal a drinking problem. Two "yes" answers show overwhelming odds of alcoholism.

Source: *Ewing, J.A. Detecting Alcoholism: The CAGE Questionnaire. JAMA* 252: 1905, 1984.

Barrier 1. *It is not polite; the person will get angry.* The truth is that if you care, you must calmly challenge the harmful behavior. This is not the time to worry about etiquette—alcoholism can be fatal. In the words of one recovering alcoholic, "People stand around and don't say anything while you're dying."

Barrier 2. *The person will deny the problem.* This may well occur. Denial is one of the alcoholic's biggest fallbacks, but stating your concern will help anyway.

Barrier 3. *A person with a drinking problem must hit rock bottom.* We used to think this was true. But

What Are the Signs of Alcoholism?

Yes	No	
☐	☐	1. Do you occasionally drink heavily after a disappointment or quarrel or when the boss gives you a hard time?
☐	☐	2. When you have trouble or feel under pressure, do you always drink more heavily than usual?
☐	☐	3. Have you noticed that you are able to handle more liquor than you did when you were first drinking?
☐	☐	4. Did you ever wake up on the "morning after" and discover that you could not remember part of the evening before, even though your friends tell you that you did not "pass out"?
☐	☐	5. When drinking with other people, do you try to have a few extra drinks when others will not know it?
☐	☐	6. Are there certain occasions when you feel uncomfortable if alcohol is not available?
☐	☐	7. Have you recently noticed that when you begin drinking you are in more of a hurry to get the first drink than you used to be?
☐	☐	8. Do you sometimes feel a little guilty about your drinking?
☐	☐	9. Are you secretly irritated when your family or friends discuss your drinking?
☐	☐	10. Have you recently noticed an increase in the frequency of your memory "blackouts"?
☐	☐	11. Do you often find that you wish to continue drinking after your friends say that they have had enough?
☐	☐	12. Do you usually have a reason for the occasions when you drink heavily?
☐	☐	13. When you are sober, do you often regret things you have done or said while drinking?

Yes	No	
☐	☐	14. Have you tried switching brands or following different plans for controlling your drinking?
☐	☐	15. Have you often failed to keep the promises you have made to yourself about controlling or cutting down on your drinking?
☐	☐	16. Have you ever tried to control your drinking by making a change in jobs or moving to a new location?
☐	☐	17. Do you try to avoid family or close friends while you are drinking?
☐	☐	18. Are you having an increasing number of financial and work problems?
☐	☐	19. Do more people seem to be treating you unfairly without good reason?
☐	☐	20. Do you eat very little or irregularly when you are drinking?
☐	☐	21. Do you sometimes have the "shakes" in the morning and find that it helps to have a little drink?
☐	☐	22. Have you recently noticed that you cannot drink as much as you once did?
☐	☐	23. Do you sometimes stay drunk for several days at a time?
☐	☐	24. Do you sometimes feel very depressed and wonder whether life is worth living?
☐	☐	25. Sometimes after periods of drinking, do you see or hear things that aren't there?
☐	☐	26. Do you get terribly frightened after you have been drinking heavily?

Those who answer "yes" to two or three of these questions may wish to evaluate their drinking in these areas. "Yes" answers to several of the questions indicate these stages of alcoholism:

Questions 1–8:	Early stage
Questions 9–21:	Middle stage
Questions 22–26:	Beginning of the final stage

Source: National Council on Alcoholism

alcoholism is a progressive disease, and early intervention can prevent the problem from getting worse and halt the person's decline.

Barrier 4. *People with drinking problems must help themselves.* Absolutely true. But few alcoholics can change their behavior on their own. In fact, it is unlikely that the person you know can do it without your help.

Barrier 5. *You will become too involved.* You will have to guard against playing the "alcoholic's game" in which the alcoholic creates a crisis by drinking (passes out at a party, smashes up the car, loses a job), is condemned by you, then seeks and wins your forgiveness—until the cycle begins again. The drinker needs these bouts to sustain his or her behavior. As long as the game is played, alcoholism is reinforced.

Barrier 6. *No one else helps people with drinking problems; I will be in this alone.* In fact, there are millions of men and women helping people with drinking problems. Once you start helping, they will be fairly easy to find.

Barrier 7. *I don't know how to help.* You can learn how. Reading this chapter is a start. For more information, guidance and support, consult some of the resources listed at the end of this chapter.

LEARNING TO HELP

Helping an alcoholic is not an easy job, so knowing how to help is a must. Neither nagging nor pity helps the problem drinker. Indeed, emotional confrontations fuel the problem. When the drinker's family and friends have been players in the alcoholic's game, it can be very hard for them to call a halt. They, too, need outside help to break the pattern.

There are two main steps to helping. The first is to learn about the problem—about the person's drinking habits as well as about alcoholism in general. The second is to guide the alcohol abuser and provide emotional support to him or her. A third step, getting involved in community and work place activities, can benefit both of you, too.

What Kind of Drinker Are You?

A social drinker:

- Drinks slowly (no fast gulping).
- Knows when to stop (doesn't get drunk).
- Eats before or while drinking (to slow the effect of alcohol).
- Never drives after drinking.
- Respects non-drinkers.
- Knows and obeys laws related to drinking.
- Drinks for social or cultural reasons, not for reasons that lead to excessive use—to forget, escape or build courage.

A problem drinker:

- Drinks to get drunk.
- Tries to solve problems by drinking.
- Becomes loud, angry or violent.
- Drinks when he or she shouldn't—before driving or going to work.
- Causes other problems—harms himself or herself, family, friends or strangers.

An alcoholic:

- Spends a lot of time thinking about drinking and planning where and when to get the next drink.
- Keeps bottles hidden for quick pick-me-ups.
- Starts drinking without planning to, and loses track of the amount of alcohol consumed.
- Denies drinking.
- Drinks alone.
- Needs to drink before facing a stressful situation.
- May have "blackouts"—cannot remember what occurred while drinking, even though he or she may have appeared normal to other people at that time.
- Suffers from malnutrition and neglect.
- Goes from having hangovers to more dangerous withdrawal symptoms, including delirium tremens (DTs), which can be fatal.

LEARNING ABOUT THE PROBLEM: GATHERING FACTS ABOUT THE PERSON'S DRINKING

When finding out how serious the person's drinking problem is, you should gather facts based on your own observations and interactions with the person. But don't sneak around "building a case."

One tool for determining the extent of the problem is a questionnaire developed by the National Council on Alcoholism (see page 164). Although the questions refer to you, you may adapt them so that they apply to the person who concerns you.

Another way to assess the problem is to look for behaviors that signal the slide from "social drinking" to "problem drinking," or "alcoholism" (see the box on page 165).

FINDING FACTS AND HELP

Sources of information, advice and help are plentiful. You might begin by contacting some of the organizations listed at the end of this chapter. These include self-help groups like Alcoholics Anonymous and its offshoots Al-Anon and Alateen, community-action groups such as MADD (Mothers Against Drunk Driving), and information sources such as the National Clearinghouse for Alcohol Information or the National Council on Alcoholism. In addition to sending you information, many of these organizations can put you in touch with groups in your community.

It is important to learn what is available locally. Knowledgeable people in your area can give you immediate face-to-face advice to help you handle your situation, refer you to the right local agencies and bolster your morale.

In most places, you can get help from your physician or clergyman, law-enforcement agencies or a librarian. Many employers and unions sponsor employee assistance programs (EAPs). You can also contact the nearest Veterans Administration office, alcoholism information and referral service, county medical society, community mental health center or public health service.

You might also want to attend an Al-Anon meeting in your area. These families and friends of problem drinkers can often give you practical advice and support.

OFFERING HELP TO THE PROBLEM DRINKER

Once you have mastered your information and mustered your resources, it is time to approach the problem drinker. Your goal is to guide him or her to professional help and to provide support throughout treatment.

You should tell the person what you have observed and learned. You must be careful not to sound like you are charging the person with a crime. Describe your feelings about the situation, and ask how he or she feels about it.

Helping an alcoholic is not an easy job. Here are some "Dos and Don'ts" to guide you in your role.

DOs
- Get advice from local experts, and use it. These people can suggest an appropriate course of action and source of treatment.
- Speak to the person about what directly affects you. For example, if you are trying to help a co-worker, you should talk about the consequences of drinking on work performance and your relationship on the job.
- Pick your time wisely. Don't confront the person while he or she is drunk. Present the person with fresh information as soon after the incident as possible.
- Use your leverage, but use it fairly. For example, if you are a supervisor, give fair warning before threatening the problem drinker with loss of a job.
- Realize that the person may deny having a problem and that several attempts may be needed over time.
- When your patience wears thin, back off.
- Set limits. Don't get caught up in the drinker's problems.
- Let the problem drinker know that you are learning about alcoholism.

- Remain calm, detached and factual when speaking with the problem drinker about his or her behavior and its day-to-day consequences.
- Give emotional support throughout the treatment process.

DON'Ts

- Don't attempt to punish, threaten, bribe, preach or be a martyr.
- Don't make appeals to the drinker's emotions. This may only increase his or her guilt and the desire to drink.
- Don't cover up or make excuses that shield the drinker from the consequences of his or her actions.
- Don't take over his or her responsibilities, robbing the drinker of self-importance or self-worth.
- Don't hide or dump bottles, or shelter the problem drinker from situations where alcohol is present.
- Don't argue with someone who is drunk.
- Don't drink along with him or her.
- Don't accept guilt for the drinker's behavior.

TREATMENT FOR ALCOHOLISM

There are a number of worthwhile methods for treating alcoholism. Some involve physicians, but many of the most successful do not. Some temporarily use drugs, but most do not. Some insist on abstinence, while others aim to reduce drinking to acceptable limits. Individual psychotherapy, intensive counseling, group sessions and various types of behavior therapy have all been used.

The common element in all of these approaches, and the most important aspect of treatment, is a focus on changing behavior, not on finding a "medical" answer to a "medical" problem. Nothing is more futile than treating alcoholism's physical complications when the alcoholic's behavior remains unchanged.

The route to recovery pioneered by Alcoholics Anonymous (AA) has been as successful as any and more successful than most. Community based, AA uses a self-help group format to help the alcoholic face up to his or her alcoholism and then come to grips with its consequences. Al-Anon for spouses and Alateen for children help family members deal with the alcoholic while protecting themselves. Almost all clinic- and hospital-based alcohol-treatment programs refer their patients to AA, once they have gotten them off to a good start. Successful recovery requires a long-term commitment, and AA provides such sustained support.

Almost always alcoholics can be treated with good results as outpatients. After all, the recovering alcoholic's long-term success rides on the ability to control drinking in the everyday world; a "cure" achieved in a controlled, institutional setting may create unrealistic expectations that lead to a relapse once the person returns to his or her usual living patterns. Even the problems of mild-to-moderate withdrawal are handled as well out of the hospital as in. And the cost of outpatient treatment is less than one-tenth that of inpatient care.

Inpatient treatment should be reserved for three types of patients: those whose bodies are so poisoned that they require acute detoxification, those who are in severe withdrawal, and those rare people who are suffering from profound psychological problems beyond their alcoholism.

Similarly, antidepressive medications have value in treating only those alcoholics who also suffer from depression. The drug known as Antabuse (which makes people sick if they drink while taking it) has been shown to have little benefit; anyone willing to continue taking it is most likely motivated to stop drinking anyway.

JOINING COMMUNITY EFFORTS

As someone trying to help an alcoholic stop drinking, you may find support and encouragement by becoming involved in community and workplace alcoholism education and prevention activities—especially if the problem drinker is not making progress as quickly as you'd like.

A good starting place may be where you work. Alcohol abuse is costly to both employers and workers; you may be able to help your employer or union create and support clear, fair policies on drug and alcohol use that are enforced consistently.

Employee assistance programs, or EAPs, can provide confidential counseling and referral services for employees with many types of problems, including alcohol abuse. EAPs can be sponsored by employers, employee associations or unions, working together or apart. You can find out how to start an EAP from national or professional associations in your field, or from the Association of Labor Management Administrators and Consultants on Alcoholism, Inc. (see the listing in Resources below).

There are also many ways to get involved in your community. Contact your area law-enforcement agency, clergy, PTA, school district, or local chapters of AA, Al-Anon, MADD (Mothers Against Drunk Driving), or SADD (Students Against Driving Drunk). Learn what they are doing and add your creative energy.

The cardinal rule is this: Get help. Whether you're an alcoholic or someone whose life is being harmed by the alcoholism of another, don't try to go it alone: Get involved. Stay involved. You can do something about alcoholism.

RESOURCES

AA—Alcoholics Anonymous, General Service Office, P.O. Box 459, Grand Central Station, New York, NY 10163. (212) 686-1100.

Addiction Research Foundation, 33 Russell Street, Toronto, Ontario M5S 2S1, Canada. (416) 595-6059.

ADPA, Alcohol and Drug Problems Association of North America, Inc., 444 North Capitol Street, N.W., Suite 706, Washington, DC 20001. (202) 737-4340.

Al-Anon Alateen, Family Group Headquarters, P.O. Box 862, Midtown Station, New York, NY 10018-0862. (212) 302-7240.

AHHAP, Association of Halfway House Alcoholism Programs of North America, 786 East 7th Street, St. Paul, MN 55106. (612) 771-0933.

EAPA, Employee Assistance Professional Association, 4601 N. Fairfax Drive, Suite 1001, Arlington, VA 22203. (703) 522-6272.

American Council for Drug Education, 204 Monroe Street, Rockville, MD 20850. (301) 294-0600.

American Council on Alcohol Problems, Inc. 3426 Bridgeland Drive, Bridgeton, MO 63044. (314) 739-5944.

ASAM, American Society on Addiction Medicine, 12 West 21st Street, 7th Floor, New York, NY 10010. (212) 206-6770.

Christopher D. Smithers Foundation, P.O. Box 67, Mill Neck, NY 11765. (516) 676-0067.

CSPI, Center for Science in the Public Interest, 1501 16th Street, N.W., Washington, DC 20036. (202) 332-9110.

Families Anonymous, P.O. Box 528, Van Nuys, CA 91408. (818) 989-7841.

Hazelden Educational Materials, Pleasant Valley Road, Box 176, Center City, MN 55012. (800) 328-9000.

ICAA/American, International Council on Alcohol and Addiction, American Foundation, P.O. Box 489, Locust Valley, NY 11560. (516) 676-1869.

Johnson Institute, 7151 Metro Boulevard, Suite 250, Minneapolis, MN 55435. (612) 944-0511.

MADD, Mothers Against Drunk Driving, 669 Airport Freeway, Suite 310, Hurst, TX 76053-3944. (817) 268-6233.

Multicultural Training Resource Center (prevention, intervention or treatment issues among blacks, Hispanics, Asian Americans, Native Americans and other minorities), 1540 Market Street, Suite 320, San Francisco, CA 94102. (415) 861-2142.

NADAC, National Association of Alcoholism and Drug Abuse Counselors, Inc., 3717 Columbia Pike, Suite 300, Arlington, VA 22204. (703) 920-4644.

NALGAP, National Association of Lesbian and Gay Alcoholism Professionals, 204 West 20th Street, New York, NY 10011. (212) 713-5074.

NASADAD, National Association of State Alcohol and Drug Abuse Directors, Inc., 444 N. Capitol Street, N.W., Washington, DC 20001. (202) 783-6868.

NBAC, National Black Alcoholism Council, 53 West Jackson Boulevard, Suite 828, Chicago, IL 60604. (312) 663-5780.

NCA, National Council on Alcoholism, Inc., 12 West 21st Street, 7th Floor, New York, NY 10010. (212) 206-6770.

NCA, National Council on Alcoholism, Washington Office, 1511 K Street, N.W., Suite 926, Washington, DC 20005. (202) 737-8122.

NCADI, National Clearinghouse for Alcohol and Drug Information, P.O. Box 2345, Rockville, MD 20852. (301) 468-2600.

NIAAA, National Institute on Alcohol Abuse and Alcoholism, Parklawn Building, 5600 Fishers Lane, Rockville, MD 20857. (301) 443-3885.

NIDA, National Institute on Drug Abuse, Parklawn Building, 5600 Fishers Lane, Room 1004, Rockville, MD 20857. (301) 443-4577.

NNSA, National Nurses Society on Addiction, 2506 Gross Point Road, Evanston, IL 60201. (312) 475-7300.

NSC, National Safety Council, 444 N. Michigan Avenue, Chicago, IL 60601. (312) 527-4800.

Rutgers University, Center of Alcohol Studies Library, Piscataway, NJ 08855-0969. (201) 932-4442.

SADD, Students Against Driving Drunk, 277 Main Street, Marlboro, MA 01752. (508) 481-3568.

Veterans Administration, Alcohol and Drug Dependency Services, 810 Vermont Avenue, N.W., Washington, DC 20420. (202) 233-4000.

MIND ↔ BODY

THE MIND DIRECTS THE BRAIN.
THE BRAIN MINDS THE BODY.
THE BODY MENDS THE MIND.
MIND ↔ BODY.

The title of this chapter is a symbol for the interaction between mind and body. Until recently, the title would have been stress, and much of the advice that is offered here may still be understood as stress management. But we are gaining new understanding of the relationship between mind and body that goes beyond the usual notions of stress. The new concepts include:

- The importance of positive approaches to healthy thinking, such as optimism and hardiness.
- The interaction of the mind and the immune system (psychoneuroimmunology).
- Understanding that healthy mind ↔ body practices go beyond relaxation and coping techniques to include the healthy pleasures of humor, entertainment and sensuality.
- The advantages of expanding personal control, stability and support.

Defining a healthy mind-body interaction is not easy. Clearly, there should be an absence of mental illness and a minimum of mental discomfort. But mental fitness goes beyond the absence of disease. Perhaps the best way to define it is indirectly, by describing the person who is mentally fit: Happy, satisfied, serene and hardy. The first three of these characteristics probably need little explanation, but the fourth, hardiness, may be a new concept. Research has suggested that heart disease is less likely in persons with three key attitudes:

1. *Commitment* to the idea that life has meaning, and the individual has a purpose
2. *A feeling of control*, or the ability to influence events through knowledge, skills, imagination and choice
3. *An appreciation of challenge*, or the belief that change is normal and good—an opportunity for growth.

Together these attitudes are referred to as hardiness.

Psychoneuroimmunology

Psychoneuroimmunology is a new branch of science that studies the relationship between the mind, the brain and the immune system. Two separate types of research gave birth to this new field. First was the discovery that cells in the immune system could respond directly to hormones controlled by the brain. The most prominent of these hormones is adrenocorticotropic hormone (ACTH), which also plays a major role in the body's response to stress. It is now well established that the nervous system can "talk" directly to the immune system. So, because the mind directly influences the nervous system, the nervous system acts as a channel through which the mind can influence the immune system.

The second type of research has focused on changes in the immune system associated with important psychological events. Here are some of the major findings of that research:

• Women who rated their marriages as unsatisfactory had poorer immune function than women who rated their marriages as good.

Likewise, women who were recently separated or divorced had poorer immune function than women in stable marriages.

• Students studying for final examinations had significantly lower immune function than they had six weeks earlier. However, in a second study, students who practiced relaxation techniques during the study period avoided much of the decline in immune function.

• The immune cells from highly distressed psychiatric patients are unable to repair X-ray damage as well as the immune cells from psychiatric patients with low distress. This suggests that high levels of distress might make cells less resistant to the kinds of changes associated with cancer.

• In one study, older adults who received relaxation training showed greater improvement in immune function than men and women who did not receive such training.

Science has now firmly established the connection between mind, nervous system and immune system, but we have only begun to understand its power and complexity.

Stress and the Mind ↔ Body Interaction

The stress model of Dr. Hans Selye has long been the most popular tool for understanding the interaction between mind and body. This chapter's emphasis on attitudes, environment and physical activity does not contradict this model, but expands upon it.

Simply stated, the stress model says that we react in a particular manner (called the fight-or-flight response) to certain events (stressors). In the fight-or-flight response, adrenaline and other hormones flood the system. The body prepares for strenuous physical activity—to fight or flee. When physical danger is actual—let's say you are being attacked by an animal—this response has real advantages, because it increases your strength and speed. (Every once in a while you read in the newspaper of a grandmother who lifts a car off her grandchild, or

some other superhuman feat made possible by the fight-or-flight response.) But if this response is continual, it leads to the ravages of "chronic stress"—everything from heart attacks to ulcers to depression.

There are three main factors involved in stress and, therefore, in the development of chronic stress. These are the event, the perception of the event and the reaction to it.

In this chapter, events that cause stress are discussed as part of control and stability in the environment. Perception is in large part a matter of attitude, which is discussed extensively here. Finally, our reactions depend on how we have prepared the body and mind and what we do when we feel stressed; this is discussed under optimism, relaxation and using the body to mend the mind.

Effects of Mental Health on Physical Health

In a landmark study of both mental and physical health, researchers have followed a group of Harvard graduates for more than 40 years. The subjects' mental health has been assessed every two years by means of a psychological test. Physical health has been determined by history and physical examination. Of the men who remained in the study, 185 were in good physical health at the age of 42. Over the next 11 years, 100 of the men remained in excellent physical health, 54 acquired minor problems, and 31 acquired serious chronic illnesses or died.

The men's mental health before the age of 42 (while they were still physically healthy) had an astonishing effect on their physical health after that age. Of the 59 men with the best mental health, only two became chronically ill or died by the age of 53. Of the 48 men with the worst mental health, 18 became chronically ill or died before the age of 52. This very strong relationship between mental health and later physical health remained true even when the effects of alcohol, tobacco use, obesity and family longevity were accounted for.

Good mental health clearly helps prevent loss of physical health. A healthy mind is very important for a healthy body.

The brain's first priority is tending to the body. More than two-thirds of the brain is devoted to monitoring and managing body functions. At the same time, this part of the brain has millions of connections with the part that thinks, the cerebral cortex. Thus, it should come as no surprise that our thinking can influence virtually all body organs and systems—the heart, stomach, intestines, muscles, immune system and so on.

The mind ↔ body connection is a two-way street. Relaxing your muscles may relieve anxiety, just as relieving anxiety may relax your muscles. Feeling good about yourself makes for a happy body, and making your body feel good makes your mind happy. From exercise to massage to sex to food, you can do things to your body that affect your mind.

HAPPINESS, SATISFACTION, SERENITY AND HARDINESS

Sounds great. So how do you get there? Although you cannot control all of life's circumstances and events, you can control the major influences on your mind-body interaction—attitudes, environment and body feedback. In the following pages, you will learn how to influence your attitudes, create a healthy environment for the mind, and use the body to nurture the mind.

You will find that many key concepts—optimism, control, challenge, stability, relaxation, physical fitness, etc.—overlap. This is as it should be. Interaction is the name of the game when it comes to mind and body, and the overlaps simply reflect this.

ATTITUDES

Optimism

What's the use of thinking that, by and large, things are pretty good? For one thing, you may live longer. Several studies have shown that "health optimists," people who believe that they are in pretty good health, live longer than "health pessimists," who rate their health as fair or poor. This is true even when doctors rate the optimists' health as fair or poor. And the health pessimists don't live as long even when the doctors rate their health as good or excellent!

Optimism relieves you of the enormous burden of worry and guilt. It is a burden that you create for yourself, as the pessimists have proven. Carrying this burden is a form of chronic stress.

There are several ways to practice optimism. The most popular is called "thought stopping," and it is just that. Negative thoughts like, "I should have," "I'm supposed to" or "Why always me?" lead to pessimism. It is this negative approach to life events that creates the burden, not the events themselves. Telling yourself that you are bad, other people are bad and things are bad in general is referred to as negative self-talk. Thought stopping means mentally shouting "Stop!" whenever negative self-talk occurs. After stopping your thought, quickly replace it with one that puts things in a better light, such as, "Will this be important five days, five months or five years from now?" or "Is this something to get sick over?" or "Why should I feel guilty when there is no reason for it?" Thought stopping requires some practice, but it's well worth the effort.

Thought stopping applies to negative thoughts about others, also. You can't be an optimist, even if you like yourself, if you hate everyone else. For example, if a teenager cuts you off in traffic, give him or her—and yourself—a break. Stop the thoughts of killing and cursing and replace them with something gentler and more constructive: "I was a teenager once, and I drove as if I was always in a hurry. What can I do to help teenagers be more careful?" (Maybe you can do nothing. But accepting that fact is a lot better than thinking that teenagers are monsters out to make your life miserable.)

Practice telling yourself a good story. Getting caught in a traffic jam may be regarded as a disastrous loss of time or a precious opportunity to think things over. Moving to a new city can be seen as losing friends and familiarity or gaining new friends and fresh experiences.

You have a choice. While looking for the silver lining, expecting good things to happen and not worrying are often put down as being unrealistic or naive, they aren't. They're smart, and good for your mind and body.

Humor

A sense of humor, good humor, lots of laughs—anything that brings a smile to the face brings relief to the mind and lightness to the heart. A good laugh exercises the lungs and massages our attitudes. (Author Norman Cousins has said that laughing is "internal jogging.") And humor may even improve immunity by increasing antibody

Serious Illnesses May Require Large Doses of Laughter

In *Anatomy of an Illness*, Norman Cousins tells how he prescribed large doses of laughter for himself when he was hospitalized with a serious illness. His preferred drug was old Marx Brothers movies. He found that several doses of this medicine each day not only reduced the signs and symptoms of his illness, it even improved the results of his laboratory tests. He gives this treatment much of the credit for his recovery from an illness for which traditional medicine had little to offer.

It may seem odd to seek out fun when you're ill. Laughter and feeling bad don't seem to go together. But after all, that's the point.

levels, according to a study by Kathleen Dillon and her colleagues.

Indeed, laughter may be the best medicine. And it is one that you can prescribe for yourself. Seek out that which makes you laugh, be it a movie, comics, a book or TV. And don't forget to laugh at yourself, too. The next time things aren't going well, step back and look at what you are doing. See yourself as playing a role in a comedy. You'll see that life isn't nearly as serious as you thought. And you're pretty funny, too. Finally, humor yourself. Give yourself a good time—just for the fun of it.

Relaxation

Freedom from tension is good for mind and muscle, heart and soul—not to mention the stomach. Those who regularly use meditation or other techniques to reduce tension have lower blood pressure, lower heart rates and fewer stomach problems; indeed, they seem to have fewer physical problems of all types. Even quick-acting techniques can moderate the impact of events likely to cause stress.

The Quieting Response

The Quieting Response requires only six seconds. Its developer, Charles F. Stroebel, M.D., emphasizes that it is a part of an overall program to reduce stress.

The four steps of the Quieting Response are:

1: Recognize when you feel worried, annoyed or anxious.
2: Smile inwardly with your mouth and eyes, and say to yourself, "Alert mind, calm body."
3: Inhale easily and naturally.
4: Exhale, letting your jaw, tongue and shoulders go loose. Feel a wave of limpness, heaviness and warmth flow to your toes as you let your breath out.

Reprinted by permission of the Putnam Publishing group from *QR: The Quieting Reflex*, by Charles F. Stroebel, M.D. Copyright 1982 by Q.R. Institute, Inc.

There are many relaxation techniques. The easiest to learn are those meant for immediate use whenever you feel stressed. The Quieting Response (above), popularized by Dr. Charles F. Stroebel, and the Instant Calming Sequence of Dr. Robert K. Cooper (at right) are among the most widely used.

Relaxation techniques that are practiced every day are often referred to as meditation. These include transcendental meditation and often require some instruction. The relaxation response, a simplified form of meditation, has been defined by Dr. Herbert Benson (see next page).

Tension describes a state of both mind and muscles, and the connection is no accident. You have a "muscle barometer"—the tension in your muscles reflects the tension in your mind. Often people who think they are relaxed are not, and the evidence can be found in their tense muscles—rigid posture, tight fists, clenched jaws. Indeed, many of us are in a constant state of tension that slowly eats away at us. The good news is that relaxing the muscles also relaxes the mind. Progressive relaxation is a technique that combines muscle relaxation with meditation (see page 176). It can be practiced daily, like other forms of meditation, and can also be used to reduce tension as needed.

Biofeedback is another method that uses the mind-body connection to relax both mind and body. Its advantage is implied by its name—instant feedback on how well you are relaxing your body as indicated by changes in skin temperature, pulse or other measurements. Although it requires some training and equipment, it is well worth considering, especially if you have trouble concentrating on other relaxation techniques.

The Instant Calming Sequence

Dr. Robert K. Cooper recommends five steps to take when faced with a stressful situation:

1. Don't hold your breath; this is common during the first moments of a stressful situation. Continue natural, uninterrupted breathing.
2. Put on a positive face. In other words, smile.
3. Assume a balanced posture—head up, chest out, shoulders loose, hips level, back straight and abdomen relaxed.
4. Let a wave of relaxation sweep through your body and release tension, starting with the scalp, jaw, tongue and face, and moving on down to the finger tips and toes. Take mental control by stopping such negative thoughts as "Not another problem!" or "Not now! I can't handle this!" Replace these with a key thought: "What's happening is real, and I'm finding the best possible solution right now."

More information can be found in *Health and Fitness Excellence: The Scientific Action Plan*, by Robert K. Cooper, Ph.D. Boston: Houghton Mifflin Company, 1989.

The Relaxation Response

The relaxation response requires four components:

- A comfortable position. Lie down or sit in a relaxed position with arms, feet and head supported comfortably.
- A quiet environment. Silence is not required, but changes in noise level and distracting sounds should be avoided. As you practice the relaxation response, you will be able to tolerate a noisier environment without being distracted.
- Repetition of a prayer, word, sound or phrase. The sound "OM" comes to us from Eastern meditative techniques and can be recommended, but anything will do so long as it is comfortable for you and easily repeated.
- A passive attitude when other thoughts come into consciousness. This is the part that requires some practice. It simply means letting any thought pass through your mind without trying to explore it, analyze it or deal with it in any way. Just let it go and return to concentrating on your repetitive phrase or sound.

Dr. Benson describes this response further in *The Relaxation Response* (New York: Avon Books, 1976).

Commitment

People who are hardy believe that there is meaning in their lives. Again, this seems to be an attitude that is chosen rather than a reflection of their situations. Given similar circumstances, some will choose to believe that what they're doing is meaningful, while others will not. But those who choose meaning are more likely to derive the benefits of hardiness, such as a lower risk of heart disease, and to gain those other attributes of a healthy mind and body—happiness, satisfaction and serenity.

Unfortunately, there are no studies that show us an easy way to gain commitment. It seems to me that commitment requires a personal philosophy of life. This may be formal or informal; it is often religious or spiritual. Indeed, in *The Road Less Traveled*, Dr. Scott Peck suggests that all of us have a religion, because we all have some overall view of the world and our life in it; this world view, or religion, can be one of either meaning or despair. Whether it is called commitment or a religion of hope, the critical element seems to be rather simple: a belief that life and your part in it make sense even if you don't understand exactly how.

Control

Feeling helpless is bad news. People who believe that they have little influence on the course of their lives are probably at higher risk for heart disease, cancer and other serious illnesses. People who give up in the face of this helplessness are in serious trouble.

Surprisingly, feeling helpless or continually frustrated is not a matter of circumstance. Given the same situation, some people will feel helpless while others will exert some control. Hardy people, those who feel in control, use several techniques that you can practice as well:

- Communication. Tell others, especially family members and fellow workers, of your desires and concerns.
- Assertiveness. State your objectives clearly and make certain that they are considered and addressed by others.
- Planning. Develop alternatives. Even if they are not used, they can help you feel in control.

Challenge

The third key attitude in hardiness, challenge, means viewing change as a good thing. As indicated below, all change creates stress. But how much stress it creates and how you react to it depend on how you perceive it. At one extreme, if a person views all change as threatening, disrupting and offering only heartache, then change will be

Progressive Relaxation

Go off by yourself for half an hour. Find a private space with carpeting on the floor where you can lie down or a comfortable easy chair. Wear loose-fitting clothes—no need for ties or belts or anything that restricts movement.

If you have any kind of back problem, put a pillow or cushion under your bent knees or the small of your back to provide added support.

Turn down the lights and lie with your arms at your sides and your legs uncrossed.

This exercise involves tensing and relaxing specific muscle groups. For each muscle group, hold the tension for six seconds and then release it. At the count of six, let go. The letting-go phase will make you sensitive to the difference between tension/work and the absence of it.

You can ask someone to lead you through the exercise or record it on a cassette tape for ongoing use.

- **Feet.** Beginning with your toes, tense your feet (point your toes). Count: One, two, three, four, five, LET GO. Repeat: One, two, three, four, five, LET GO.

- **Calves.** Tense your calves. Count: One, two, three, four, five, LET GO. Repeat.

- **Thighs.** Tense the tops of your thighs. Count: One, two, three, four, five, LET GO. Repeat.

Remember: Breathe easily. No tension, no mind, only passive attention to procedure.

- **Buttocks and hips.** Tense the buttocks and hips. Count: One, two, three, four, five, LET GO. Repeat.

- **Hands.** Raise your hands, but keep your arms on the floor. Count: One, two, three, four, five, LET GO. Repeat.

- **Shoulders.** Raise your shoulders up toward your chest, but keep your head on the floor. Count: One, two, three, four, five, LET GO. Repeat.

- **Head.** Tense your forehead. Count: One, two, three, four, five, LET GO. Repeat.

- **Jaw.** Gently place your tongue between your teeth, just touching the tips. Feel the jaw relax. Stay still for one minute.

- **Face and neck.** Make a distorted face, stick out your tongue and hold the tension in your face and neck. Count: One, two, three, four, five, LET GO. Repeat. Now back down the body to the toes.

- **Shoulders.** Tense. Count. LET GO. Repeat.

- **Hands.** Raise hands. Count. LET GO. Repeat.

- **Buttocks and hips.** Tense. Count. LET GO. Repeat.

- **Thighs.** Tense. Count. LET GO. Repeat.

- **Calves.** Tense. Count. LET GO. Repeat.

- **Feet.** Tense toes and feet. Count. LET GO. Repeat.

Return to normal breathing.

Source: *FOCUS* on Stress, Reston, VA: Center for Corporate Health Promotion, 1986.

threatening, disruptive and heartbreaking. At the other extreme, someone who accepts change as the only constant and relishes its opportunity is unlikely to be scarred by life's ups and downs. Few of us will reach a point where we greet every change with enthusiasm. But if you like a challenge, you are ahead of the game.

Again, studies do not tell us how to accept a challenge easily. Clearly, this is related to optimism and humor, so it seems logical that practicing those attitudes will foster an attitude of challenge as well. In addition, a dedication to and pleasure in learning seem to be essential. There really is something new just around the corner, something you did not know, understand or appreciate before. Philosophers, both ancient and modern, have often cited a lifelong habit of learning as the key to a long and happy life.

Friendship and Love

A life without satisfying relationships with other human beings is empty and unhealthy. Some people use the term "support network" or "support system" to describe these relationships (see below). I have included them here because it is important to understand that there is an attitude of friendship and love, of trust and concern that goes beyond specific relationships. It requires a willingness to view others as valuable and important in your life without requiring them to prove that they are worthy of your love.

While almost everyone believes in the value of friendship, the practice of friendship is often overlooked. It requires some work. Yes, you do have to be a friend to have a friend. Showing affection, be it with hugging or listening, flowers or phoning, is the habit of a healthy heart. More importantly, on a regular basis, you must be able to detach yourself from your own concerns and open yourself to others on their terms, accepting their loves, fears, jealousies and happiness. You have to be completely on their side.

THE ENVIRONMENT OF THE MIND

A healthy environment for the mind makes it easier to develop healthy attitudes. Actions taken

A Place of Your Own

Everyone needs a place of his or her own, an island of peace away from the rest of the world, a place for dealing with thoughts and attending to feelings. Sometimes this place is physical—a mountain cabin, a lonely stretch of beach, a den or a sewing room. Sometimes it exists in the mind as a vision or a memory into which your thoughts can retreat. The two are not separate. The memory of the tranquil mountain cabin becomes the place in the mind where thoughts retreat to find that same feeling of peace.

Indeed, the greatest advantage of the place in the mountains is the place it helps you create in your mind. Build a place for yourself. Use peaceful thoughts, visions and memories as mental building blocks. Use the physical world—the cabin, the photo, the book—to make its construction easier.

to create this environment often overlap with practices designed to develop these attitudes, but it is worthwhile looking at these actions as a more tangible and concrete way of creating a good place for your mind to live.

Control

Control is one of the key attitudes for hardiness. With respect to the environment, taking control means using practical methods to increase your options and your ability to choose among them. Career planning and time management are two methods for taking control.

Career planning is a continuous process, not something that you do once or twice in your life. When planning, consider several options, and don't overlook any that require further education or training. By broadening your horizons and increasing your confidence, education or training may yield benefits even if you don't select the option most closely related to them.

Time management is a skill that goes to the heart of being in control. Courses in time management can be worthwhile, but picking up even a few "tricks of the trade" can make the difference between feeling efficient and feeling out of control. Here are some basics of time management:

- Conduct a time-management study:
  1. For three to five days, keep a log of your activities and the time they take.
  2. Categorize activities such as phone calls, projects, meetings, driving and eating, and list the total time spent on each one.
  3. Rank each task or activity as a #1 (high priority), #2 (medium priority) or #3 (low priority).
  4. Identify those #3 items that consume more time than they merit.
  5. Reduce the time spent on your #3 activities, or eliminate them altogether.
  6. Use the same process to assess your #2 items.
- Use a calendar or log as a "time planner" to organize your schedule by days, weeks and months.
- Set realistic schedules on projects at work and home.
- Organize your work space in the office and at home. Know where things are: files, tools, equipment, etc.
- Set realistic goals.
- Rank your goals. What is really important?
- Learn to delegate tasks.
- Do things right the first time!
- Get away from your work; schedule relaxation and leisure into your day.
- Whenever possible, save your phone messages for a certain time of the day.
- Don't over-commit yourself. Learn to say no!

Stability

Most of us feel that we need a stable foundation and equate this with minimal change, even though an attitude of challenge allows us to see change as acceptable and non-threatening. However, few of us will learn to accept challenge to the degree that we welcome any and all changes. Most of us will benefit from practical steps to produce a feeling of stability.

As indicated by the Holmes Scale (see Life-Score, Chapter 1,), the impact of change can be measured. The implication of your Holmes score is straightforward: Do what you can to keep major changes from piling up on you. There are three basic skills for doing this:

(1) Planning a reasonable schedule for changes that you can foresee and influence.
(2) Asserting yourself when others are planning changes that affect you.
(3) Learning to say no to some changes even if you want to consent to them.

Support

Few things are as important as feeling that there are people who care for you and who will help when needed. Numerous studies have shown that support is important to both mental and physical health. The benefits range from specifics, such as a reduced risk of heart attack, to the general, such as increased life expectancy. The main source of support is often the family, but friends are essential, too.

Similarity makes for support. Similar interests, hobbies, jobs and locations encourage interactions that evolve into support. Similar problems —from alcoholism to Alzheimer's disease—have led to the formation of many support, or self-help, groups. Such groups may be more important than formal medical care for certain problems.

Everyone needs someone to talk to, someone who will listen without judging and be completely on your side. If you think that this sounds as if you need a friend, you're right. Professional counselors are often good listeners and can offer help without passing judgment. They can be very helpful over the short term for people dealing with difficult transitions. For the long term, look to friends and family for the support you need.

Pleasure

Most of us fail to plan for pleasure. Some of us simply fail to set aside the time because we are pressured by day-to-day events or imprisoned by our own work ethic. Pleasure simply has a low priority. But a life of little pleasure is not a happy one, and our minds and bodies suffer for it.

For others, there is confusion about what actually brings pleasure. We all need to be entertained, but endless hours of television, movies, rock concerts, shows, etc., do not mean endless hours of pleasure. Sensual activities—touching, caressing, sex—are important sources of healthy pleasure, if they are part of healthy relationships. A drink may be a part of a pleasurable experience, but an eye opener never brings pleasure. To be pleasurable, an experience must please us, and not just during the experience itself. The anticipation and the memory of the experience must please us as well. Pleasure is not sinful. It is a necessary part of a happy life. Make sure that you choose activities that are truly pleasurable, and then make time for them.

THE BODY MENDS THE MIND

You can take advantage of the intimate connections between body and mind to think and feel better. Exercise, fat control and nutrition all have benefits.

The most dramatic impact of body on mind is demonstrated with exercise. In fact, the mental benefit of exercise—feeling better and more energetic—is the reason most regular exercisers continue their programs.

Exercise benefits the brain and the mind in a number of ways. Through improved cardiovascular conditioning, the brain is more likely to receive plenty of oxygen. Atherosclerosis is less likely to impede blood flow. Endorphins, pain-relieving chemicals produced by the brain, often create a feeling of well-being in regular exercisers. They are not broken down as quickly in the bodies of exercisers as they are in non-exercisers. In fact, endorphins have been called "the brain's own morphine."

Also, a recent study supports the observation that exercise helps prevent depression. Aerobic exercise has even been used to treat mild to moderate depression; it appears to work as well as the most popular drugs used for this condition.

Good nutrition and fat control are part of a healthy mind ↔ body interaction, too. The mechanisms are not well understood, but they are both direct (supplying nutrients to the brain) and indirect (an improved self-image). Use your nutrition and fat-control skills to improve the fitness of both mind and body. Remember that nothing tastes as good as being fit feels.

Insight and Instinct

Each day brings new insight into the interactions of mind and body. Their complexity is astounding, yet our new knowledge confirms simple truths: The mind and body are closely connected; the health of one influences the health of the other.

The more we learn, the more we know to trust our instincts. A healthy mind and a healthy body go together. People who are happy, satisfied, serene and hardy are likely to have healthy bodies. People with healthy bodies are more likely to be happy, satisfied, serene and hardy.

RESOURCES

QR: The Quieting Reflex, by Charles F. Stroebel, M.D. New York: G.P. Putnam's Sons, 1982.

Health and Fitness Excellence: The Scientific Action Plan, by Robert K. Cooper, Ph.D. Boston: Houghton Mifflin Company, 1989.

The Relaxation Response by Herbert Benson, M.D. New York: Avon Books, 1976.

The Road Less Traveled, by M. Scott Peck, M.D. New York: Simon and Schuster, 1978.

Healthy Pleasures, by Robert Ornstein, Ph.D. and David Sobel, M.D. Reading, MA: Addison-Wesley, 1989.

Anatomy of an Illness, by Norman Cousins. New York: Bantam Books, 1981.

Minding the Body, Mending the Mind, by Joan Borysenko, Ph.D. Reading, MA: Addison-Wesley Publishing Company, 1987.

Take This Job and Love It, by Dennis Jaffe, Ph.D. and Cynthia Scott. New York: Simon and Schuster, 1988.

Self-Evaluation Program

The following UnStress evaluation is designed to help you discover your strengths and weaknesses as a stress manager. Just circle the number for each question which best describes your situation in the past 2 months. If the question doesn't apply, circle 1.

1	2	3	4	5
Rarely		Sometimes		Frequently

PHYSICAL

1. I have tightness in my back, shoulders or neck.   1 2 3 4 5
2. I have trouble either getting to sleep or staying asleep.   1 2 3 4 5
3. I have less energy and zip than I think I should.   1 2 3 4 5
4. I feel pain in some part or another of my body.   1 2 3 4 5
5. Considering what the normal weight is for my height, I am over-weight as follows:

1	2	3	4	5
+0 to 6 lbs.	+7 to 10	+11 to 18	+19 to 24	+25 lbs. or more

TOTAL PHYSICAL SCORE _____

EMOTIONAL

6. I am anxious or nervous.   1 2 3 4 5
7. I have a feeling of the blues.   1 2 3 4 5
8. I feel dissatisfied or down on myself.   1 2 3 4 5
9. I feel uneasy about people or situations   1 2 3 4 5
10. It's easy for people to get on my nerves.   1 2 3 4 5
11. People around me seem to enjoy themselves more than I do.   1 2 3 4 5
12. Sometimes I snap at people and later regret it.   1 2 3 4 5
13. It's hard for me to really enjoy activities.   1 2 3 4 5

TOTAL EMOTIONAL SCORE _____

PERFORMANCE

14. I feel I am meeting my potential.   1 2 3 4 5
15. My boss is satisfied that I am meeting my potential in my work.   1 2 3 4 5
16. I am satisfied with the quality of my social and family life.   1 2 3 4 5
17. My family and friends are satisfied with my relationship with them.   1 2 3 4 5
18. I believe my energy and time are well balanced between work, family, leisure and private time.   1 2 3 4 5
19. I have short- and long-term goals and am working toward them.   1 2 3 4 5
20. I believe I am where I should be in terms of meeting my goals at this point in my life.   1 2 3 4 5
21. I believe I make good use of my time.   1 2 3 4 5

TOTAL PERFORMANCE SCORE _____

Self-Evaluation Program, continued

1	2	3	4	5
Rarely		Sometimes		Frequently

HARD DRIVEN
22. I tend to eat, walk and/or talk rapidly.   1 2 3 4 5
23. I am frustrated by the inefficiency or incompetence of others.   1 2 3 4 5
24. I feel a sense of anger when I'm in a competitive situation.   1 2 3 4 5
25. Time and not wasting it is very important to me.   1 2 3 4 5
26. I find myself competing even when the situation doesn't call for
    competition.   1 2 3 4 5

TOTAL HARD DRIVEN SCORE _____

LIFE CHANGE

1	2	3	4	5
None	Few	Some	Quite a lot	Many or Major

27. There have been changes (good or bad) in my: (give each category a score of 1 to 5)

A. Job in the past year   1 2 3 4 5
B. Living circumstances   1 2 3 4 5
C. Family members' lives   1 2 3 4 5
D. Moods and habits   1 2 3 4 5
E. Financial income and commitments   1 2 3 4 5

TOTAL LIFE CHANGE SCORE _____

1	2	3	4	5
Rarely		Sometimes		Frequently

SUBSTANCES
28. I drink more than one alcoholic drink (wine, beer, liquor) in a day.   1 2 3 4 5
29. I take prescribed medication to help me relax or sleep.   1 2 3 4 5
30. I use mood-altering drugs.   1 2 3 4 5
31. I smoke more than one cigarette a day.   1 2 3 4 5
32. I drink more than 2 cups of coffee containing caffeine per day.   1 2 3 4 5

TOTAL SUBSTANCES SCORE _____

ATTITUDES
33. The stress in my life is caused by factors out of my control.   1 2 3 4 5
34. I tend to worry more than a situation really deserves.   1 2 3 4 5
35. Certain situations always make me anxious.   1 2 3 4 5
36. I don't feel responsible for who I am or for what I do.   1 2 3 4 5

TOTAL ATTITUDES SCORE _____

Self-Evaluation Program, continued

1	2	3	4	5
Rarely		Sometimes		Frequently

TIME MANAGEMENT

37. I need more hours in my day.   1 2 3 4 5
38. I accomplish about half of what I think I should.   1 2 3 4 5
39. I have trouble keeping my priorities straight.   1 2 3 4 5
40. I allow the situations which arise determine how I spend my day. 1 2 3 4 5

TOTAL TIME MANAGEMENT SCORE _____

EXERCISE

41. Season, location and my schedule tend to determine whether I exercise or
    not.   1 2 3 4 5
42. The exercise I do is more of a chore or a "have to" than something I really
    enjoy.   1 2 3 4 5
43. I exercise actively (enough to work up a sweat) for 20 minutes or more:

0	3	8	15
5+ times/week	3 to 4 times/week	1 to 2 times/week	Less than 1 time/week

TOTAL EXERCISE SCORE _____

RELAXATION

44. It's difficult for me to just stop doing things and relax mentally and physi-
    cally.   1 2 3 4 5
45. I feel guilty any time I sense I haven't accomplished anything.   1 2 3 4 5
46. I stop everything for 5–10 minutes and do a relaxation exercise, medita-
    tion or just coast before resuming my activity:

2	4	6	8	10
More than once/day	1/day	2-3/week	1/week	Less than 1/week

TOTAL RELAXATION SCORE _____

COMMUNICATION

47. I am able to shut out other thoughts and really listen when family or friends
    talk to me.   1 2 3 4 5
48. I spend five minutes or more telling someone close to me about my day:

2	4	6	8	10
Once/day	Once/2 days	Once/3–5 days	Once/week	Less than once/week

49. Considering the one or two people I'm closest to, I would rate our communication as:

2	4	6	8	10
Excellent	Good	So-so	Poor	Terrible

TOTAL COMMUNICATION SCORE _____

Personal UnStress Profile

Your UnStress Profile can tell you a lot about you and your stress. It will help you identify current problem areas and potential problem areas, and it will show you where you are already doing a good job of stress management.

All you need to do is go back through the self-evaluation you just took and total the section scores. For example, the first section was called "Physical Signals." There were five questions and for each question you circled a number from one to five. Add each of these circled numbers together to get your "Physical" section score.

The next step is the fun one. On the profile below you will find each of the section headings listed across the top of the profile. Just below the heading is an empty box. Write each section score in the box below the appropriate heading.

Now look down the column of numbers below the box and find the number that most closely corresponds to your section score and circle it.

The final step is to draw lines to connect each circle so you can see your whole UnStress Profile at a glance. The scores in the white area are your strong areas, and those in the shaded area not labeled are where you may want some help.

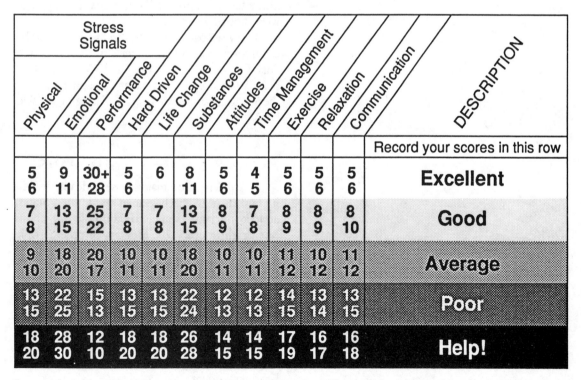

Physical	Emotional	Performance	Hard Driven	Life Change	Substances	Attitudes	Time Management	Exercise	Relaxation	Communication	DESCRIPTION
											Record your scores in this row
5 / 6	9 / 11	30+ / 28	5 / 6	6 /	8 / 11	5 / 6	4 / 5	5 / 6	5 / 6	5 / 6	**Excellent**
7 / 8	13 / 15	25 / 22	7 / 8	7 / 8	13 / 15	8 / 9	7 / 8	8 / 9	8 / 9	8 / 10	**Good**
9 / 10	18 / 20	20 / 17	10 / 11	10 / 11	18 / 20	10 / 11	10 / 11	11 / 12	10 / 12	11 / 12	**Average**
13 / 15	22 / 25	15 / 13	13 / 15	13 / 15	22 / 24	12 / 13	12 / 13	14 / 15	13 / 14	13 / 15	**Poor**
18 / 20	28 / 30	12 / 10	18 / 20	18 / 20	26 / 28	14 / 15	14 / 15	17 / 19	16 / 17	16 / 18	**Help!**

Source: Adapted from *The UnStress Express* by Whit Jones, Ph.D., Sun Valley Health Institute, 1987. Reprinted with permission.

SAFE AND SOUND

Each year Tom and Sally Clark throw a huge Christmas party. Last year's is one they will never forget. With the first guests due to arrive in minutes, Tom headed for the garage, just off the kitchen, where cases of soda were cooling. He opened the door and recoiled. Facing him was a wall of flames.

He pulled the door shut, yelled to his family, and raced to phone 911. Tom, Sally, their five children and three caterers tumbled out of the house. In minutes the first of the fire engines rolled up. So did the first of the hundred guests, who joined neighbors on the broad suburban lawn and watched in disbelief as firefighters struggled and flames raced. By the time the fire was out, the house had been gutted and the cars in the garage were destroyed.

In years past, Christmas fires were sparked by candles on trees. In the inner city they are often linked to space heaters. The Clark's was from fireplace ashes swept into a paper bag and stashed in the garage. Bad luck? Yes. Poor judgment? You bet.

ACCIDENTS IN THE UNITED STATES

Accidents are a major cause of death, disability and damage. Each year in the United States, accidents claim some 100,000 lives—about one death in every 20. Millions of other people sustain injuries, many serious enough to haunt them for life. The young are at special risk: Accidents are the greatest killer of those under the age of 45. These deaths seem doubly tragic—the beautiful toddler who dies in agony after drinking drain cleaner, the debutante mangled beyond recognition in the wreck of her car, the young man at the height of his physical prowess swept away in a boating accident.

Between the ages of one and four, deaths due to accidents occur about equally in the home and automobile. For the 40 years that follow, the automobile has no equal as a grim reaper. Cars and trucks are involved in almost half of all fatal accidents, as well as more than 2 million disabling injuries each year.

But the automobile is hardly the only problem. About 15 percent of all accidental deaths occur on the job—an alarming percentage considering that only a portion of the population spends only a part of its time in the workplace. And because many jobs carry little or no risk, those recognized as hazardous are likely to be very hazardous indeed. Mining tops the list, but construction and heavy industry are not far behind. Accidents on the job account for more than 14,000 deaths and 2.5 million disabling injuries each year.

In the home, falls, fires, power tools and poisons are a hazardous quartet. According to the National Safety Council, home accidents account for almost half as many deaths (more than 20,000 a year) and more than twice as many disabling injuries (3.1 million) as the automobile. Although most victims are young children, many adults find that starting a house fire is as easy as falling off a ladder.

The most important single factor in accidents is alcohol use. More than half of the people killed in auto accidents have been drinking, and often heavily. So have more than half of those who die in recreational accidents—while swimming, boating, fishing and hunting. Alcohol plays a major role in deaths due to falls and injuries to pedestrians. About 10,000 people die each year from alcohol-related overdoses. One-third of the nearly 30,000 persons committing suicides each year have alcohol in their blood. And each year about 10,000 murders occur in situations involving alcohol.

Cigarettes, for their part, not only kill through cancer, emphysema, heart disease, stroke and diabetes, they cause more than half of the nation's fatal house fires. (Alcohol is often involved in these deaths. In a Maryland study, two-thirds of the people between the ages of 30 and 59 killed in home fires were legally drunk.) The Consumer Product Safety Commission tried to mandate cigarettes that would go out if more than a few minutes went by between puffs, but its efforts were foiled by the tobacco lobby. Smokers also have a higher rate of automobile accidents.

ACCIDENT INSURANCE

The makings of accidents are all around us, every minute and every day. We have little control over some, such as earthquakes, plane crashes and falling trees. But many others can be foreseen and avoided by following a few basic rules:

- Minimize your risks.
- Become more safety conscious.
- Accident-proof your environment.
- Learn to handle emergencies.

Minimizing Risks

Reducing risks doesn't mean spending your life in a rocking chair. After all, some people earn their living doing such risky things as flying fighter jets or putting out fires. But it does mean knowing your limits. So if you are bent on climbing Mount Everest, be sure to start out well-conditioned, well-trained and well-equipped—mentally as well as physically.

On the other hand, people take unnecessary risks every day. Lots of these risks—jaywalking, leaving the car with the motor running "just for a minute," carrying a huge mound of laundry down the stairs, juggling four cups of steaming coffee, ignoring seat belts, running a yellow light—are seen as timesavers. You can do yourself a favor by learning to slow down. Make it a habit to allow enough time for the tasks at hand. Bandaging a sprained ankle or icing down a burned hand also eats up precious time. Haste makes waste, and it may waste you.

Two risks that are not only unnecessary but also deadly are drinking and smoking. If you drink, do so in moderation, and never drink and drive. If you smoke, quit.

Traffic deaths occur more often in the evening and nighttime hours, when visibility is poor and drivers tend to be tired. Alcohol-related traffic fatalities are nearly twice as numerous on Friday and Saturday nights as on other nights, and they tend to peak a few hours later than fatalities that do not involve alcohol.

Figure 12.1
Alcohol-Related Traffic Deaths

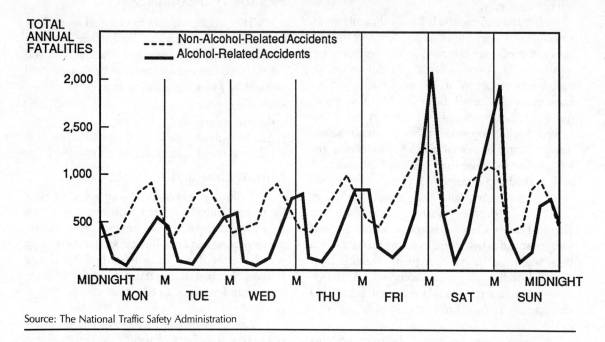

TOTAL
ANNUAL
FATALITIES

- - - - Non-Alcohol-Related Accidents
───── Alcohol-Related Accidents

2,000

2,500

1,000

500

MIDNIGHT   M   M   M   M   M   M   MIDNIGHT
        MON   TUE   WED   THU   FRI   SAT   SUN

Source: The National Traffic Safety Administration

Becoming More Safety Conscious

How many accidents are followed by, "If only ... "? If only I had seen the broken step. If only I had turned the iron off. If only I knew where they kept the fire extinguisher. Many, many accidents result from carelessness. Just as many could be prevented through alertness and care.

Pay attention to what you are doing. Learn to look before you leap—before you head down the stairs, step up on a curb or cross the parking lot. Don't get distracted when you are using a knife, wielding a chain saw or driving a car. (How often have you seen—indeed, been frightened by —drivers who are engrossed in conversation on their car phone, reading a newspaper in stop-and-go traffic, or putting on make-up in their rear-view mirror?) Drive defensively; don't depend on the other guy always to follow the rules. (And this goes double for bikers.) Having the right of way has never saved anyone's life.

Be extra alert when you are under stress.

Problems with your job, spouse or children, a recent death in your family, or financial worries can make you easily distracted. Make a special effort to keep your mind on the task at hand during times of stress, particularly when you are behind the wheel or in the kitchen.

Develop safety reflexes. Whenever you go to a theater or hotel, note the location of exits and fire escapes. (Count the number of doors between your hotel room and the nearest exit so you can find your way out even if the hall is dark or filled with smoke.) At a pool or on a boat, notice where the life preservers are stored. At the office, find out where the first-aid equipment and the fire extinguisher are kept. Know where the closest hospital is, and how to get there. At home, when cooking, turn the pot handles away from the stove edge; be sure to unplug the iron. When in a car, buckle your safety belt. These practices don't need to become a morbid preoccupation, but something you do automatically.

ACCIDENT-PROOFING YOUR ENVIRONMENT

On the Road

- Don't drive if you have been drinking or if you're taking drugs that cause drowsiness or dull your reflexes.
- Wear your seat belt. Seat belts cut the risk of injury by an estimated two-thirds. Get approved safety seats for younger children, and insist that older children—and all other passengers—wear seat belts.
- When you are in the market for a new car, look for one equipped with air bags.
- Keep your car in good repair. Don't rely on worn tires, old hoses and faulty brakes. Promptly replace burned-out headlights.
- Carry emergency gear in your car, including flares. If you need to perform roadside repairs, be sure you are well out of the path of traffic, and that oncoming drivers can see you.
- Know and observe the laws. Drive within the designated speed limit. When weather conditions are bad, slow down.
- Drive defensively.
- Show courtesy to other drivers. Everyone is safer when frustrations are at a minimum.
- Know your limits. If you have poor night vision, don't drive at night. If you're afraid to drive on the highway, take some lessons or stick to the side roads. If your reflexes have slowed down with age, consider giving up your license.
- Wear a helmet when you ride a bicycle, moped or motorcycle.

In the Home

Home accidents cause 3 million disabling injuries a year. One reason that so many accidents occur in the home is that we spend so much time there. Another is that we are not always as careful as we could be. Also, we let dangerous situations develop: We leave paper bags near the stove, toxic cleansers in unlocked cupboards, and rumpled throw rugs in hallways.

It is important to build safety into your everyday surroundings. Make a thorough safety inspection of your home, keeping alert to the four main sources of danger: falls, fires, power tools and appliances, and poisons.

Go through your house one room at a time. Try to step back and look at your surroundings and habits objectively, as if seeing them for the first time. (You might try imagining that you are a prospective home buyer.) Make a note of any hazards. Then work out a schedule for making changes, and check them off as you take care of them. Making home a safer place isn't something to be postponed. There's a lot to be done right now.

PREVENTING FALLS

Home-survival tactic number one is learning to prevent falls. Each year 1 million people are injured by falling, and falls account for as many as half of all home-accident deaths. The most frequent victims are the young and the old, but people of any age can trip or tumble.

Safe Stepping

Each year some 700,000 people are treated in emergency rooms because they fall on steps or stairs. Perhaps they couldn't see where they were stepping, they were running, or the stairs were slippery.

Make sure the stairs in your home are safe:

- Don't store objects on stairs. Your mop and bucket don't belong on the basement or back-porch steps. And if something needs to be put away upstairs, don't store it on the stairway until you're ready to go up—carry it up right away. It's not only safer, it's good exercise.
- Don't hang pictures on walls next to stairs. They may look pretty, but they can distract and disorient.
- Cover stairs with rubber treads, abrasive strips or skid-resistant paint. Slippery wax

Falls and Older People

Each year one of every three persons over age 75 can expect to fall. It's not bad enough that falls cause injuries and deaths (some 9,500 a year in persons over 65), the fear of falling causes many older people to curtail vital and healthful activities. And it's a vicious cycle: The less exercise they get, the more infirm they become.

The high likelihood of an older person's falling is partly a reflection of failing health. Chronic illness often affects mobility. Poor vision, problems with hearing or balance, and the use of medications all increase the chances of a fall. But falls also have environmental causes—such as objects left where they can be tripped over, poor lighting, slippery surfaces, and the wrong kind of furniture—chairs that are too deep to get out of easily, beds that are too high or too low, high-sided bathtubs, and kitchen cabinets that can be reached only by climbing. Older people can also be tripped up by ill-fitting shoes or a robe or pants that are too long.

finishes are a real hazard. Carpeting can be treacherous, too, if it develops worn spots or, if it's thick, catches people's heels.

- Make sure handrails are securely fastened. Building codes require a single handrail, but two would be better. Make sure that handrails and stairs end at the same point.
- See that stairs are well lighted. Put lights and switches at both top and bottom.
- Maintain a clear field of vision when carrying things up and down stairs. Avoid the temptation to carry everything at once. If you can't see where you're placing your feet, make more than one trip.
- Alert people to surprise steps, those that are unusually low, deep or steeply turning, and to a change in level between rooms. Use bright, contrasting tape or paint, or special lighting.

- Keep outdoor steps cleared of snow, ice and slippery leaves.

WATCH WHERE YOU WALK

In addition to the 700,000 people who hurt themselves on the stairs each year, another 300,000 fall on level surfaces—floors, sidewalks and streets. Although some of these falls result from hurrying and carelessness, most are due to slippery conditions and other changes in traction.

- Be alert to spills. If you see one at home, wipe it up. If you're at the grocery store, inform the manager.
- Keep the garage floor cleaned of oil, grease and mud. Absorbent chemicals available in hardware stores can take care of oily spills.
- Be on the lookout for icy patches on streets and sidewalks.
- Clean slippery soap film off of tub and shower surfaces. Use a rubber mat or non-skid decals in the tub or shower, and a non-skid rug on the bathroom floor.

LOOK OUT FOR WINDOWS

Lots of people compound their injuries by falling against, and breaking, a glass door or window.

- Make sure that sliding glass doors, large windows, and shower and bath enclosures are made of safety glazing materials.
- If a sliding glass door is so clean you can't tell it's there, you'll want to do something to keep people from walking into it. Try a sticker, an outdoor thermometer or some kind of ornament.

LEARN ABOUT LADDERS

Ladders let us clean fallen leaves from gutters, trim branches, paint ceilings and crown the Christmas tree. But 60,000 times a year, what goes up comes tumbling down. If you need to use a ladder, learn to do it the right way, before you take your feet off the ground.

- When you buy a ladder, learn its *maximum load rating* (usually between 200 and 250 pounds), which includes the total weight of you and your materials—and don't exceed it.

- If you will be working near power lines or with electrical tools, choose a ladder made of wood or fiberglass.

- Make sure your ladder is long enough for the job. There's a difference between *total* length and *usable* length. The top three rungs of a straight or extension ladder, or the top step and top platform of a stepladder, should not be used to support your weight.

- Inspect your ladder for wear and damage. Look for rotting or splitting wood rungs, or stress marks on metal.

- Position your ladder correctly. The distance between the base of a straight or extension ladder and the wall should be one-fourth of the *usable* length. Secure the base in firm, flat ground, or have a helper firmly hold the bottom of the ladder. If you're using a stepladder, place it on a flat surface with its legs fully extended and locked.

- Use both hands for climbing or descending. Carry tools in your pockets or belt —not your hands. Hoist a bucket with a rope, or have someone hand it up to you. While standing on the ladder, keep your body between the side rails, and don't reach to the right or left—instead, get down and move the ladder.

SAFETY IN THE NURSERY

Babies are so small and helpless that they can be endangered by many seemingly safe items and situations. Even their cribs must be carefully chosen! A baby's crib should have no more than 2.5 inches of space between the slats, so the infant's head cannot become wedged between them. For the same reason, crib mattresses and bumpers should be the correct size and snugly fastened. (A recent study found that parents' waterbeds can pose a hazard, too; infants who get caught face down may be unable to move their heads enough

Safety Glazing Materials

Several types of safety glazing materials are in wide use. They include:

- **Tempered glass,** the safety glass most often used in homes, crumbles when broken, eliminating the dangers of sharp shards of glass. You can recognize it by a permanent label etched into its corner.

- **Laminated glass** consists of two sheets of glass with plastic bonded between them. The plastic bonding will keep pieces of glass from scattering if the pane breaks.

- **Rigid plastic** is made from one or more layers of heated plastic. It is more difficult to break than glass, and won't produce the ultra-sharp pieces that ordinary glass does.

to breathe.) Also, keep the crib area free of all cords (from Venetian blinds, mobiles, etc.) that could become tangled around the baby's neck.

Toys pose danger, too, for toddlers as well as infants. They should not have sharp edges, nor should they have small parts that can easily be removed and swallowed. Check even soft stuffed animals to make sure hard pieces, such as eyes, are firmly attached.

Never leave a baby on a raised surface, such as a changing table, bed or sofa, that doesn't have sides to prevent the baby from rolling off. As the baby grows more mobile you must grow more cautious. When the baby is old enough to move around, be sure that all stairways are closed off, and that there's nothing the child can pull over onto himself or herself. See to it that no household products, sharp objects or poisonous plants are left within range. Keep the toilet lid shut. When the infant reaches the climbing stage, raise your sights: Be sure that all windows are closed or protected, that tables are free of dangling cloths or purse straps, that dishes, food and soap are not left near the edge of a table or counter. Eternal vigilance is the price of parenthood.

When Children Are on Their Own

Teaching children safety skills not only increases their self-confidence, it helps you feel better when they are left alone after school. Use the following suggestions from the National Safety Council to set guidelines that can help children cope with emergencies.

- A child who carries a house key should wear it so that it can't be seen. The key can be worn around the neck so it's hidden beneath clothing, or pinned inside a pocket.
- If your child comes home to an empty house, establish strict rules for unsupervised after-school hours. Let your child know which activities are permitted and which are not—whether playing with friends and cooking are allowed. Also, have your child check in with you by phone at a set time.
- Prepare a list of important telephone numbers for your child. Show him or her how to report an emergency by dialing 911 (if that service is available in your area) or "O" to call the operator.
- Decide how the child should handle callers at the door. Some parents teach children to ignore the doorbell. Children should never tell callers, either at the door or on the phone, that no adult is at home.
- All children need to know how to deal with adults. Tell your child never to talk to strangers or accept rides or gifts from *anyone* without your permission. (Unfortunately, many assaults on children are committed by people they know.)
- Teach your child to recognize whether the house is safe to enter. Are there any signs of a break-in—a broken window, a door left ajar or a ladder under a window? If the child spots anything like this, he or she should phone the police from a neighbor's house.

Fires: Prevention and Preparation

Nearly 3 million fires occur in the United States each year, taking 7,600 lives and leaving 200,000 people with burns and other injuries. Though major fires in high-rise hotels may capture the headlines, home fires claim more victims. Many could be avoided if people took preventive steps or knew what to do when a fire occurred.

Smoking: The Number-One Killer

It's sad but true: Most fire-related deaths are caused by smoking. Stray ashes or a fallen cigarette can easily ignite upholstered furniture, bedding or sleepwear. Sleepiness and alcohol or drug use make it more likely that a cigarette will be dropped or forgotten.

The number-one solution, of course, is to quit smoking. Short of that, smokers and their families can take several steps to make their homes safer.

- Have plenty of large, steady ashtrays with central grooves for holding cigarettes —and use them. Don't rest cigarettes on a countertop, sink edge or any other place from which they may roll.
- Check chair and sofa cushions for smoldering cigarettes before going to bed.
- Wait until the next day to empty ashtrays. Never dump ashes that could still be hot into plastic waste baskets or paper bags, or on top of other trash.
- Never smoke in bed.
- Keep matches, lighters and other smoking supplies out of children's reach.

Caution in the Kitchen

The best way to keep stove tops, ovens and broilers from starting a fire is to keep flammable materials from coming into contact with them. The same holds true for toasters, toaster ovens and counter-top broilers.

- Keep curtains, wall hangings and paper towels away from the stove area.
- Don't wear loose-fitting or flowing garments while cooking.

- Never lay towels, pot holders or other combustible items on top of the stove, even when the burners are turned off.
- Turn pot handles inward. This keeps children from reaching for them and adults from knocking them over.
- Keep burners and ovens clean and grease-free.

Electrical Know-How

Electricity is a powerful source of energy, and of danger. It needs to be handled with respect.

- Guard against overloading electrical outlets. This can cause wires to overheat, damaging their insulation and sparking fires. Blown fuses and circuit breakers warn of this problem, so take the hint. Luckily, the remedy is simple: Switch some appliances to another outlet.
- Inspect electrical cords and outlets periodically. And while you're at it, check the area around your television set. Heat from the back of a TV can ignite accumulated dust or papers stored nearby.
- Replace frayed cords. To minimize wear on wires, don't run them alongside door jambs or across high-traffic areas. (You'll also guard against falls.)
- Block unused outlets with plastic plugs, especially if you have children in the house.

Fireplaces and Wood Stoves

The warmth and coziness of a fireplace or wood stove are mighty appealing, but using fire to heat your home requires special precautions.

- Have your fireplace or wood stove installed by a professional. A stove should sit on a fireproof base, away from combustibles.
- Watch out for loose bricks and the buildup of creosote, a flammable substance produced when wood burns. If creosote isn't cleaned away periodically, it can cause a chimney fire. Have all fireplaces, chimneys and wood stoves cleaned and checked yearly by a reputable servicing company.

Help! Fire!

How would *you* extinguish a fire on the stove? The National Safety Council recommends turning off the burners and covering the flames with a pot or pan lid. It helps to keep the correct size lids handy while you cook.

Baking soda can also put out a fire, but you might not have enough on hand to do the job. Never try to douse flames with flour; it may *look* like baking soda, but it burns.

- Use a fire screen to keep sparks from spitting out into the room.
- Be careful of what you put in your fireplace. Don't burn substances that create excessively hot fires, such as dried Christmas tree limbs. And don't burn plastics or chemically treated materials that can give off noxious fumes.
- Never stack newspapers or magazines near the fireplace or stove.
- It's fine to pull upholstered furniture close to the fire for a while, but push it back when you're no longer using it.
- Never let a fire burn unattended or overnight.
- Let the embers die down completely before you clean the fireplace. Put the ashes in a metal (not paper) container and place it outside.

Using Space Heaters Safely

To save money on heating bills, many people are turning to portable electric and kerosene heaters. While they don't require costly installation and can be moved easily from room to room, they can be risky if handled improperly.

- Keep them at least three feet away from children, and vice versa. Children's hands can fit between the protective bars of some portable electric heaters—and the coils can reach 500 degrees Fahrenheit. Protective covers help, but they do not eliminate the danger.

- Don't let heaters come into contact with such combustibles as papers, curtains and upholstered furniture.
- Place the heater away from busy areas.

Today's kerosene heaters have safety features designed to prevent them from tipping over easily or leaking fuel. Automatic flame cutoffs activate if the heaters are bumped or knocked over. Still, these features are no guarantee against a fire. If you plan to use a kerosene heater, follow these safety guidelines:

- Know the correct way to refuel the heater. Let it cool first. Remember that kerosene expands with heat—if you add too much, some will overflow.
- Use only high-quality kerosene. Never use gasoline, which is highly volatile.
- Open a nearby window one inch or more to permit air to circulate.

Attention All Pack Rats!

Don't foster a fire in storage areas. Clean out your basement, attic and garage, and get rid of anything that you don't intend to use—old papers, clothes, dirty rags, chemicals and cleaning agents, and boxes and empty containers. They could fuel a blaze. Store whatever you do keep away from sources of heat.

Storing a gasoline-powered lawn mower presents special concerns. Ideally, it should be stored in a garage or, even better, in a shed or other building separate from the house. If your only option is to store it in the basement, make sure the fuel tank is thoroughly drained and washed out. Do not chance a gasoline leak near your heating system.

Smoke Detectors Save Lives

According to U.S. Fire Administration statistics, smoke plays a role in three-fourths of all fire deaths. Smoke and poisonous gases can quickly render victims unconscious. Then, as the fire spreads, they suffocate or burn to death.

The Center for Fire Research of the National Institute of Standards and Technology (formerly the National Bureau of Standards) estimates that by alerting residents early, before escape becomes impossible, smoke detectors could prevent more than half of all fire deaths.

Smoke detectors are inexpensive, easy to install and battery-operated. In most major metropolitan areas, landlords are required by law to maintain working smoke detectors in all rented dwellings. See that your family has adequate smoke-detector protection:

- Place at least one smoke detector on each level of your house.
- Install the detector on the ceiling or on a side wall 12 inches below the ceiling. Never place it in a corner where walls and ceilings come together—air doesn't circulate there. Be sure that it is at least three feet from heat registers and air vents, so that drafts don't make it less effective.
- Test your detectors periodically to make sure they are working. Many have a test button for this purpose. Alternatively, you can hold a lighted, smoking piece of paper or other substance nearby. (Be ready to extinguish it safely!) Or, as too many of us know, you can burn the toast.

Home Fire Extinguishers

Except for very small fires, the point of using a fire extinguisher is not to put the fire out. Rather, it is to slow the spread of flames to give people more time to escape.

Experts recommend a *dry chemical extinguisher* for home use. It should be "triple rated" for use on fires of class A (wood, textiles or paper), class B (flammable liquids), and class C (electrical equipment). The Underwriters' Laboratories (UL) or Factory Mutual (FM) seal of approval ensures that a fire extinguisher meets rigid standards of construction and performance.

- Store your extinguisher in a handy place, and *remember* where you put it. It's easy to get flustered in an emergency.

- Know how to use it. Even the best fire extinguisher won't help if you can't operate it. You won't have time to read the instructions if you are actually faced with a fire, so read them now, carefully, and be sure you understand them.
- Check it every few months to make sure it's in working order. Many fire extinguishers have a *gauge* that shows whether they are full and properly pressurized, or charged. If yours doesn't, *weight* is a reliable indicator: Compare its present weight to the weight when fully charged. (This is marked on a metal plate attached to the extinguisher.) If either the gauge or the weight tells you the extinguisher is not fully charged, have it recharged at a fire station.
- Make sure the nozzle is unobstructed. And check to see that the seal or plastic wire holding the pin in place is still intact. If it's not, someone may have used the extinguisher, and it may no longer be charged.

In the Event of a Fire

If a fire breaks out, the National Fire Protection Association recommends these steps:

- Follow the procedures and routes you've established and practiced beforehand (see "Prepare Yourself to Handle Emergencies," page 200).
- When escaping a fire, stay low—on hands and knees, if possible—to avoid breathing smoke or heated air, which rises.
- Before you open a door, feel it's temperature. If it's hot, leave it closed. If it's cool, open it slowly, but be prepared to shut it again quickly at the first sign of smoke or heat.
- If smoke is leaking in around a closed door, block it with clothing or blankets.
- Never re-enter a burning building for valued possessions or even pets.
- Call the fire department from a neighbor's house.

POWER TOOLS AND APPLIANCES: DO-IT-YOURSELF DANGER

Power tools are a boon to homeowners and hobbyists, but the combination of sharp, rapidly moving parts and electricity can be treacherous. Each year chain-saw and power-saw accidents cause 100,000 injuries. Slip-ups with other home workshop tools lead to another 25,000 accidents, and improper use of power mowers and hedge trimmers add 42,000 more.

Still, millions of people use these tools regularly and don't get hurt. The difference is that *they know what they are doing*.

To use electrical power tools safely:

- Read the owner's manual *before* you begin.
- Make sure the tool's safety guards are in place.
- Wear approved safety goggles.
- Check the tool for faulty insulation or wiring.
- See that your work area is dry.
- Be sure the tool has a three-pronged, grounded plug. Insert it into a three-pronged socket. (Do not cut off the third prong in order to use a 2-hole socket.)

Chain Saws

Two types of chain-saw injuries are common. Fast-moving chains can cause serious cuts and even amputations, and flying wood fragments can cut or bruise skin, or injure the eyes.

To prevent a chain-saw accident, heed these suggestions from the U.S. Consumer Product Safety Commission.

- Buy a saw that is easy for you to control. If possible, choose one with a low kickback chain or a plastic cover on the guide bar.
- Test the saw to see that the chain stops as soon as the trigger is released.
- Wear sturdy shoes, heavy pants and safety glasses.
- Place logs firmly on the ground. Hold the saw parallel to the ground.

A Word to the Not-so-Wise

The detailed safety instructions that come with most electrical tools may strike you as a prime example of overkill. Who could be so stupid as to lift a running power mower from the bottom, or plunk a radio on the edge of the bathtub? Who indeed? Ask the manufacturers or any emergency personnel. They've probably heard it all.

- Turn off the motor before walking around with the saw, or when leaving it unattended.
- Use a lightweight hand saw, not a chain saw, for trimming branches.
- Keep children away from your work area.

Portable Power Saws and Table Saws

Most injuries that involve power saws and table saws come from contact with the blade. Here are some guidelines for working with these tools:

- Always keep blade guards and other safety devices in place.
- Employ a plush block when making straight cuts with a stationary saw. This is a piece of wood used to push the item being cut.
- Allow the saw to operate at its own speed —don't try to force it forward.
- Unplug any saw before cleaning or repairing it.

Lawn Mowers and Hedge Trimmers

People can suffer severe cuts and even amputations when working with power lawn mowers and hedge trimmers. Two-thirds of the injuries from power mowers, and almost all of those from hedge trimmers, occur when hands or feet come into contact with moving blades. Many of the rest are caused when the blades throw rocks, twigs and other objects.

When you're buying a power lawn mower, look for one with safety features. It should have a guard that shields hands and feet from the blades, as well as a "dead man" control—a handle that must be held in place in order for the blades to turn. The grass-discharge chute should aim downward and have a shield to block thrown objects. The safest hedge trimmers have two handles, one for each hand, as well as pressure-sensitive switches that shut off power when finger pressure is removed.

When mowing:

- Pick up rocks and other debris before you begin cutting the lawn.
- Wear heavy boots and close-fitting garments.
- Turn off the mower before cleaning it or making adjustments.
- Keep others away from your work area.
- If your mower is gasoline-powered, allow the engine to cool before refueling. Don't take a chance on igniting flammable vapors.
- When operating a hedge trimmer, always use both hands.

Kitchen Appliances

Even though they may be small, kitchen appliances can still pack a wallop, and they deserve the same respect as large power tools. Thousands of people are injured every year while operating blenders, garbage disposals and food processors. The major cause? Contact with rapidly moving blades.

When using kitchen appliances, take these precautions:

- Make sure all parts are properly connected before you turn on the appliance.
- Do not insert utensils into the blades of mixers, blenders, or food processors, or the slots of a toaster.
- Never adjust parts while the machines are turned on or even plugged in.
- Keep your hands away from moving blades.

Microwave Safety

Microwave ovens have popped up in 75 percent of American homes and most offices. While there has been some worry about radiation leaks in older models, all recent models test well within government safety standards. In addition to snug door seals, they have at least two interlocks that prevent them from working if the door is not tightly closed.

When using a microwave oven, make sure the seals are clean and tight. If you have reason to think the oven may be leaking, get it evaluated by a professional from an appliance company or contact your local health department.

And don't forget that even though microwaves don't heat plates and cups directly, dishes can pick up plenty of heat from the food they contain; using a pot holder is usually a good idea.

• Avoid operating portable appliances near sinks or wet areas. Unplug machines for cleaning, and never immerse them in water.

POISON PATROL

Each year more than a million Americans are accidentally poisoned; of these, 4,000 die. Usually the poisons are swallowed, but they can also be absorbed through the skin or inhaled. Poisoning's symptoms depend on both the poison and the part of the body that is affected. Injury to the lung leads to shortness of breath, clear sputum production or rapid breathing. Damage to the gastrointestinal tract can cause nausea, vomiting, abdominal cramps or diarrhea. If the nerves are affected, the person can develop excessive fatigue, sleepiness, headache, muscle twitching or numbness. Some poisons affect many body systems. The effects of certain pesticides, for instance, can progress in minutes from minor vision problems to a paralyzed diaphragm that makes it impossible to breathe.

Most **oral poisonings** occur in the home, and most victims are children younger than five. Clearly the best way to prevent poisoning is to child-proof your home. Even if you don't have young children, you never know when a youngster may visit.

• Store medicines, cosmetics, and household chemicals out of the reach of little hands. These substances include insecticides, caustic cleansers and organic solvents such as kerosene, gasoline and furniture polish. The most damaging are strong alkali solutions used as drain cleaners (Drano), which will destroy any tissue with which they come in contact. *Never* store toxic liquids in soda bottles. Use safety latches on cupboards in which you keep toxic cleansers, especially low ones, like those beneath sinks. Storing dangerous substances in high places is not a good solution, though; young children can be champion climbers. Also, there is a risk that bottles can fall, shatter and spill their contents.

• If children are in the house, take any hazardous substances you are using with you when you answer the telephone or door. It only takes a moment for a child to swallow a fatal dose.

• Avoid taking medicine in front of children, and never refer to medicine or vitamins as "candy." But don't be lulled into complacency by child-proof containers. Often the best way to open a troublesome child-proof cap is to ask your child to do it for you.

• Keep the number of your local poison control center on your list of emergency phone numbers, next to the telephone. You can get the number from your physician or local hospital.

• Keep a bottle of syrup of ipecac in your first-aid chest. Syrup of ipecac is used to induce vomiting, which is the remedy in *some*, but not all, poisonings. In the event of a poisoning emergency, the poison control center will tell you what type of first aid to administer.

If a Poisoning Emergency Occurs

Poisonings are governed by three basic principles:

1. **Poisoning always requires professional help.** If you suspect that poisoning has taken place, even if you're not sure, contact a poison control center, emergency room or doctor's office immediately.

2. **The longer a poison remains in the body, the more damage it does.** Speed is of the essence.

3. Different types of poisoning call for different types of treatment, so **it is vital to identify the substance correctly.**

Inhaled poisons cause about 1,800 deaths a year. The usual culprit is carbon monoxide, the colorless, odorless gas found in motor-vehicle exhaust and fumes from faulty heating systems and burning charcoal. The first signs of carbon monoxide poisoning are dizziness and headache, followed by drowsiness and difficulty moving, and then unconsciousness.

To keep carbon monoxide from reaching dangerous levels:

- Open the garage door before warming up or tuning up your car engine.
- Have your heating and ventilation systems checked yearly by a certified heating and cooling specialist.
- Never burn charcoal in a garage or other enclosed area.
- Carbon monoxide is not the only inhaled poison. Mixing one kind of cleaning product with another can also produce toxic fumes.
- Use household products according to directions.
- Don't mix substances.
- Keep work areas well ventilated.

Poisons that enter the system **through the skin** include insecticides, rat poisons and corrosives, such as oven cleaner and gasoline. Their damage is not limited to the skin, however. Signs and symptoms of contact poisoning include nausea and vomiting, difficulty breathing, and burned skin. The eyes, which absorb toxins more quickly than any other outside part of the body, are especially vulnerable to damage.

- Wear a mask, gloves and long sleeves when working with toxic substances.
- Don't let children play in areas that have recently been sprayed or treated.

In the event of a poisoning emergency:

- Don't panic.
- If the victim's skin is blue or he or she has stopped breathing, begin artificial respiration and then *call the rescue service* for help.
- If the poison was inhaled, immediately carry or drag the victim into fresh air, but take care not to be overcome yourself. If you don't think you can rescue someone safely, call the fire department. (Even if the victim appears to recover quickly, he or she should seek medical attention to prevent complications.)
- Call the nearest poison control center and follow their instructions.
- If it's possible, get the victim to tell you what the poison was.
- Look around for open containers that might help poison control personnel identify the toxin and determine correct treatment.
- Check for burns around the mouth or a petroleum odor on the breath, signs that a corrosive substance has been swallowed.
- If you go to the hospital, bring any evidence that might help identify the poison, such as bottles, boxes or vomited material. But keep the substance out of the car's passenger space.

Home Treatment

When the poison is a plant or medication, the goal of home treatment is to get the toxin out of the body as quickly as possible. Vomiting is more effective and safer than using a stomach

Figure 12.2
Oral Poisoning

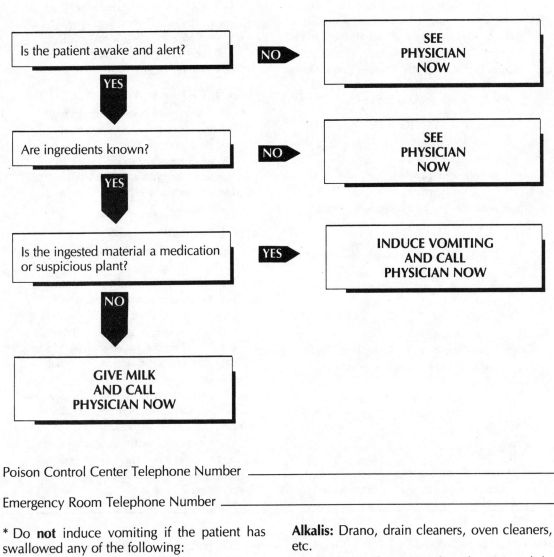

Poison Control Center Telephone Number _____

Emergency Room Telephone Number _____

* Do **not** induce vomiting if the patient has swallowed any of the following:

Acids: battery acid, sulfuric acid, hydrochloric acid, bleach, hair straightener, etc.

Alkalis: Drano, drain cleaners, oven cleaners, etc.

Petroleum Products: Gasoline, furniture polish, kerosene, oil, lighter fluid, etc.

Adapted from *Take Care of Yourself: Your Personal Guide to Self-Care and Preventing Illness* by Donald M. Vickery, M.D., and James F. Fries, M.D. Reading, MA: Addison-Wesley, 1990 (available from the Center for Corporate Health Promotion, 1850 Centennial Park Drive, Suite 520, Reston, VA 22091.)

Safeguarding Against A Break-In

The first step you can take to protect yourself against a burglary and possible assault is to make it hard for the criminal to break in. An unlocked door or window is an invitation to crime. The National Sheriffs Association recommends using the following checklist to make sure your home is secure.

Doors and Windows

- Can all your doors (including basement, porch, balcony and French doors) be securely locked?
- Do your basement doors have locks that allow you to isolate that part of your house?
- Are your locks in good repair?
- Do you know everyone who has a key to your house, or are some keys still in the hands of previous owners or tenants?
- Are window locks properly and securely mounted?
- If you live in a high-hazard area, do you use window bars or ornamental grills?
- Are you as careful with basement and second-floor windows as you are with those on the first floor?

Garage

- Do you lock your garage door at night and when you are away from home?
- Do you have good, secure locks on garage doors and windows?
- Do you lock your car and take the keys out even when it is parked in your driveway or garage?

When You Go Away on a Trip

- Do you stop all deliveries or arrange for neighbors to pick up papers, mail and packages?
- Do you leave some shades up, so that the house doesn't look deserted?
- Do you arrange to keep the lawn and garden trim?

Safe Practices

- Do you plan so that you don't need to "hide" a key under a doormat?
- Do you have a list of the serial numbers of watches, cameras, televisions, typewriters and similar items?
- Do you have a description (or photographs) of other valuable property that cannot be identified by serial number?
- Have you recorded credit card numbers, as well as the numbers to call if cards are lost or stolen?
- Have you told your family to leave the house undisturbed and call the police if they discover a burglary has been committed?

---

pump and can be induced by anyone. (Of course, vomiting should never be induced in a person who is unconscious or having convulsions.) Vomiting can usually be achieved immediately by stimulating the back of the throat with a finger (don't be squeamish!). In a child, two to four teaspoons of syrup (*not* extract) of ipecac may be used, followed by as much liquid as the child can drink. Vomiting usually follows within 20 minutes, but because

time is important, using your finger is quicker. Or you can try both. Mustard mixed with warm water also works. If there is no vomiting within 25 minutes, repeat the dose of syrup of ipecac. Collect the vomitus so that it can be examined by the physician.

Vomiting can be very dangerous if the poison contains strong acids, alkalis or petroleum products. These substances can destroy the esophagus or damage the lungs as they are vomited. Neutralize them with milk while contacting the poison control center or physician. If you don't have milk, give the person some milk of magnesia or water.

When a poison is spilled or splashed on the skin, it should be thoroughly rinsed off with running water. The victim should then be dried off and wrapped in a blanket. Remove any contaminated clothing. (Either throw it away or wash it separately from other laundry.)

If a poison gets in the eye, hold the eyelid open and wash the eye quickly and gently with clean, running water for five minutes or more. Do not use eye drops or any chemicals or drugs in the wash water.

Major poisoning is best managed at the emergency room. Treatment of the conscious patient depends on the particular poison and whether the victim has vomited. If needed, the stomach will be emptied with a stomach pump. Patients who are unconscious or have swallowed a strong acid or alkali will require admission to the hospital. Persons who are not admitted will require close observation at home.

On the Job

People who work in offices must be ready for the same types of dangers they encounter at home. Falls are common, and fires are a threat. In addition, the office environment can offer some new arenas for risk—escalators, elevators and slick terrazzo floors, as well as office machines and noxious fumes from supplies or equipment.

For many industrial workers, the risk of accidents comes with the territory. Just doing one's job can mean daily contact with heavy machinery, fast-moving conveyor belts, powerful tools, high-voltage electricity, toxic substances, extremes of temperature, heights, caverns, radiation or infectious agents. In situations like these, safety precautions have to be second nature.

- Be fully knowledgeable about your job and fully familiar with the equipment.
- If no one on your work team is trained in cardiopulmonary resuscitation (CPR), get that training yourself.

- Make sure you know how to handle any toxic chemicals in your workplace, and that you would recognize signs of exposure.
- Reduce wear-and-tear on your body. Take breaks, vary your position and maintain good posture.
- When lifting, let your legs, not your back, do the work. Keep the weight close to your body, your knees somewhat apart and one leg slightly forward. Bend your knees, not your back.
- Keep your equipment well-maintained, and check it before each use.
- Wear clothing that fits close to the body and is unlikely to catch in a machine.
- Use personal protective equipment, such as safety goggles, a face shield, a hard hat, gloves and aprons, as needed.
- Don't mix alcohol or drug use with work.
- Learn and *follow* the rules for fire safety on the job. Learn the location of all exits and fire extinguishers (and how to use them); review the regulations about smoking, waste disposal and use of flammable materials. Ask your supervisor to explain any aspects of fire safety that are unclear.
- Keep your mind on your job. When you're tackling a risky procedure, give it your full attention. Don't take on dangerous tasks when you are drowsy.
- Speak out about hazards you encounter on the job.

At Ease

Leisure time can be fraught with peril, too. This is especially true when we are trying something new, or seeking out adventure. White-water rafting is indeed more dangerous than being a couch potato (in the short run, anyway). But danger also lurks in everyday leisure activities. People who have a back-yard pool or weights in the basement need to develop special skills as well as "house rules" to safeguard family members and guests.

Remember, exercise is not risk-free. As discussed at length in Chapter 6, it's always important to warm up and stretch your muscles before exer-

Water Safety

It doesn't take very much water or time for someone to drown. In 1988, 5,000 Americans drowned. Eight hundred of them drowned at home, mostly in pools or tubs—and almost half of these were children under five.

- Learn how to swim and see that your children do, too.
- Never leave a young child unsupervised in or around water.
- All backyard pools require *constant adult supervision* when they are in use.
- A portable poolside phone is a good idea, both for emergency use and so you won't be tempted to go inside to answer calls.
- A flotation device and a long pole should be handy, in case someone gets into trouble in the water. When not in use, the pool should be inaccessible—behind a fence and a locked gate.
- Don't mix alcohol and water sports.
- Be prepared to give artificial resuscitation.

cise and to cool down afterward. Drink plenty of fluids and avoid extremes of temperature.

Most sporting activities are covered by certain basic principles.

- Know the rules.
- Learn the skills—and don't rush it. Avoid the advanced ski slope or the spirited horse until you know what you're doing.
- Get into condition. There's almost no surer recipe for a sports injury than throwing yourself into a game, race or climb when you're not in shape.
- Quit before you're exhausted. Many a mishap can be traced to fatigue.
- Make sure your equipment is in good working order. Check the snorkeling mask for cracks, the bike for broken spokes, or the motorboat's fuel tank for a full supply.

- Get good professional advice, guidance and coaching. But before you sign on with a guide, outfitter or balloonist, check out the person's or company's reputation for safety.
- Don't disdain safety equipment. Wear a helmet when riding a bike or a horse, a life preserver when paddling a canoe, and an orange vest and hat when hunting. If you run at night or twilight, wear reflectors and light-colored clothing.

Prepare Yourself to Handle Emergencies

Despite our best efforts, accidents sometimes happen. When they do, we have to be ready to meet them and minimize their damage. Such readiness requires information and skills.

The first and easiest step is to gather emergency phone numbers—fire and police, poison control center, hospital, ambulance, doctor. Post these numbers in an easy-to-locate spot near the telephone, and make sure that everyone in the family is familiar with them. (Put *your* home address with the emergency numbers. Kids and panicked adults may need it.) Even young children can be taught the proper use of 911. And all drivers in the household should know where the closest hospital is, and the best route to reach it.

Second, keep first-aid supplies stocked and handy, but out of children's reach. Every house should have syrup of ipecac on hand. You should also stock a fever and pain reliever (aspirin, acetaminophen, ibuprofen, etc.) a thermometer, Band-Aids, gauze dressing, elastic bandages, and hydrogen peroxide. (Along with soap and water, peroxide will help clean out most dirty wounds.) A soothing lotion such as calamine can ease the itch of poison ivy and other rashes. A copy of *Take Care of Yourself* will tell you when and how to use them.

Third, drill your family in how to survive an emergency. The main concern is fire safety.

- Plan an emergency escape route. If possible, all rooms should have two escape routes (two doors or one door and one window). Place a portable escape ladder in each upstairs bedroom, loft or den.

- Plan an alarm system—for instance, a special whistle or bell to be used only in case of fire.
- Agree now on a post-escape meeting place.
- Hold fire drills, both announced and unannounced. Schedule some between 11 p.m. and 6 a.m., hours when fires often occur.

If you live (or vacation) where tornados, hurricanes or earthquakes are a threat, develop and practice strategies for surviving those emergencies, too.

Finally, you and your family should learn lifesaving skills. These include cardiopulmonary resuscitation (CPR) and the anti-choking abdominal-thrust (Heimlich) maneuver. If your house or apartment has a pool or you spend summers at the shore, you should also learn water rescue and resuscitation techniques. All of these skills require intensive hands-on instruction. To find out when classes are scheduled, contact community organizations such as the American Heart Association and the American Red Cross, or your community hospital.

Can Accidents Be Treated?

This century has seen enormous strides in the treatment of accidental injuries. However, it appears that these strides have been less successful in reducing fatalities. It also appears that in the past few decades we have made little progress in preventing accidental disability. Most of the past improvements were due to improved care once the patient was in the hospital.

Now we have turned our interest to what happens *before* the patient arrives at the emergency-room door. Our belief that treatment should be more effective if begun earlier (which is not illogical) has led communities to invest hundreds of millions of dollars in sophisticated ambulance systems—some of them airborne. There is hardly a more dramatic or exciting image than highly trained paramedics racing to save lives through a combination of skill and advanced technology. (Indeed, it's an image TV projects repeatedly on dramatic series, the soaps and the nightly news.) Un-

All-Terrain Vehicles

Lots of sports, hang gliding and skiing among them, are risky. Riding all-terrain vehicles (ATVs) is risky, too; these unwieldy bikes can flip over and pin the rider beneath them. In this "sport," however, the risk is borne largely by children. Each year more than 300 Americans die in ATV accidents, half of them under 16.

In recent years, the U.S. Consumer Product Safety Commission (CPSC) battled successfully to halt the manufacture of three-wheelers, and to get dealers to agree not to sell adult-sized four-wheelers to kids. Although there's been a drop in injuries (from a high of 90,000 hospitalizations a year to 60,000) as well as in sales, deaths have not decreased proportionately. In 1989, CPSC, suspecting that adult-sized bikes were still being bought for youngsters, sent a safety alert to every school in the country.

fortunately, these high-speed, high-tech systems may have less impact than we would like. It may be that most accidents will either be fatal regardless of how quickly help appears, or be survived as long as help arrives within a reasonable time. This leaves a fairly small number of accidents for which a very quick ambulance response is critical.

When it comes to decreasing the toll taken by accidents, prevention is the name of the game.

What Can Be Done About Accidents?

Perhaps the most disturbing thing about accidents is that so many could be prevented and we have known how to prevent them for so long. Lowering speed limits reduces deaths. So do TV spots against drunk driving, home-safety campaigns, poison control centers and occupational safety programs.

So what are we waiting for?

The answer raises a basic question: Can peo-

Firearms

Hardly a day goes by that we don't read of a new tragic accident—children shooting brothers and sisters, teens killing their friends, adults maiming their companions or themselves. Some 1,400 such senseless shootings occur each year, mostly when people are cleaning or playing with a weapon. If you own a gun, you are more likely to shoot someone you know than an intruder. If you keep a gun in your house, take these precautions:

- Make sure it is not loaded.
- Keep it under lock and key.

ple's habits be changed? Time and time again, those who prefer to do nothing have argued that people cannot change their ways and that accidents must happen.

Yet it is clear that behavior can be changed, and it has been changed without resorting to oppressive methods or loss of basic freedoms. But our approach has been haphazard and uneven. We lowered speed limits only to raise them again. (Of course we lowered them to save energy, not lives. A 1989 study by the Insurance Institute for Highway Safety found that when the rural interstates posted a 65 mph limit, deaths rose dramatically — about 30 percent in 1988.) As of mid-1989, 34 states had enacted seat-belt laws; 16 still had not. Mines are safer than they were 50 years ago but are still a treacherous place to work. Poison control

centers are more common, but the most fundamental approach to poison control, public education, has been neglected.

So it is a question of will rather than way. We are not waiting for any new discovery, drug or technology. We are waiting for ourselves.

Additional Resources

Books to Read

Safety: A Personal Focus, by David L. Bever, Ph.D. St. Louis, MO: Times Mirror/Mosby, 1987.

Take Care of Yourself: Your Personal Guide to Self-Care and Preventing Illness, by Donald M. Vickery, M.D., and James F. Fries, M.D. Reading, MA: Addison-Wesley, 1990 (available from the Center for Corporate Health Promotion, 1850 Centennial Park Drive, Suite 520, Reston, VA 22091).

Organizations

American Association of Retired Persons, 1901 K Street, NW, Washington, DC, 20049.

International Association of Firefighters, 1750 New York Avenue, NW, Washington, DC, 20006.

International Rescue and Emergency Care Association, 8107 Ensign Drive, Bloomington, MN 55438.

International Society of Fire Service Instructors, Box 88, Hopkinton, MA 01748.

National Institute of Standards and Technology, Center for Fire Research, Commerce Department, Washington, DC 20036.

National Safety Council, 444 N. Michigan Avenue, Chicago, IL 60611.

U.S. Consumer Product Safety Commission, 1111 18th Street, NW, Washington, DC 20207.

DEALING WITH DRUG ABUSE

ocaine and crack; heroin and marijuana; PCP, crank and ecstasy. These have become household words in America. According to a survey by the National Institute on Drug Abuse (NIDA), more than 70 million Americans have tried illicit drugs, more than 23 million have used them within the past year and nearly 6 million within the past month.

Drugs have led to the death of athlete Len Bias and the disgrace of countless other sports figures; drug use has derailed not only Amtrak trains but also the nomination of a Supreme Court justice; the drug trade has triggered a flood of murders in our large cities and frightened people even in small towns. Drugs can warp the brain and personality as well as the body; they can destroy families and careers; paying for drugs can lead to a life of crime. Pregnant women who take drugs risk the well-being of their unborn babies. Intravenous drug users are at high risk of AIDS.

It's no wonder that "drugs" topped the list of major worries among American voters polled during the 1988 presidential campaign. A Gallup Youth Poll released in 1988 reported that 55 percent of teenagers named drug abuse as the biggest problem facing their generation.

WHAT IS DRUG ABUSE?

Drugs that affect the brain and the nervous system—so-called mind-altering drugs—are known as psychoactive substances. They include not only "street drugs" but also prescription drugs, such as diet pills and sleeping pills. Other widely available psychoactive substances are alcohol, caffeine and nicotine. A substance problem exists any time drugs interfere with a person's life—physically, personally or socially, at work or in the community.

Psychoactive substances can act as stimulants, depressants, narcotics or pain killers. Some others act as hallucinogens. More and more, drug abusers are using drugs in combination or with alcohol.

Table 13.1
Symptoms and Signs of Drug Abuse

CENTRAL NERVOUS SYSTEM STIMULANTS:
(Amphetamines, cocaine, methylphenidate, phenmetrazine, phemylpropanolamine, most anti-obesity drugs)

Signs of Severe Intoxication:	Pupils dilated
	Rapid pulse
	Shallow breathing
	Hyperactive, easily excitable behavior
	Rapid speech
	Dry mouth
	Sweating
	Impulsive behavior
Symptoms of Withdrawal:	Muscle aches
	Abdominal pain
	Chills and tremors
	Intense hunger
	Extreme depression
	Anxiety
	Increased sleep
	Suicidal behavior

CENTRAL NERVOUS SYSTEM SEDATIVES:
(Barbiturates, chlordiazepoxide, diazepam, flurazepam, glutethimide, meprobamate, methaqualone)

Signs of Severe Intoxication:	Decreased blood pressure
	Reduced breathing rate
	Slow motor reflexes
	Drowsiness or coma
	Loss of muscular coordination
	Slurred speech
	Delirium
Symptoms of Withdrawal:	Trembling
	Sweating
	Collapse of cardiovascular system
	Delirium
	Hallucinations
	Disorientation
	Inability to sleep

OPIOIDS AND NARCOTICS:
(Heroin, morphine, codeine, meperidine, methadone, hydromorphone, opium, pentazocine, propoxyphene)

Signs of Severe Intoxication:	Pupils constricted
	Reduced breathing rate
	Decreased body temperature
	Reflexes diminished or absent
	Decreased blood pressure

Table 13.1
Symptoms and Signs of Drug Abuse, continued

Symptoms of Withdrawal:	Abdominal cramps Muscle jerks Flu symptoms Vomiting Diarrhea Trembling Anxiety
In overdoses:	Stupor or coma Convulsions

HALLUCINOGENS:
(LSD, psilocybin, mescaline, PCP, STP, MOMA Bromo-DMA)

Signs of Severe Intoxication:	Pupils dilated Rapid pulse Elevated blood pressure Face flushed Visual hallucinations Distorted vision and sense of time Slurred speech Increased heart rate
With PCP:	Extreme hyperactivity Drooling Impulsive, often violent behavior
Symptoms of Withdrawal:	None

CANNABIS SUBSTANCES:
(Marijuana, hashish, THC, hash oil)

Signs of Severe Intoxication:	Bloodshot eyes Increased appetite Euphoria or anxiety Dreamy, fantasy state Time-space distortions Increased heart rate
Symptoms of Withdrawal:	Irritability Anxiety Nausea Inability to sleep Restlessness

Source: *The Medical Letter on Drugs and Therapeutics*, Vol. 27, September 1985. Published by the Medical Letter, Inc. New Rochelle, NY.

STIMULANTS

Stimulants, or "uppers," activate the central nervous system, increasing energy and alertness. Caffeine in coffee, tea or cola drinks and nicotine in cigarettes are examples of widely used stimulants. Although there are concerns that drinking too much coffee (more than five cups per day) may cause heart problems, and the risks of tobacco use are well known, the stimulants most often discussed are cocaine and amphetamines:

- **Cocaine** is derived from coca leaves. It can be snorted as a white powder or injected in liquid form. Contrary to earlier beliefs, cocaine is powerfully addictive; it seems to act directly on "pleasure centers" in the brain. There is increasing evidence that it can also cause irreversible damage to the central nervous system. Cocaine use has soared in the 1980s; street consumption more than doubled between 1982 and 1985, and NIDA estimates that each day several thousand Americans try cocaine for the first time.

  Crack is a potent cocaine derivative that can be smoked. It reaches the brain quickly and is not only highly addictive, but cheap, making it affordable to young people.

- **Amphetamines** can be pills, powders or liquids. They can be swallowed or injected. Prescribed to increase alertness, in quantity or over time they can create a high level of physical and psychological dependence.

  Methamphetamine, a long-acting "upper" commonly known as "crank" or "speed," is easily made in makeshift labs. Recent reports show that it is growing more popular in blue-collar populations and rural areas of the country, especially along the Pacific Coast and in the Southwest.

  Ecstasy is a methamphetamine derivative originally used to suppress appetite. It is also known as MDMA, an abbreviation for its chemical name. It has recently become popular in nightclubs; users claim it makes them feel alert, yet relaxed. Psycho-logically but not physically addictive, ecstasy is thought to damage the brain.

DEPRESSANTS

Depressants, also known as "downers," slow the activity of the central nervous system. They narrow a person's field of perception and act as sedatives. In addition to alcohol, depressants include sleeping pills and tranquilizers. Certain gases, including fumes from solvents (glue), aerosols and nitrous oxide, also fall into this group.

Barbiturates, which contain phenobarbital or a related chemical, induce sleep and can help control convulsions. Drug abusers take them to reduce anxiety or produce a sense of euphoria. They produce moderate to high physical and psychological dependence.

Narcotics affect centers in the brain that register pain and are used medically for pain relief. They appeal to the substance abuser because they produce a sense of euphoria. Narcotics can be highly addictive, creating severe mental torment and physical discomfort when they are stopped. Heroin, morphine, codeine and opium are narcotics derived from the opium poppy. Synthetic narcotics include hydromorphone (Dilaudid), oxycodone (Percodan), meperidine (Demerol) and propoxyphene (Darvon).

Heroin, the opium derivative most widely abused in this country, comes in powder form. It can be injected, snorted or smoked. It causes a high degree of physical and psychological dependence; withdrawal causes nausea, cramps, chills, sweating, tremors and panic.

HALLUCINOGENS

Hallucinogens affect and distort a person's perceptions of reality. They are so named because they can produce mild to strong hallucinations. Hallucinogens include LSD, magic mushrooms and today's favorite, PCP.

Also known as angel dust, PCP is a synthetic drug used as an anesthetic for animals. It comes in a variety of forms that can be smoked, snorted or swallowed. Frequent users like to mix it with leaves of something such as parsley, mint or marijuana, and smoke it. Recent studies show that PCP acts as both a stimulant and a depressant, producing a state similar to schizophrenia. It can also trigger violent behavior.

CANNABIS SUBSTANCES

Cannabis substances are exemplified by marijuana, hashish and THC. These are products of the infamous five-leafed cannabis plant; the plant's leaves can be either smoked or eaten. These drugs alter users' perceptions, leading them to believe, incorrectly, that their field of perception has "expanded." Occasionally, they cause hallucinations, panic attacks, depression or rage. These drugs are taken to relax or heighten awareness; they often produce a sense of euphoria. Contrary to widespread belief, marijuana can be harmful—and the marijuana available today is much more potent than "grass" was in the 1960s. Studies show that it can cause lung disease, weaken immune responses, impair memory, hamper judgment and diminish motor skills. Moreover, it can affect attitude, leading to apathy, loss of ambition and a decline in school or work performance.

SUBSTANCE DEPENDENCE

All psychoactive substances can create dependence, even if it is only a strong habit. All of these drugs work by acting on receptor sites in the brain, which become accustomed to their presence. Over time, it takes more and more of the substance to produce the desired effect. If the nervous system is then deprived of the substance, it rebels, and the person experiences the mental and physical discomforts—even agonies—of withdrawal.

Dependence on the Substance Experience

People can become hooked not only on the drug but also on the lifestyle associated with it. This is known as "dependence upon the substance experience." A cocaine abuser, for instance, can get pleasure from and develop dependence on the status of being a user, the risks involved in securing the drug and the party atmosphere associated with

it. As Richard Miller, Ed.D., of the University of Rochester explains, "Getting hooked on the cocaine effect is quite possible, but it's the substance experience that intensifies that possibility."

Dependence as a Disease

Substance dependence is considered a disease because it is a primary, progressive, chronic and, in many cases, fatal behavior. *Primary* means that the person cannot function without the drug. A *progressive* problem is one that grows worse. As a compulsive, chronic and self-defeating way of thinking and behaving, dependence overrides willpower and prevents a person from making healthy decisions on his or her own behalf.

What Triggers Substance-Abuse Problems?

Some experts believe that certain people inherit a susceptibility to the effects of alcohol or the "high" from marijuana. Coupled with a substance-oriented lifestyle, this increases the risk of a drug-abuse problem. According to another school of thought, dependency is largely a matter of lifestyle and negative response to a stressful world. But both groups of experts agree that a learning process takes place: The person learns to reduce physical or emotional discomfort by using drugs. This turns into a vicious circle, causing more pain that requires more relief.

Why Today?

Availability is part of the answer. More drugs can be purchased today than at any other time in U.S. history. Early in this century, our society restricted narcotic use and made a vain attempt to ban the manufacture and sale of alcohol. Synthetic stimulants and depressant pills entered the market mid-century. During the 1960s and 1970s, when the number of young adults reached an all-time high, marijuana and other hallucinogens became symbols of discontent and defiance. Today, cocaine, crack and heroin are available throughout the country. In short, laws against drugs have not stopped their distribution.

But there must be a demand to sustain this illegal supply. It is clear that many people have

Do You Have a Substance Abuse Problem?

Do you use any of these psychoactive substances?

Stimulants	Depressants	Hallucinogens	Cannabis Substances
Caffeine	Alcohol	LSD	Marijuana
Nicotine	Narcotics	PCP	Hashish
Amphetamines	Barbiturates	Psilocybin	THC
Antidepressants	Tranquilizers		
Cocaine	Inhalants		

If yes, does your substance use:

- Make you forget your problems?
- Usually occur when you feel troubled?
- Make you feel good about yourself and life?
- Prevent you from fulfilling responsibilities?
- Discourage you from trying new things?
- Prevent you from interacting with non-users?

- Have to be done regularly?
- Make you uncomfortable when you stop using the substance?
- Make you intolerant of schedule changes that affect your use?
- Lead you to ignore changes and events in your life?
- Lessen in effect with time?
- Make you annoyed at the thought of stopping?

The more "yes" answers you gave, the more likely it is that you have a substance-abuse problem. The wise thing is to find out for sure: Seek professional advice from a counselor in your community or at work, or through your church or synagogue.

---

learned to use drugs to produce desired psychological effects. This is as true on the job as off. For example, some managers have begun to use cocaine to enhance feelings of effectiveness and control. Other workers use drugs to counter the boredom, stress or lack of fulfillment they experience in their jobs. At least 20 percent to 30 percent of the work force has relied on substance experiences at one time or another.

THE FAR-REACHING EFFECTS OF SUBSTANCE ABUSE

The impact of substance use and abuse—on the individual, family life and work—is alarming.

- From 5 percent to 13 percent of adults heavily abuse or depend on some kind of psychoactive substance other than alcohol.
- Between 50 percent and 85 percent of our youth have at least experimented with

drugs such as alcohol, marijuana, LSD, cocaine and prescription pills. According to NIDA's most recent (1985) survey, nearly one-fourth of American youngsters between 12 and 17 had used an illicit drug in the preceding year.

- At least one-half of all spouse-abuse cases and one-third of all child-abuse cases are related to substance abuse. In 1988, there were more than 2.3 million *reported* cases of child abuse.
- The nation's bill has been put at $60 billion for substance abuse and $175 billion for alcohol abuse. Altogether, this is about $1,000 for every man, woman and child in America. This includes the costs of medical care, decreased productivity, lost employment, welfare payments and prisons.
- Employee assistance counselors report that nearly half of their clients have problems

with alcohol, cocaine or other drugs of abuse.

- More than one-third of all suicides are drug related.
- Hospital admissions due to adverse cocaine reactions have risen dramatically. In 1987, more than 46,000 persons sought help in emergency rooms for cocaine-related problems—nearly double the number from 1986.
- There are more than one million intravenous drug users in the United States. A recent survey of heterosexual intravenous drug users showed that 19 percent of daily heroin injectors and 35 percent of daily cocaine injectors carried the AIDS virus.

TACKLING THE PROBLEM

Fortunately, something is being done to prevent and reduce substance abuse in our society. More people are learning how to recognize substance abuse and where to seek help. Young people are receiving drug education in the classroom. Parents are learning that "hugs are better than drugs." Employees are being trained to aid fellow workers who may be drug troubled.

Drug use among teenagers, which rose steadily through the 1970s, has declined in the 1980s, according to two major surveys, one by NIDA and the other by the University of Michigan. However, the surveys predate a sharp upswing in the use of crack in the late 1980s. And they do show the continuing popularity of the so-called "gateway" substances, which may lead to drug abuse: alcohol and nicotine. Two-thirds of the high-school class of 1986 described themselves as "current" drinkers, while about one of every three smoked cigarettes—a statistic unchanged since 1984.

HOW TO RECOGNIZE SUBSTANCE ABUSE

By their very behavior, substance abusers make both subtle and direct appeals for help. If you suspect that someone near to you has a substance-

Steroids: A Special Case

The last couple of years have seen the rise of a different type of drug-abuse problem —drugs that target the muscles rather than the brain. A nationwide survey published in the *Journal of the American Medical Association* in 1988 showed that one out of 15 male high school seniors reported taking bodybuilding anabolic steroids. Two-thirds had begun taking these drugs by age 16, almost half were taking more than one type at a time and 38 percent took them both orally and by injection. Nearly half of these seniors said they took the drugs to bolster athletic performance, but more than a quarter said they were mainly trying to improve their appearance. Ironically, these young men risk stunting their growth, impairing their fertility and developing psychological problems.

abuse problem, here are some signs to look for:

- Unhealthy lifestyle. Dependent persons neglect their health and lose interest in their appearance. Cocaine users often develop a chronic runny nose and frequent colds.
- Secretive behavior. Drug use must be hidden, especially in the school or work setting.
- Frequent absences from school or work. Hangovers and drug after-effects take their toll on both attendance and performance.
- Mood swings. The "high" from a drug is often replaced by depression when it wears off.
- Weight loss. Stimulants suppress appetite.
- Money problems. A drug habit is costly. Substance abusers can quickly run through their pay or allowance; some start to steal from family and friends or, at work, pad expense accounts. Many drug abusers turn to robbery or prostitution.
- Anxiety and nervousness. Drug abuse makes people less able to cope with stress.

- Impulsive behavior. The urge to use a substance can be overpowering.
- Troubled relationships. Substance abusers neglect commitments and responsibilities to others.
- Denial that a problem exists. This "Catch 22" is common to most addictive behavior. The first step in getting help is admitting there is a problem.

Getting Professional Help

If someone you care for is acting in a way that makes you suspect drug abuse, you will want to learn more about the problem and how to approach and guide the person to professional help. Although some substance abusers seek professional help on their own, most need encouragement to "find out what's wrong." However, your role is not to diagnose the problem. Let the professionals do that.

It can be very hard to admit that someone close to you has a drug problem. You must be willing to admit that his or her behavior is harming your relationship. And you must be willing to forgo "covering up" for the person.

Start by learning more about substance abuse and the services that are available. You can do this by contacting any of the resources listed at the end of this chapter. Learn what services are available in your community or through your employer. Consult the Yellow Pages.

Seeking outside help is a very important step. Work through local chapters of the "Anonymous" groups or your company's employee assistance program. Speak to your physician. Discuss the matter with a minister, priest or rabbi. You can also call an anonymous service such as one of the hotlines that are available, either locally or nationwide. You can find support for yourself, too, through groups serving the friends and families of drug abusers.

Once you have learned about the problem, you may be able to confront the drug abuser. There is nothing wrong in saying, "Look here. I am concerned about your behavior. You seem troubled. Why not speak to someone about it?"

However, it isn't easy to deliver an unpleasant message, especially one that the listener resists. The help of an experienced professional—a physician, drug counselor, social worker, or psychologist—can be crucial. Many experts recommend a method called intervention. After meeting several times with the professional advisor, family members—perhaps joined by the dependent person's friends, employer or co-workers—confront the user. Led by the professional, they express their concern and back up their claims with specific examples. If the abuser agrees, he or she promptly enters a treatment program. If the abuser refuses help, it is critical that the others get counseling to prevent their enabling the abuser to continue his or her behavior.

Treatment and Recovery

There is no cure for substance dependence; the craving can persist for life. However, it can be controlled. Successful rehabilitation or recovery can be expected for 50 percent to 70 percent of all substance abusers.

Treatment programs must be geared for the long haul: helping the drug abuser return to and maintain a healthy lifestyle. Sometimes, short-term hospitalization is necessary to prevent death from overdose or withdrawal. The hospital may also be used to hold an unstable person who is a threat to himself or herself or to others. Sometimes persons need to be hospitalized to treat certain medical complications of drug abuse, primarily infections. The average hospital stay for drug-abuse problems is 12 days, and the cost ranges between $3,000 and $15,000.

Once the immediate danger has passed, the most useful thing the hospital can do is guide the patient into a treatment program outside the hospital. Such treatment programs emphasize counseling and group support. They should also help the person restore healthy eating habits, increase physical activity and learn to cope with stress. Ultimately, the person can expect to move from a therapist-supervised support group to a self-help group such

Co-Addiction: Are You Helping a Drug User?

John uses cocaine regularly, and often can't get up and moving in the morning. Rather than confront him, his wife Joan wakes him up, pulls him out of bed and into the shower and drops him off at work. If he's late, she makes excuses to his boss.

John is the one with the drug problem, but—without realizing it—Joan is helping him stay on drugs. In fact, he might not be able to keep up his habit without her unintentional cooperation. Drug experts have only recently investigated such "co-addiction" among drug users.

In one research study, psychologist Dr. Charles Nelson identified six "styles of enabling" among the spouses, lovers, friends, and relatives of cocaine users:

- **Avoiding and Shielding**—Co-addicts may cover up for abusers or prevent them from experiencing the full impact of the harmful consequences of drug use. For example, a co-addict may say the user is working on a project and can't be disturbed so friends don't visit when the user is strung out on drugs.

- **Attempting to Control**—A co-addict may try to take control of the significant other's use of drugs personally, for instance, by withholding sex or using sex as a reward for cutting down on drug use.

- **Taking Over Responsibilities**—A co-addict may take over the user's household chores, such as grocery shopping or running errands, or may get money to pay the user's drug-related debts.

- **Rationalizing and Accepting**—Co-addicts try to understand, explain and accept their partner's drug use, telling themselves that the drugs are giving the user more energy or helping him or her be more open.

- **Cooperating and Collaborating**—The co-addict may become involved in buying, selling, testing, preparing or using the drug.

- **Rescuing**—The co-addict may be overprotective, allowing a user to use drugs at home to avoid the risk of an accident elsewhere.

Sources: Sorenson, James and Guillermo Bernal. *A Family Like Yours: Breaking the Patterns of Drug Abuse.* San Francisco: Harper & Row, 1987; H. Julia. *Letting Go With Love: Help for Those Who Love an Alcoholic/Addict Whether Practicing or Recovering.* Los Angeles: Jeremy Tarcher, 1987.

as Narcotics Anonymous or Cocaine Anonymous. Self-help groups are made up of adults involved in lifelong recovery who rely on each other for support, for the understanding that comes from sharing common fears and obstacles and for constructive criticism and encouragement.

Relapse is not uncommon, so be prepared. Expect a re-entry into therapy and recovery. If you are a friend or relative of the abuser, do not help the abuse to continue (see box above).

Substance abuse is a reality of today's fast-paced, high-tech world. Yet you can do something about this problem. Help others and help yourself: encourage a substance-free lifestyle; become healthy and stay that way.

Where Can You Get More Help?

Adult Children of Alcoholics, Central Service Board, P.O. Box 3216, Torrance, CA 90505.

Al-Anon Family Groups, P.O. Box 862, Midtown Station, New York, NY 10018-0862. (212) 302-7240.

Alcoholics Anonymous and AA hotline. Check the local phone book.

Cocaine Hotline. (800)-COCAINE (24-hour information service).

Coc-Anon Family Groups, P.O. Box 64742-66, Los Angeles, CA 90064. (213) 859-2206.

Families Anonymous, Inc., P.O. Box 528, Van Nuys, CA 91408. (818) 989-7841.

Institute on Black Chemical Abuse, 2616 Nicollet Avenue, Minneapolis, MN 55408. (612) 871-7878.

Nar-Anon Family Group Headquarters, World Service Office, P.O. Box 2562, Palos Verdes Peninsula, CA 92704. (213) 547-5800.

Narcotics Anonymous and NA hotline. Check the local phone book.

National Institute on Drug Abuse Hotline. (800) 662-HELP.

For written information:

National Clearinghouse for Alcohol and Drug Information, P.O. Box 2345, Rockville, MD 20852. (301) 468-2600.

American Council for Drug Education, 204 Monroe Street, Suite 110, Rockville, MD 20850. (301) 294-0600.

For help in starting prevention programs in your community or workplace:

National Federation of Parents for Drug-Free Youth, 1423 N. Jefferson, Springfield, MO 65802-1988. (417) 836-3709.

National Institute on Drug Abuse/The Drug-Free Workplace Helpline. (800) 843-4971.

Books:

Adult Children of Alcoholics, by Janet Woitetz. Deerfield Beach, FL: Health Communications, Inc., 1983. [201 S.W. 15th Street] (800) COCAINE.

Choices and Consequences: What to Do When a Teenager Uses Alcohol/Drugs, by Dick Schaefer. Minneapolis: Johnson Institute Books, 1987. (800) 231-5165.

Codependent No More, by Melody Beattie. New York: Harper & Row, 1988.

Kids and Drugs: A Handbook for Parents and Professionals, by Joyce Tobias, R.N. Annandale, VA: Panda Press, 1989. (703) 750-9285.

Drugs and the Whole Person, by D. Duncon and R. Gold. New York: John Wiley and Sons, 1982.

Healthier Workers: The Role of Health Promotion and Employee Assistance Programs, by Martin Shain, H. Suurvali, and M. Boutiliere. Lexington, MA: Lexington Books, 1986. [Distributed by D.C. Heath Company, 2700 Richardt Avenue, Indianapolis, IN 46219]

Hope: New Choices and Recovery Strategies for Adult Children of Alcoholics, by Emily Marlin. New York: Harper & Row, 1987.

Not My Kid: A Parent's Guide to Kids and Drugs, by Beth Polson and Miller Newton. New York: Avon Paperback Books, 1985.

When Society Becomes an Addict, by Anne Wilson Schaef. New York: Harper & Row, 1987.

White Rabbit: A Woman Doctor's Story of Addiction and Recovery, by Martha A. Morrison, M.D. New York: Crown Publications, 1988.

CREATING A HEALTHY ENVIRONMENT

*F*or better or for worse, the environment is a major influence on our health. On the one hand, we still benefit from the public health measures that eliminated so much of the contagion and early death that were common in the 19th and early 20th centuries. These include better sanitation and adequate housing. On the other hand, we are subject to smog, cigarette smoke, diesel exhaust, sick buildings, dirty beaches, microwaves, video display terminals (VDTs), the roar of jets, radon seeping into our basements and toxins spewing from smokestacks. We have witnessed the Love Canal, Bhopal and Exxon Valdez disasters. And we worry about the well-being of an "Endangered Earth"—*Time* magazine's Planet of the Year in 1988—as we face the dangers of atmospheric warming, destruction of tropical forests, a thinning ozone layer and soaring population.

Although global issues may seem beyond our control, we owe it to ourselves and our children to keep informed about these matters and to make our views known in appropriate settings —town meetings, letters to the editor and the ballot box. Moreover, there are a number of choices we can all make to improve life on our planet. We can conserve energy by driving smaller cars, taking public transportation, turning off lights and modulating the thermostat in summer and winter. We can recycle newspapers, office paper and cans, use yard clippings for mulch, and buy long-lasting tires. (Each year, the United States produces 160 million tons of solid waste —garbage.) We can opt for biodegradable and recyclable packaging over bulky and one-time-only plastics.

There are also many actions we can take to improve our personal environment. We can make sure that our homes are well-ventilated, well-lit and noise-free. We can minimize our use of household products that emit volatile fumes, shun harmful aerosols and say no to pesticides. Choosing to walk

Good Ozone and Bad

The ground-level variety of ozone, a dangerous pollutant, should not be confused with a second environmental concern, the loss of "good" ozone in the upper atmosphere. A layer of natural ozone high in the sky absorbs a large part of the sun's ultraviolet radiation. Scientists believe that this protective layer is thinning, largely as the result of chlorofluorocarbon gases (CFCs) released from spray cans, air conditioning units, refrigerators, foam insulation and solvents. It is feared that as more ultraviolet radiation reaches the earth the incidence of skin cancer and perhaps of cataracts will rise.

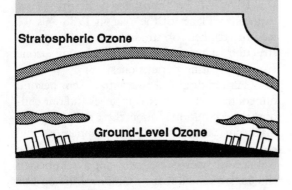

or bike instead of taking the car is not only good for the environment, it is good for our bodies as well.

Environment and Health

The effects of the environment on health are complex. Because we are exposed to so many different things over a lifetime, it is often difficult to single out the contribution of a single substance. Many of the studies showing that a certain pollutant can cause cancer, for instance, were made in the workplace, where the relationship was clearcut. This is because, in certain cases, the exposure was high. Although we may come into contact with many potentially dangerous pollutants in our daily lives, the levels tend to be very low. At the same time, these substances may be hard to avoid.

Overall, there is a good deal of evidence supporting the old-fashioned notion that clean air, clean water and "elbow room" are good for you. For example, several studies have shown that people in rural areas are healthier and live longer than city dwellers—even though there are more doctors and hospitals in metropolitan areas. It also appears that mental illness is more common in our cities. Perhaps human beings really do need some elbow room in order to keep their wits about them.

Pollution in the Air

Air becomes polluted with exhaust from cars, emissions from industrial plants and chemical fumes that emanate from countless everyday objects—carpeting, clothing, cleansers and cosmetics. When you fill up your gas tank, you inhale benzene; traces can be detected in your breath hours later. Stopping by the dry cleaner's exposes you to a lingering dose of tetrachloroethylene. Air also becomes polluted with cigarette smoke and the thousands of chemicals it contains.

Polluted air irritates the eyes and skin, and it poisons the lungs. It presents a health hazard to everyone, but especially to persons who already have breathing problems. As the air pollution index goes up, emergency rooms and doctors' offices fill with people who have asthma, emphysema and other respiratory illnesses. Medications can be of some help to these people, but the best remedy is to stay out of the polluted air.

Air pollution is known to increase a smoker's chances of getting lung cancer, and it can probably cause cancer all by itself. The death rate due to lung cancer in Los Angeles is greater than that in Chicago, apparently because of heavy air pollution in the Los Angeles basin. Airborne cancer-causing agents can enter the body through the skin as well as the lungs, and once they get in the bloodstream they can reach any organ. Polluted air can also endanger persons with diseases of the heart and blood vessels.

At times the toxicity of air pollution is dramatized by "killer smogs," such as the one that caused 4,000 deaths in London in 1952, and the one that struck Donora, Pennsylvania, in 1948, when half of the town's 12,300 residents fell ill and 20 people died.

The Major Offenders

Since the Clean Air Act was passed in 1970, the government has targeted half a dozen highly toxic airborne pollutants: ozone, carbon monoxide, sulfur dioxide, nitrogen oxides, airborne particulates and lead. Almost everyone agrees that air quality has improved in the past two decades, even in such well-known pollution pockets as Los Angeles and Denver. Still, most Americans live in areas where at least one major pollutant still exceeds federal standards.

Ozone, a form of oxygen, is a pungent and very reactive gas that interacts with almost every material with which it comes into contact. Ozone is formed by a chemical reaction, when sunlight acts on two types of pollutants, nitrogen oxides and hydrocarbons. These are both discharged by motor vehicles and industry.

Ozone is the major component of the hazy mixture of more than 100 chemicals known as smog; smog pollution is often expressed as the "ozone level." As you might expect, ozone pollution is at its worst in hot, sunny weather; levels are highest after the morning rush hour.

Because it tends to break down tissues and cells, ozone irritates the membranes lining the mouth, throat and lungs; people cough, choke, develop chest pain and have trouble breathing. When healthy people try to exercise even at low ozone concentrations, they experience a significant drop in lung function after a few hours. Like other air pollutants, ozone can aggravate chronic lung diseases, such as asthma and bronchitis. Moreover, it can be lethal for persons whose health is frail, because it reduces the lungs' ability to defend themselves against viruses and bacteria. It may also cause premature aging of lung tissue. (What's more, ozone can severely damage crops.)

The ozone standard set in 1979 as acceptable is .12 ppm (parts per million). However, more recent research has found that levels lower than .12

Urban Exercising

Running by the roadside may be less than marvelous for your health when the traffic is heavy and the weather is steamy. In summer, ozone builds during the morning rush hour and peaks late in the afternoon, so time your exercise accordingly. Run or walk in the early morning, before ozone has a chance to build.

Winter is another story. Although there is less ozone in winter, a blanket of other auto emissions—including carbon monoxide, nitrogen dioxide and sulfur dioxide—can be trapped by the cold nighttime air. In cold weather, it's better to exercise in the evening. (Whatever the weather, it always makes sense to avoid heavily trafficked areas where cars are idling and buses are belching out fumes.)

ppm can affect even healthy people, and that damage accumulates over time. Studies at the University of Arizona Medical School have shown that children with asthma lose lung power at .055 ppm, begin wheezing at .08 ppm, and at .12 ppm suffer outright asthma attacks.

The use of unleaded gasoline and catalytic converters (which transform noxious gases into less harmful forms) has cut hazardous emissions for the average automobile by at least 75 percent. But the growing number of vehicles on the road—up by about 25 percent between 1977 and 1988, according to the National Highway Traffic Safety Administration—has made it hard to pull ahead. In 1988 ozone/smog nearly doubled from 1987 levels in many Eastern cities. In sunny, car-riddled Los Angeles, levels have dropped markedly in the past two decades, but they still exceed the safe levels for more than half of the days in each year.

Carbon monoxide, a colorless, odorless, poisonous gas, forms when carbon-containing fuel is not burned completely—for instance, when cars are starting up, idling or crawling in heavy traffic. Most of this pollutant, the nation's most common, comes from gasoline-fueled cars and trucks. Al-

Acid Rain

Acid rain is the name given to rain or snow that has picked up damaging pollutants. Its main components are sulfur dioxide from older, coal-fueled power plants and smelters, and nitrogen oxides, primarily from auto engines and utility plants. These emissions interact with sunlight and water vapor in the upper atmosphere to form acidic particles. The sulfur dioxide combines with water vapor in the atmosphere to form sulfuric acid. The acid particles are carried hundreds of miles by prevailing winds, typically from plants in the Midwest to the Northeast and southeastern Canada. Once liquified, they fall as rain or snow that is 10 to 100 times more acidic than normal rain. Acid rain can also carry toxic chemicals such as arsenic and selenium.

Acid rain causes severe environmental damage. It ruins trees and kills fish and plant life in lakes and rivers. It erodes stone buildings and monuments. It is also thought to damage health, aggravate respiratory symptoms and decrease lung function. Harvard researchers participating in the federally funded Six Cities Study, which is investigating the health impact of sulfur dioxide, sulfates and particulates, have concluded that acid in the air may be responsible for as many as 100,000 deaths in this country each year. Acid rain has also been linked to unhealthy levels of toxic metals in drinking water and in fish that we eat.

though carbon monoxide does not build up in the atmosphere overall, it can reach dangerous levels in neighborhoods with high-rises, lots of traffic and little wind.

Figure 14.1

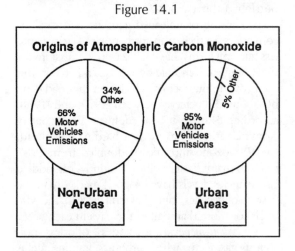

Tragic stories of families being poisoned when carbon monoxide seeped into the house from a motor that was accidentally left running in the garage illustrate all too well the danger of this gas. Inhaled, it replaces life-sustaining oxygen in red blood cells, cutting the supplies to body tissues. The brain is quickly affected; thinking slows and so do reflexes. At low levels carbon monoxide can cause fatigue in healthy persons and chest pain in people with heart disease. At higher levels, it can cause headaches, dizziness, weakness, nausea, confusion and disorientation. At very high levels it can cause heart or breathing failure.

Sulfur dioxide and its relatives cause the "rotten egg" smell enveloping many power plants and refineries that burn such sulfur-containing fuels as coal and oil. Sulfur dioxide is also released from smelting and certain other industrial processes.

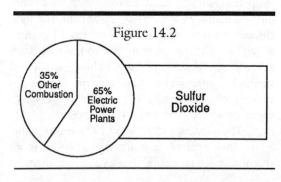

Figure 14.2

This invisible gas can make it difficult to breathe and produce a choking effect. It can cause coughing and throat irritation in healthy people, and even low levels can spell trouble for people who are highly sensitive—persons with asthma, emphysema, bronchitis or allergies, as well as heart patients, the very young, the very old and pregnant women. In people with asthma, for example, exposure to sulfur dioxide can trigger a severe reaction that lasts for an hour or more.

Government standards stipulate how much sulfur dioxide a plant can emit over a 24-hour period, but short-term bursts can be many times higher than the 24-hour average and still be "legal." As recently as 1988 the Environmental Protection Agency (EPA) declined to change the standards, since *only* 100,000 asthmatics and 200,000 allergy sufferers live near sulfur-spewing plants and refineries. And the effects of sulfur pollution are multiplied by the presence of other pollutants, such as particulates.

Nitrogen oxides, including nitrogen dioxide, are suffocating, highly reactive gases that are formed from nitrogen, which is abundant in the air, when fossil fuels are burned at high temperatures. Fossil fuels are coal, oil and natural gas. Most nitrogen oxides come from power plants and other industrial boilers, and gasoline engines.

At lower levels nitrogen oxides work like ozone, irritating the eyes, nose and lungs. Prolonged or high exposure can trigger bronchitis and lower resistance to respiratory infections, such as influenza. Animal studies show that exposure may also contribute to emphysema, and perhaps pose a threat to people with liver, hormone and blood

The Greenhouse Effect

A number of gases, including carbon dioxide, CFCs, methane (released from natural gas and decomposing garbage), and nitrous oxide, have increased dramatically in the atmosphere, creating a blanket that traps heat and sends it back to earth. Scientists are concerned that temperatures inside this global "greenhouse" are rising, setting off major changes in sea level, rainfall patterns and agriculture. The greenhouse gases are released by the burning of fossil fuels and industrial processes. They also result from the widespread cutting of trees in developing countries; whereas living trees soak up excess carbon dioxide, trees that are burned or left to rot release it.

Table 14.1
U.S. Sources of Carbon Dioxide

Electric Power Plants	33%
Motor Vehicles	31%
Factories	24%
Buildings (Heating)	12%

disorders. At high levels, nitrogen oxides can be fatal. Importantly, nitrogen oxides and their by-products are major ingredients in smog.

Particulates are bits of dust, soot, smoke or other substances—often toxic—that are small

Figure 14.3

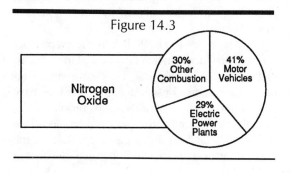

Nitrogen Oxide

41% Motor Vehicles
30% Other Combustion
29% Electric Power Plants

Table 14.2
Primary Sources of Particulates

Agricultural Burning and Wood Stoves
Windblown Dust
Factories
Motor Vehicles
Power Plants and Waste-Disposal Incinerators

enough to remain suspended in air and be inhaled. The smaller the particles, the more deeply they can penetrate the lungs, where they lodge.

Some particles simply clog lung structures. For instance, the black lung of coal miners and the asbestosis of workers exposed to asbestos fibers are caused in this way. Other particles undergo a chemical change and pass through the lung into the bloodstream; this can happen with inhaled lead and other metals. Certain cancer-causing substances, including radon (see below) and benzopyrenes, attach to particles and get a free ride deep into the lung. What's more, particulates are often found in the company of sulfur oxides, a combination that is, according to many studies, a peril to respiratory health.

Lead in the air comes from vehicles that burn leaded gasoline and smelters of industries that process lead. Inhaled and absorbed into the bloodstream, particles and fumes of this toxic metal can cause brain and nerve damage in children and unborn infants. Lead has also been linked to slowed growth, low birth weight and minor hearing impairment. In adults, high blood levels of lead can cause kidney disease, and even minor lead exposure appears to raise blood pressure. Today, thanks to the catalytic converter, which cannot work with leaded fuel, lead levels in the air have dropped dramatically. (Lead can also contaminate drinking water, as discussed below.)

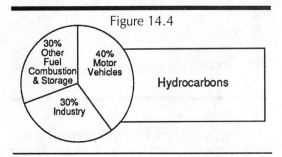

Figure 14.4

30% Other Fuel Combustion & Storage

40% Motor Vehicles

30% Industry

Hydrocarbons

Hydrocarbons are the gaseous form of unburned fossil fuels, such as gasoline, which are made up of various combinations of hydrogen and carbon. Most of the hydrocarbons in the air come from gasoline vapors that seep from gas tanks or fuel lines or escape from tail pipes. Others are released from the gas pump, while yet others come from solvents, paints and dry-cleaning fluids.

While hydrocarbons are not one of the major airborne pollutants, the government monitors their emission because of their role in the formation of ozone/smog.

Then there is the thorny issue of so-called *hazardous pollutants*. These poisons, which include such toxic metals as cadmium, mercury and beryllium, and toxic organic compounds, such as vinyl chloride and benzene, come from many sources, including industry, waste disposal and motor vehicles. They are primarily inhaled, but you can also encounter them in produce or fish that has become contaminated.

Although the Clean Air Act calls for the regulation of more than 300 such contaminants—including scores of substances that can cause cancer, birth defects and miscarriages—emissions are regulated for just a handful. Ironically, industries that now comply with emission standards for such pollutants as particulates may still be venting tons of other toxins.

A prime example of a hazardous pollutant (one that *is* regulated) is the family of organic compounds known as *PCBs* (polychlorinated biphenyls). PCBs, which take several decades to decompose, have leaked into the environment from faulty electrical equipment and from materials such as inks. They can be absorbed through the skin, inhaled or eaten in contaminated food. Once PCBs start moving along the food chain from plants and small aquatic animals to birds and larger animals, they become increasingly concentrated. Within the human body they accumulate in high amounts in fatty tissue and breast milk and in lesser amounts in many organs.

Even at low levels, PCBs can affect reproduction and produce stomach disorders, skin problems and cancers in lab animals. They can reduce supplies of commercial fish. At high levels they have been found to cause serious health problems. Although their manufacture has been banned since 1976 and their uses are being phased out, some 400 million pounds are still being used or stored in the United States, and they continue to be produced as byproducts during the manufacture of certain organic chemicals.

The environment is already loaded with PCBs. Some 150 million pounds have permeated soil, water, fish, and human milk and tissue, and virtually every person in the country has "trace" amounts of PCB in his or her body. A 1987 study showed that the milk of nursing Eskimo women in northern Quebec, women who eat large amounts of fish and animal fat, contained the highest levels of PCBs in the world (an average of 3.59 ppm, with some as high as 14.7 ppm, compared to 0.76 ppm for other Canadian women who were tested).

The greatest risk of PCB exposure today is through fires involving electrical transformers made with the chemicals. Everything used to control such fires—water, foam and hoses—as well as everything the smoke touches can become contaminated. One 18-story office building in upstate New York needed such extensive cleaning that the building had to be closed for years after the fire, with cleanup costs outstripping the original construction cost.

Another hazardous pollutant that has been regulated is *asbestos*, a fibrous mineral that has been widely used in insulation, automobile brake linings and many industrial processes. Too fine to see, asbestos fibers float in the air. Breathed in, they accumulate in the lung where they trigger disease, most notably cancer—as many as 12,000 cases a year, almost all of them fatal. Asbestos is the only known cause of a cancer of the membranes lining the chest and abdomen called mesothelioma. It can also cause lung cancer. The dangers of asbestos are greatest for smokers: Asbestos insulators who smoke have a lung-cancer risk more than 50 times that of non-smokers without asbestos exposure. About 65,000 Americans suffer from asbestosis, a gradual scarring of the lungs that makes it hard to breathe and eventually kills.

Asbestos-related diseases have been most evident among workers exposed to high levels of asbestos on the job, including shipbuilders and auto mechanics. However, no level of exposure is considered safe, since some people have developed

Asbestos in the Home

Asbestos products can show up in many parts of your house—vinyl floor tiles, textured paints, ceilings, furnace or pipe insulation, roofing, or siding. Often such products don't pose a problem unless they are damaged or severely worn. If it becomes necessary to remove or repair asbestos-containing materials, take these precautions:

- Get help from a contractor trained and experienced in working with asbestos. (Most home-repair contractors do not meet this requirement.)
- Keep in mind that removal, which stirs up and releases asbestos fibers, is a last resort; covering the material is preferred.
- Never dust, sweep or vacuum particles suspected to contain asbestos; this just sends them into the air. Asbestos fibers are too tiny to be trapped by ordinary vacuum cleaner filters. The dust should be removed by a wet-mopping procedure or with specially designed vacuums used by trained asbestos contractors.

mesothelioma after brief or low-level exposure. Moreover, families of asbestos workers are at risk from fibers carried home or into the car on clothing and hair.

The dangers of asbestos are greatest with products that are easily crumbled; a prime example is the fluffy, sprayed-on asbestos used in many buildings for fireproofing, insulating and soundproofing. This use is now banned, and precautions must be taken whenever asbestos is being handled. However, asbestos continues to be used. It is still a part of brake linings, for instance, and during brake and clutch servicing asbestos fibers are readily released. This poses a hazard not only for the mechanic, but for everyone in the garage, including the customers.

Indoor Air Pollution

The newest frontier in pollution control is the great indoors. Our homes and offices, increasingly air-tight in an energy-conscious society, are loaded with potential pollutants. These include fumes from typewriter correction fluid, clothes from the dry cleaner, bathroom cleanser, moth cakes, hair spray and bug spray. Pollutants come from tobacco smoke, gas ranges, space heaters, chlorinated water, furniture and air fresheners. The risk is not minor: Most people spend about 90 percent of their time in enclosed structures, including their cars; the people most susceptible to pollution—the very young, the old, and the ill—spend nearly all of their time indoors. It is estimated that such pollution may cost several hundred lives each year.

Volatile Chemicals

A recent EPA study shows that in terms of potentially toxic volatile chemicals (chemicals that release vapors into the air), many Americans encounter more pollution within the walls of their own homes than outdoors—even if they live in big cities or along industrial corridors. EPA researchers measured the concentration of about 20 potentially toxic substances in the blood, breath and urine of several hundred volunteers, and also in the air outdoors. The chemicals included *formaldehyde*, which is used in furniture, foam insulation and pressed wood; *perchlorethylene*, used by dry cleaners; and chemicals from cosmetics. Other common indoor pollutants are *benzene* (a known carcinogen), which we encounter in stored fuels and paint supplies as well as tobacco smoke and auto emissions, and *methylene chloride*, which enters our lives in paint strippers, aerosol spray paints and pesticide "bombs."

The EPA study found that levels of all the chemicals tested were much higher indoors than outdoors—sometimes 100 times higher. This was equally true in heavily industrialized cities in New Jersey, a light industry area in North Carolina, and a rural section of North Dakota.

Further EPA studies of air samples from public buildings (offices, hospitals, homes for the aged and a school) disclosed more than 500 chemicals. They were emitted by many sources—building materials, furnishings, paint and so on. And many of the sources emitted several chemicals. Brand-new office buildings were the biggest offenders; in general the levels of the chemicals dropped markedly by the end of the first year, but they still exceeded outdoor levels.

Such chemicals can produce a number of health effects, including irritation of the eyes, nose and throat; blurred vision; and memory impairment. Many cause cancer in animals; some, such as benzene, cause cancer in people. The long-term effects from the levels found in houses are not known. When using household chemicals, be sure to follow instructions carefully, and keep your work area well-ventilated. Store products in a place that is well-ventilated and safely out of children's reach.

Environmental Tobacco Smoke

Environmental tobacco smoke, which comes from the burning end of a cigarette and smoke exhaled by smokers, contains thousands of compounds, including benzene, styrene, xylene and ethylbenzene. Not only can benzene be detected in the breath of smokers, benzene levels are 30 percent to 50 percent higher in the homes of smokers than in those of non-smokers.

Environmental tobacco smoke irritates the eyes, nose and throat, and it can trigger a variety of respiratory symptoms. Its adverse effects are especially evident in the children of smokers. And the more the parents smoke, the worse the problems. The children of smokers risk such symptoms as wheezing and coughing, as well as such infections as pneumonia and bronchitis, and perhaps chronic ear infections. There is also evidence that parental smoking may affect the rate of children's lung growth, and perhaps their growth in general. And non-smoking pregnant women married to men who smoke have been reported to give birth to babies with lower birth weights than babies born to non-smoking couples. An excess of leukemia has also been reported among the children of smokers.

Exposure to environmental tobacco smoke also makes lung cancer more likely. The lung-cancer risk is about 30 percent higher for the non-smoking spouses of smokers than for non-smokers married to non-smokers. Environmental tobacco smoke may also contribute to heart disease.

Ventilation reduces, but does not eliminate, exposure to tobacco smoke. And because tobacco smoke is loaded with pollutants, ventilation systems can't clear them out of the air as quickly as they build up. The moral: Don't smoke, and discourage others from smoking in your home (or office or car).

Where There's Fire ...

Many other pollutants enter the air in our homes from things we burn. Whenever we turn on a gas stove, light a fireplace or woodstove, or use an unvented kerosene or gas space heater, we can be exposed to carbon monoxide, nitrogen dioxide and particulates. The problem can be worsened by chimneys and flues that are not working properly.

Here's what you can do to reduce exposure:

- Use exhaust fans over gas cooking stoves, and keep the burners properly adjusted. (The flame tip should be blue, not yellow.)
- Have furnaces, flues and chimneys inspected yearly, and promptly repair cracks and damage. Change filters often.
- If you use an unvented space heater, use the proper fuel, keep the heater properly adjusted, and air the room well.
- When using a wood stove, make sure its doors fit tightly and keep emissions to a minimum.

Radon

Radon is a serious indoor pollutant. An invisible radioactive gas produced by the breakdown of naturally occurring uranium in rocks and soil, radon can seep into buildings through cracks in basement floors and walls and through floor drains. It can also be released into the air from water drawn from radon-contaminated wells while the water is being used—for showers, baths, laundry or washing dishes. Outdoor levels are low, but once it is trapped within a building, radon builds to dangerous levels.

Like the radiation in X-rays, uranium and nuclear reactions, radon can cause cancer. Inhaled,

Radon Testing

Two types of radon detectors are popular for home use; both are exposed to the air in your home for a certain period and then sent to a laboratory for analysis. Charcoal canisters are exposed for two to seven days and cost between $10 and $25 per canister. Alpha track detectors are set out for several weeks, and cost $20 to $50 apiece.

You can do your own testing or have it performed by a private firm. Canisters are sold at many supermarkets and hardware stores, and in some areas local governments provide radon detectors. If you choose a private firm, be wary: Some dishonest persons have entered the radon-testing business, using everything from Geiger counters to divining rods to mayonnaise jars.

The first step is to take a short-term "screening" measurement, to get an idea of the highest radon level in your home. This measurement should be made in the lowest livable area of your house—the basement, if there is one. All windows and doors need to be closed for at least 12 hours prior to the test and throughout the testing period. If the reading exceeds 4 picocuries per liter, you will want to take further tests throughout the house.

it can trigger cancerous changes in the lungs. Radon is by far the single largest source of radiation for the average person, and it is thought to cause some 5,000 to 20,000 lung-cancer deaths in the United States each year. The higher and longer one's exposure, the greater the risk, but the greatest risk of all is among smokers.

The government's "action level" (the point at which some changes are warranted) is 4 picocuries per liter of air. In surveys made by the EPA, between one-third and one-fifth of the thousands of houses that were sampled exceeded that level; in some houses readings reached 200 picocuries per liter—1,000 times the outdoor level, and a greater lung-cancer risk than smoking four packs a day.

All told, EPA estimates that as many as 8 million American homes may have a radon problem. However, no one knows just which houses are affected. Certain regions of the country have more of the types of rocks or minerals that might release radon, but radon levels can vary widely even within the same community. You can check with your state radiation protection office to see if high levels have been discovered in your area, but the only way to know for sure is to have your house tested.

If these test results show high levels, you'll want to take corrective action. And the higher the level, the more quickly you should act. If levels exceed 200 picocuries per liter, you should get the problem fixed within a few weeks. If you cannot, consider temporarily moving out.

When radon levels are high, permanent solutions sometimes require major remodeling and professional advice. One solution is to install a ventilation system below the basement "slab." Another approach is to improve house-wide ventilation by putting in an air-to-air heat exchanger.

In the short-term, here are some quick and inexpensive steps to take:

- Stop smoking and discourage smoking in your home. Studies show that smoking may increase the risk of cancer associated with radon.
- Spend less time in areas that have higher levels of radon, such as the basement.
- Open windows and turn on fans to increase air flow—especially in the basement. (To prevent drawing in more radon, keep windows open when using outdoor-vented exhaust fans. Open windows evenly on all sides of the home.)
- If your house has a crawl space, keep all the vents fully open.
- Seal cracks and other openings in the basement floor.
- Aerate radon-contaminated well water or filter it through granulated activated charcoal.

Bugs, Molds and Other Mementos of Nature

The air in homes and offices can pick up a variety of biological contaminants capable of causing allergy or illness. For instance, plants can produce pollen, pets can import germs, air conditioners and humidifiers can become breeding grounds for mold, mildew and the bacteria that cause Legionnaire's disease. House-dust mites, a potent cause of asthma and other allergic reactions, also thrive in dampness.

The best way to curb the growth of these contaminants is to control the humidity. The recommended relative humidity for homes is between 30 percent and 50 percent. Use exhaust fans in kitchens and bathrooms, and vent clothes dryers outdoors. Ventilate your attic and crawl spaces. Promptly dry water-damaged carpets and furnishings. And if you use cool-mist or ultrasonic humidifiers, clean water trays daily. Do the same for evaporation trays in air conditioners, dehumidifiers, and refrigerators. And be mindful of water trays under houseplants.

PESTICIDES

Crawly critters inside the house are not very popular: Nine out of 10 American households use chemicals to kill pests. The most obvious danger of pesticides comes from accidental spills and ingestion. However, these chemicals can also pose a long-term threat to both the environment and human health by infiltrating air, water and land.

Scientists have found traces of as many as 12 different pesticides in a single home, so it is not surprising that most exposure to pesticides in the air occurs indoors—some during use, some during storage and some from vapors that float in from outdoors.

More than 34,000 pesticides, derived from about 600 basic ingredients, are currently registered for use, and new ones come on the market each year. Both active (bug-killing) ingredients and "inert" carrier agents, such as methylene chloride, can pose dangers to human health. Many have been shown to cause cancer in animals, and some

The Sick-Building Syndrome

The sleek white marble walls that encase the Library of Congress's James Madison Memorial Building give little clue to trouble within. Yet ever since the early 1980s, when the massive annex opened in the nation's capital, workers have complained of headaches, rashes and sinus problems. This is a textbook case of the sick-building syndrome, in which many of the people who work (or, less frequently, live) in a certain building develop a variety of symptoms—eye, nose and throat irritation, a stuffy or runny nose, fatigue or lethargy, headache, dizziness, nausea, irritability and forgetfulness. The problems typically clear up when the person gets away from the building.

Of course, these symptoms are very common and only rarely will be caused by the sick-building syndrome. This makes it hard to investigate the possibility that this problem exists. In fact, at times just asking about these symptoms has convinced a building's residents that they had them and that the cause was the sick-building syndrome, when in fact there was no problem with the building. Some of these cases may have been due to the power of suggestion.

In contrast to individual "building-related illnesses" that can be traced to specific causes, such as Legionnaire's disease or humidifier fever, the complaints that characterize the sick-building syndrome don't fit the pattern of any single illness and are difficult to trace to any one source. Poor indoor air quality seems to be a major culprit, along with poor lighting, noise, vibration, temperatures that are too high or too low, and stress. Vapors can come from an array of sources—building materials, paint, furnishings, cleaning materials, pesticides, copy machines and tobacco smoke. Pollutants can also be drawn in from parking garages or vents from rest rooms or the boiler room. The problem can be aggravated if the ventilation system is poorly designed or if, in the interest of saving energy, it is run below capacity.

Methods to diagnose and cure sick-buildings are evolving. For example, new technology now makes it possible to detect a pollutant that is present in the amount of not one part per million, but one part per quadrillion (1 followed by 15 zeros). In 1989 the government, taking advantage of all the latest methods, launched a study designed to serve as a model for the entire country as well as to clear the air at the Library of Congress.

If you suspect you are a victim of the sick-building syndrome, here are some things you can do:

- Consider other causes of your symptoms. These symptoms are common and usually are *not* caused by the sick-building syndrome.
- Discuss your symptoms with your doctor, and report your problems to the company doctor or nurse.
- Check with your supervisor, other workers and union representatives to see if others are in the same boat—and urge that a record of complaints be kept. But remember that just asking about symptoms sometimes convinces people that there is a problem.
- If the sick-building syndrome seems likely, see if an experienced company can be hired to identify possible sources of the problem and solutions.
- Contact your local health department or air pollution control agency.

Integrated Pest Management

The latest word in pest control is a kinder, gentler strategy called integrated pest management (IPM). IPM is an ecological approach that combines new technology with old-fashioned methods, tailoring solutions to fit the nature of the pest and how it lives. Although IPM can include the use of pesticides, it emphasizes non-chemical alternatives. Controlling cockroaches, for instance, starts with lowering the temperature, removing food, eliminating moisture, reducing clutter and caulking hiding spaces, such as cracks and crevices. Only if these methods fail are pesticides called upon—and for cockroaches the most effective, least toxic and cheapest one is 99 percent boric acid dusted into cracks.

in people. For example, a 1987 National Cancer Institute study showed that Kansas farmers who used the chemical 2,4-D—a popular herbicide in agriculture and home lawn-care products—were more likely to develop cancer than farmers who did not.

Several older pesticides, as was belatedly learned, can remain in the environment for many years. A buildup of DDT threatened the survival of many birds in the 1970s, including ospreys and bald eagles. A group of chemicals popular for zapping termites in their underground lairs—chlordane, heptachlor, aldrin and dieldrin—were found to seep into the air in treated houses; traces could still be found a year later. Although the use of these chemicals has been either banned or restricted, even DDT continues to make its way into the environment in several ways, notably as a byproduct of another pesticide ingredient, dicofol.

In high levels, such chemicals can produce headaches, dizziness, muscle twitching, weakness, tingling and nausea. They may also cause long-term damage to the liver and central nervous system, and increase the risk of cancer.

Not only do pesticides pose risks to health and the environment, heavy use of these chemicals is creating hundreds of "super pests" that are resistant to their effects. (Meanwhile "beneficial" insects, natural enemies of the pests, continue to succumb.) Moreover, several dozen species of weeds have grown resistant to herbicides. It appears that chemicals can actually alter the physiology of desirable plants, making them *more* vulnerable to insect damage.

To minimize your exposure to toxic chemicals, use pesticides only when necessary. Learn to live with a few weeds, some less-than-perfect garden vegetables and an occasional mosquito attack. Discourage pests by cutting off their supplies of water and food: fix leaky plumbing; remove empty glasses; put food away—your pet's as well as your own; and cover garbage tightly. Get rid of their shelter and breeding sites: caulk cracks; remove wood piles; clear away fallen fruit; and clean up pet feces, litter and standing water.

Try non-chemical alternatives. Encourage natural predators—purple martins, lady bugs and praying mantises. Fight pests with pests: A bacterium called *Bacillus thuringiensis*, for instance, is an important weapon in the battle against the leaf-devouring gypsy moth. Choose hardy, disease-resistant plants. Exploit tricks of landscape design, spacing and crop rotation. (Experiments at the Pennsylvania State University have shown that harmful rootworms can be tempted out of corn crops by planting borders of squash and sunflowers.) Attack weeds with a hoe or by hand. Try mousetraps, mosquito netting and a fly swatter.

If you decide a pesticide is needed, take these precautions:

- Read the label carefully, and exercise both caution and restraint.
- Buy or prepare only as much as you will need.
- Air out your house well.

When applying pesticides to your lawn or garden, remember to:

- Choose a day that is not windy.
- Use coarse-droplet nozzles to reduce misting.

- Apply the spray as close to the target as possible.
- Shower and shampoo thoroughly afterwards.

TOXINS ON THE TABLE

Over a lifetime, the major source of pesticides for most people is diet. Fruits and vegetables, grains, meat, poultry and eggs are all likely to contain measurable pesticide residues. Our drinking water often contains low levels of pesticides, too. Some trickle down into water supplies from farms and lawns; others are discharged into lakes and rivers by industry.

The amounts of most pesticides in our food are very small. The government sets allowable limits, generally more than 100 to 1,000 times lower than the level that has been found to have any effect on test animals. And in 1987 only 1 percent of the food products sampled by the government had residues exceeding these limits. (Three percent contained residues of pesticides for which no limits had yet been set.)

Still, potentially harmful chemicals creep into the food chain in various ways. Sometimes it takes years or decades for the government to get rid of suspected sources of trouble. Four years after animal tests suggested that daminozide (trade name Alar) and one of its breakdown products might cause cancer, the EPA was unable to decide on a ban. Though apple growers had promised to stop using it, residues showed up in 30 percent to more than 50 percent of the apples and apple juice on grocers' shelves.

Sometimes contaminants follow an indirect route to the table. For instance, in 1986 it was discovered that an Arkansas firm was using discarded seed treated with heptachlor and other pesticides to make fuel-grade alcohol, then selling the leftover "mash" as animal feed to dairy farmers. The feed contained heptachlor levels more than 1,000 times higher than the allowable limits. Cows that ate it produced milk in which the pesticide exceeded 120 times the allowable level.

Contaminated fish are another source of

Pesticide Poisoning

According to the U.S. Consumer Product Safety Commission, pesticides are second only to medicines as a cause of poisoning in young children. In 1985, an estimated 20,000 people were rushed to emergency rooms due to suspected or actual exposure to toxic levels of pesticides—and one-tenth of them were admitted to the hospital for further treatment.

Before you use a pesticide, read the label carefully. For one thing, it's illegal to use a pesticide except as specified. Should the substance be accidentally swallowed, inhaled or absorbed through the skin, the label states what type of treatment is appropriate. ("Danger" on the label means the chemical is highly poisonous, "warning" means moderately poisonous, and "caution" means least dangerous.)

Should pesticide poisoning occur, you need to apply speedy first aid. If the poison was inhaled, get the victim into the fresh air. If it was splashed or spilled onto the skin or into the eye, wash the chemical off with water. If the pesticide was swallowed, the person should rinse his or her mouth with water, then drink up to a quart of milk or water to dilute the poison. (Vomiting should be induced *only* if the label specifically says so.)

Then get medical help immediately. And remember to bring the container with you, so the doctor can see what chemicals are involved.

You can get help in an emergency by calling a 24-hour toll-free hotline run by the federally funded National Pesticide Telecommunications Network: (800) 858-7378.

chemicals in the diet, although this contamination is more likely to come from industrial waste than pesticides. Many fresh-water fish, especially those from the Great Lakes, have been contaminated

Lead Paint

The use of lead-based paints in housing has been banned since the 1970s, but most houses built before 1960 contain some lead paint. Lead can be present in household dust, and children are sometimes drawn to eat sweet-tasting paint flakes. One study found that more than 780,000 cases of lead poisoning occurred in American children between 1976 and 1980. If you live in an older house, be careful about your children's exposure to lead. It is probably a good idea to have your child's blood level tested. (Remember that lead can also leach into food from lead-glazed ceramic dishes, especially imports.)

with PCBs as well as *dioxin*, of Agent Orange fame and a byproduct of chemical manufacturing and the processing of paper products. (Just about all of us have dioxin in our bodies, too.) In Japan, fish have caused mercury poisoning; the U.S. Food and Drug Administration now routinely detains swordfish imports until they have passed muster, because they are especially likely to concentrate toxins in their bodies.

The possible risk of eating contaminated fish can be seen in a 1987 study that looked at the babies born to more than 300 American women who had eaten PCB-tainted fish from the Great Lakes two to three times a month during their pregnancy. These babies, the researchers found, weighed seven to nine ounces less at birth than babies born to women who had not eaten contaminated fish; at five months they showed some developmental delays, and at seven months they did not score as well on memory recognition tests.

Here are some things you can do to reduce your intake of pesticides:

- Thoroughly rinse and/or scrub fruits and vegetables. (However, many pesticides are inside these foods and cannot be washed off.)

- Remove the outer leaves of leafy vegetables, such as lettuce.
- Trim the fat from meat and poultry, and discard fats from cooking. This will not only get rid of pesticides, which can concentrate in fat, it will also be good for your arteries.
- Eat fish from a variety of sources, and select smaller fish, which are usually younger and less apt to be polluted.
- Avoid eating fish skin and trim visible fat from fish. Skip the fish liver or the liver-like organs in lobsters or crabs: They concentrate harmful chemicals to very high levels.
- Avoid hunting or fishing in areas where pesticide use is high.
- Pregnant women should limit their consumption of fatty fish (bluefish, salmon, striped bass and swordfish) and fish from fresh waters, especially the Great Lakes.

TOXINS ON TAP

Travelers to the Third World quickly come to appreciate something Americans take for granted —water that is safe to drink, cook with and bathe in. Still, American water supplies contain many potential toxins including asbestos, metals, radioactive substances and industrial chemicals. Some seep into water supplies from natural sources in soil or rocks; some are introduced or created in the process of treating water or piping it; some derive from years of using our rivers as sewers, letting pesticides contaminate groundwater, and burying hazardous wastes in porous landfills.

About half the people in this country get their water from groundwater via wells or springs. This is water that naturally seeps through the soil and is stored in rocky reservoirs below ground. The rest comes from freshwater sources, such as streams and lakes. Water sources can become contaminated in many ways—from pesticides, industrial discharges, underground storage tanks, septic tanks, leaking sewers and landfills. As many as 10 million underground tanks store fuels and other hazardous chemicals; experts predict that 75 percent of them will begin to leak over the next decade unless corrective action is taken. In some parts of Nebraska, the widespread use of fertilizers has polluted the drinking water with nitrate; infants must drink bottled water, and people who use wells must have them tested every month.

Drinking water can also be contaminated by lead, usually from plumbing. Most public water supplies, household faucets and many water fountains contain lead parts. When the plumbing becomes corroded—by too-soft water, for instance, or as a result of grounding electrical equipment such as telephones to water pipes—lead seeps into the water. On the homefront, lead contamination is most likely in houses that are very old (built before 1930, when lead pipes were common), or very new (before mineral deposits from the water have had a chance to build up a protective coating over the lead solder often used on copper pipes).

If you suspect you have too much lead in your water (the recommended limit is 20 parts per billion), get your water tested by a qualified laboratory; your local health department or water utility can steer you in the right direction. In the meantime, don't drink water that's been sitting in the pipes for more than six hours; flush the faucet until the water runs cold. And never drink or cook with water from the hot-water tap; hot water dissolves lead more quickly than cold water.

Water supplies can also become contaminated with disease-causing germs; waterborne illnesses strike an estimated 10,000 Americans each year. In recent years the most common known cause of community-wide waterborne disease has been a parasite called *giardia*, which causes severe diarrhea that can last for months. In a 1988 outbreak in Pittsfield, Massachusetts, *giardia* infected some 3,800 people; for six months in 1984, about 250,000 Pennsylvanians were advised to boil drinking water because of *giardia* contamination. Nor is the threat limited to cities: *giardia* has struck skiers at Vail and Aspen, and so many hikers and campers have fallen ill after drinking from seemingly pristine mountain streams that *giardiasis* has been nicknamed "backpacker's diarrhea."

One of the most common ways to purify community water supplies is to use chlorine as a disinfectant. (Another common disinfectant is ozone.) Unfortunately, chlorine can cause problems of its own; when it reacts with certain compounds in the water, a type of chemical called trihalomethanes, or THMs, can form. Some studies have suggested that the levels of THMs found in many city water supplies may increase the risk of cancers of the gastrointestinal and urinary tracts. A study by the National Cancer Institute found that people who had been drinking chlorinated water for 40 years or more had an increased risk of developing bladder cancer. Some cities filter water so that they don't need to use so much chlorine.

Chlorinated water—especially in the form of a hot running shower or bath water—can also give rise to chloroform. Chloroform, like many other contaminants, can be absorbed through the skin as well as inhaled. If you are partial to long showers or soaks in the tub, you may want to invest in a water filter that removes chlorine from hot running water.

RADIATION

Radiation—vibrating electromagnetic energy traveling invisibly at high speeds—is all around us. We are exposed to natural sources such as the sun's rays and radon; we encounter many other sources that are man-made, such as X-ray machines and microwave ovens.

High frequency or *ionizing radiation*, including X-rays and atomic radiation, alters the body's molecules, producing changes that can cause genetic mutations and many kinds of cancer. Because the effects of ionizing radiation add up, it behooves us to minimize exposure.

There is much evidence that we are not nearly as cautious as we should be with X-rays. "Routine" X-rays taken during physicals and dental examinations and upon admission to the hospital are often not justified. Equally important, the amount of radiation delivered in any particular X-ray depends on the equipment used and the skill of the person using it. For example, in the American Cancer Society's breast cancer screening project, some women received *60 times* more radiation than others. Don't be afraid to question the need for any X-ray procedure, or to ask about the amount of radiation involved.

A number of consumer products also expose us to ionizing radiation. Avoid them. Skip glow-in-the-dark dials, switch plates and automobile instrument panels. Choose smoke detectors that have photoelectric cells rather than radioactive cells.

Low frequency or *non-ionizing radiation* includes visible light, radio waves and microwaves. Scientists are increasingly concerned that non-ionizing radiation may also pose dangers to health.

Microwaves of the type emitted by ovens and VDTs have been found to produce vibrations that can cause significant changes in cell structures and functions. Scientists at New York University have reported that workers in industries where microwaves are used experience an increase in cataracts.

To be on the safe side, use only microwave ovens of recent vintage. Newer models have been designed to limit emissions and maximize safety. Make sure the seals are clean and tight. If you think the oven may be leaking, get it evaluated by a professional from an appliance company, or contact your local health department.

There have also been reports of clusters of miscarriages or birth defects among women who work with VDTs. While one study of 4,000 women by researchers at the University of Michigan found no increased risk in women working fewer than 20 hours a week, a 1988 study by California scientists found that women who spent at least 20 hours a week at VDTs were almost twice as likely to suffer a miscarriage in their first trimester as non-VDT users. Still, the connection was not clear-cut; clerical workers, for instance, had more miscarriages than professional women regardless of whether they used VDTs.

Several studies to get better answers are under way. In the meantime, it seems prudent for pregnant women to limit their hours in front of a VDT and take frequent breaks. (This also is a good way to prevent other VDT complaints—back pain, eye strain and the painful hand-wrist-arm damage known as repetition strain injury.)

The lowest-wave energy in the radiation spectrum is called *extra-low frequency*, or ELF. ELF radiation is produced by electric power lines, electric subways, electric wires and phone lines, and even electric blankets. ELF and the electromagnetic fields associated with it are suspected of interfering with delicate electromagnetic force fields within the body. It appears that such low-level radiation may impair the ability of cells to communicate with one another, making them unable to function properly. Animal and laboratory studies have shown that ELF stimulates cancer growth and lowers resistance to disease. People exposed to electromagnetic fields from power lines and transformers on the job, or those who live near such structures, may have an increased risk of cancer, according to some studies.

NOISE POLLUTION

The gradual hearing loss that often accompanies aging appears to be yet another product of our environment. Scientists in the early 1960s showed that African tribespeople living in very quiet surroundings could hear as well at age 70 as most Americans in their 20s. (They also ate a diet low in animal protein, were not overfat, had low blood pressure and experienced few tension-related diseases.)

Twentieth-century Americans, in contrast, are regularly exposed to a welter of loud noises —screams, whines, roars and throbbing from power tools, household appliances, industrial machinery, airplane engines and amplified music. At first the damage may be a temporary ringing in the ears or inability to hear certain sounds. However, continued exposure to loud noise results in permanent hearing loss.

Moreover, noise exerts a negative effect on behavior. Studies have shown that children living in noisy environments don't do as well in school, and that people living or working in noisy surroundings are less helpful and friendly, than folks in quieter areas. Noise reduces workers' concentration and accuracy, and increases fatigue.

Here are some ways to minimize noise in your corner of the world:

- Install materials to absorb sound—padded carpeting, curtains, acoustical ceiling tiles, foam pads under small appliances and vibration mounts under big appliances.
- Buy appliances that are quiet.
- Keep the stereo from blasting.
- Wear ear protectors when running noisy equipment.

POPULATION PRESSURES

Our health depends not only on whether or not we contaminate ourselves with poisons and chemicals that cause cancer, but also on whether there is enough food, clothing and living space to go around. Historically, there has been no better correlate of poor health than a high birth rate.

Furthermore, health and population growth are closely tied to economic health. Birth and death rates are highest in the poorest nations and lowest in the richest nations. Within our own society, a similar pattern prevails. The poorest American families have the most children while the richest have the fewest.

Researchers from the University of Virginia ran into a classic example of this principle in a poor area of Brazil in the late 1980s. They wanted to study the relationship between economic status and the severe diarrheal diseases that kill many children in developing countries; they planned to observe and compare the experience of poor and "well-to-do" families. (In this case, affluence meant only that the people had a piped water supply.) However, the study ran into an unexpected stumbling block: The American doctors had trouble finding enough well-to-do families who had at least two children under the age of 12. The poor families often had six children in this age group, and during the course of the two-year study most of the poor women became pregnant again. What with tuition and other expenses, the better-off parents explained, they simply could not afford to have more than a couple of children. As for disease, the scientists found diarrhea to be much more common among the poor, especially those who did not have even pit toilets.

There can be no healthy solution to the world's problems when an ever-increasing number of persons competes for ever-decreasing resources. Yet today's global census of 5 billion is expected to double in the next century. The final determinant of our ability to conserve the environment is population.

FUTURE OPTIONS

There is no doubt that our civilization has the capacity to re-create the Middle Ages in terms of environment and health. It *is* possible to create an environment that can overwhelm our best efforts to put it right.

Technology can provide some solutions. It is possible to clean up automobile emissions, to burn industrial fuel more thoroughly, and so on. But every technological solution brings on another technological problem. For example, many people have advocated a switch from gasoline to methanol (methyl alcohol, or wood alcohol). While methanol emits about half the hydrocarbons, carbon monoxide and nitrogen oxides of gasoline, it produces carbon dioxide and formaldehyde instead. It is much less efficient (it provides just about half the miles per gallon), and is often made from coal in a process that itself dirties the environment.

More important, it is unlikely that technology can keep up with the problems created by an ever-growing population. For example, in the Washington, D.C., area, more than $1 billion has been spent to clean up the Potomac River, long used as the capital's sewer. Thanks in part to an ultramodern sewage treatment plant, the river is no longer the "national disgrace" that President Lyndon Johnson deplored in 1965. Aquatic vegetation, a hallmark of clean water, is thriving, and fishing has made a remarkable comeback. Nonetheless, the Potomac may always be polluted. The reason: extensive pollution from so-called nonpoint sources—rain run-off from building sites, roads and suburban lawns heavily contaminated with debris, dirt and chemicals—which has nothing to do with sewage-treatment facilities. Combine this with the likelihood that the demand for water will soon be so great that it will at times exceed the entire river flow, and you have a problem for which technology has no answer: A growing population creating more demand for water while increasingly polluting it.

In the long run, we will have to learn to use less and to use it better. Our future health will depend on our ability to conserve and recycle. We must be willing to pay a price, in both dollars and convenience. But we must stop being a throwaway society before we throw away our future.

ADDITIONAL RESOURCES

The United States Environmental Protection Agency (EPA) is charged with protecting the nation's land, air and water. It runs a number of hotlines and publishes a variety of booklets.

EPA phone numbers include:

Asbestos Hotline: (800) 334-8571, extension 6741, 8:15 a.m. to 5 p.m., Monday through Friday

National Pesticides Telecommunications Network: (800) 743-7378, 24 hours a day, seven days a week

National Response Center Hotline (operated by the U.S. Coast Guard to respond to accidental releases and chemical spills): (800) 424-8802, 24 hours a day, seven days a week

Public Information Center: (202) 382-2080

EPA publications, available from the Agency's Public Information Center, 401 M Street, S.W., Washington, DC 20460, include:

The Inside Story: A Guide to Indoor Air Quality

A Citizen's Guide to Radon and *Radon Reduction Methods: A Homeowner's Guide*

A Consumer's Guide to Safer Pesticide Use and *Termiticides: Consumer Information*

Asbestos in the Home

Lead and Your Drinking Water

The American Lung Association, 1740 Broadway, New York, NY 10019: (212) 315-8700, publishes:

Air Pollution in Your Home?

Facts About Radon: The Health Risk Indoors

Formaldehyde Fact Sheet

SECTION IV

PREVENTION AND THE DOCTOR'S OFFICE

- ❏ Understanding Screening Tests
- ❏ Immunizations: Protection from Infections
- ❏ Medicines: Key Concepts

UNDERSTANDING SCREENING TESTS

There are very good reasons to avoid screening tests. But some tests are worthwhile. So, which tests should you have? And when? This chapter will help you answer those questions, because it presents the pros and cons of the most frequently recommended tests. What's more, these tests have been graded as follows:

A+

A+bsolutely recommended. As it turns out, there is only one test that receives the highest grade because it meets all of our criteria.

A

Acceptable. While the evidence for these tests is not perfect, they are widely considered to be among the best screening tests.

B

Be selective. These tests are not for everyone and should be used only when there is a higher-than-usual risk of a problem.

C

Caution. These tests are borderline. Their benefits are uncertain and there are risks, mostly from false positives.

D

Don't seek these. While these tests are often touted as part of a good "checkup," they produce far more mischief than benefit.

F

Forget these. Primarily because of problems with false positives, these pose a real threat to your health and should not be used for screening.

Using this rating scale, here are our rankings for the tests discussed in this chapter:

A+

Blood pressure

A

Cholesterol test (a special case)
Mammography
Pap smear
Physician examination of breasts

B

AIDS test
Gonorrhea, syphilis and chlamydia tests
Tuberculin skin tests

C

Breast self-examination
Dental examination
Hearing and vision tests
Occult blood in stool
Ophthalmoscopy and tonometry for
    glaucoma
Physical examination
Rectal examination of the prostate
Sigmoidoscopy
Testicular self-examination

D

Blood cell counts (including hematocrit, he-
    moglobin and CBC)
Blood chemistries (tests for liver and kidney
    function, gout, etc.)
Blood glucose
Urinalysis

F

Carotid sonogram
Chest X-ray
Electrocardiogram, resting
Exercise stress test
Pulmonary (lung) function tests

A+

WHO: Everyone
WHEN: Every one to two years, beginning at
           age three
WHY: To detect high blood pressure

The ideal screening test is risk free, simple to perform, accurate, informative, inexpensive, widely available and able to detect a significant disease that can be treated effectively. With luck, it doesn't even hurt.

Only one test meets all of these criteria. It is blood pressure measurement. The test takes only a few minutes and can be done easily and cheaply, often free of charge. Organizations from fire departments to personnel departments offer free screening, and some studies indicate that the testing machines available in many drug stores are fairly accurate. Importantly, this test detects a disease that is without symptoms but which, if not detected and treated, can cause a major stroke or heart attack.

Blood pressure is the amount of force the blood exerts against artery walls as it flows through the body. It is measured at two moments, when the heart beats and pressure is greatest (the systolic pressure), and when the heart rests between beats and pressure is least (the diastolic pressure).

Blood pressure is measured with a *sphygmomanometer*, an instrument that consists of a cuff with a pressure gauge attached, and is used along with a device for detecting pulsations in the artery. The cuff is wrapped tightly around the upper arm and inflated until the pressure in the cuff exceeds the pressure in the large artery in the arm, cutting off blood flow. As the cuff is slowly relaxed, a small amount of blood squirts through the artery, and the artery snaps open and closed, making a sound.

There are three types of sphygmomanometers. In mercury column devices, a column of mercury, encased in a clear tube marked with units of measurement, rises and falls with pressure; a stethoscope is used to detect arterial sounds. Aneroid devices display pressures on a circular dial with a needle, and also require a stethoscope. Electronic devices—often found in pharmacies and department stores—detect the artery's pulsations with a microphone, and display the pressure as a number or on a dial.

Pressures can fluctuate greatly throughout the day. They drop with sleep, rise with activity and soar with stress. For many people, the stress of visiting the doctor can trigger a rise. (This is called "white-coat hypertension.") While a single high reading does not mean a person has high blood pressure, it does signal the need for repeat tests.

Blood pressure is expressed in terms of millimeters of mercury (mm Hg), because the first equipment (like some modern devices) used a column of mercury as a measure. A systolic reading of 120 mm Hg and a diastolic reading of 80 mm Hg are recorded as 120/80, and read as "120 over 80."

Classifications for various blood pressure readings are given in Chapter 18. Usually the diastolic and systolic readings move in the same direction. If one is high, then the other is usually high; if one is low, then the other is also low. However, there are exceptions, most frequently "isolated systolic hypertension." Older people whose blood vessels have grown rigid with age are most likely to have this condition. (As discussed in Chapter 18, many physicians are reluctant to treat isolated systolic hypertension vigorously in older adults.)

One often hears that a reading of 120/80 is "normal" or that anything below 140/90 is considered OK. There is more to it than this, and the issues of normality and treatment are discussed in Chapter 18. As for screening, here are some fairly simple guidelines:

1. If your diastolic pressure remains above 115 in repeated measurements or your systolic pressure remains above 180, you should see a physician without delay.

2. If your diastolic pressure remains above 90 but less than 115 on repeated readings or your systolic pressure remains above 140 but less than 180, then an urgent visit to the physician is not necessary, but you do need to visit your physician and begin a program to lower your blood pressure within a few weeks.

There is no reason to withhold blood pressure measurement from anyone. Even among youngsters, any of the few positives are apt to be true positives. Starting at age 15, blood pressure should be measured each year.

A

CHOLESTEROL TEST

WHO: Everyone

WHEN: Every three to five years starting at age 21, or starting at age two for children in families in which heart attacks have occurred before age 50

WHY: To promote a healthier lifestyle

Cholesterol, a fatty substance that is essential to cell structure and function, is both made in the body and eaten in foods. Cholesterol levels that are too high contribute to the development of atherosclerosis, the major cause of clogged arteries and, consequently, of heart disease and stroke. The higher the cholesterol level, the higher the risk.

Cholesterol testing is performed on a blood sample, and levels are expressed in terms of milligrams of cholesterol per deciliter (mg/dl) of blood. The results may be reported in several ways. This is because there are two main types of cholesterol: high-density lipoprotein cholesterol (HDL-C), which may be thought of as "good" cholesterol, and low-density lipoprotein cholesterol (LDL-C), the "bad" cholesterol. (See Chapter 18 for more information on the different kinds of cholesterol.) Tests that measure both kinds of cholesterol or total cholesterol are the oldest and most widely used in screening. Because most of the total is LDL-C, a high total usually means a high LDL level, and that means trouble.

Current scientific information suggests that total cholesterol and HDL-C are independent risk factors for heart disease and stroke. This means that they separately influence risk and suggests that HDL-C should be measured in addition to total cholesterol, because a low level of HDL-C is cause for concern, as is a high total cholesterol. Further, the balance between these good and bad types of cholesterol can be expressed by using the ratio of total cholesterol to HDL-C. Table 15.1 relates these measurements to the risk of heart disease in the American population. Please note that the levels classified as moderate or even low risk are only relative to "average" and are not the best you can do. A reasonable goal for all Americans is a total cholesterol under 180 and an HDL-C above 60.

There is some controversy as to whether a total cholesterol test, which is quicker and cheaper to do, is adequate for initial screening. In my view, the basic issue is to decide how often an acceptable total cholesterol level will hide a dangerously low HDL-C level. I don't think this is very likely unless there is a strong family history of heart disease. Furthermore, the risk of this problem is further decreased by interpreting total cholesterol according to desirable levels (total cholesterol below 180, HDL-C above 60) rather than "normal" levels, which are higher for total cholesterol and lower for HDL-C. Therefore, I advocate a rule of convenience and cost: If you can get the total cholesterol and HDL-C done as easily and for about the same price as the total cholesterol alone, fine. Otherwise, get the total cholesterol and don't worry about HDL-C on the first test. If your total cholesterol level is below 200, you should get an HDL-C measurement if: 1) You have a strong family history of heart disease (heart attacks before age 50) or (2) your other risk factors (smoking, obesity, fatty diet, inactivity) don't go along with this low reading. In other words, if your total cholesterol seems too good to be true based on your family history or your habits, it probably is.

The value of cholesterol testing as a screening measure does not lie in getting people to a doctor for drug treatment. As explained in Chapter 18, there is only a small chance of finding someone who will need to be treated with cholesterol-lowering drugs. In fact, drugs have been proven to be effective only in middle-aged (age 35 to 59) men with very high total cholesterol levels (higher than 250); they are of no proven benefit in women, older people, young men or children as yet. Exer-

Table 15.1
Cholesterol Levels and the Risk of Heart Disease in the United States

Person Tested	Cholesterol Level (mg/dl)		Ratio of Total Cholesterol to HDL Cholesterol
	Total Cholesterol	HDL Cholesterol	
Low Risk			
Male			
Age 20–39	162–179	>51	3.6–2.3
Age 40–59	186–209	>52	4.2–2.6
Age 60+	189–213	>60	4.0–2.5
Female			
Age 20–39	157–176	>63	2.8–1.9
Age 40–59	186–209	>69	3.0–2.0
Age 60+	205–227	>74	3.2–2.0
Moderate Risk			
Male			
Age 20–39	180–202	37–51	5.1–3.7
Age 40–59	210–233	37–52	6.0–4.3
Age 60+	214–240	40–60	6.0–4.1
Female			
Age 20–39	177–197	45–63	3.6–2.9
Age 40–59	210–235	49–69	4.0–3.1
Age 60+	228–252	50–74	4.8–3.3
High Risk			
Male			
Age 20–39	203–225	<37	6.1–5.2
Age 40–59	234–257	<37	7.4–6.1
Age 60+	241–262	<40	6.9–6.1
Female			
Age 20–39	198–220	<45	4.2–3.7
Age 40–59	236–259	<49	4.9–4.1
Age 60+	253–276	<50	5.5–4.9
Very High Risk			
Male			
Age 20–39	>226	—	>6.1
Age 40–59	>258	—	>7.4
Age 60+	>263	—	>6.9
Female			
Age 20–39	>221	—	>4.2
Age 40–59	>260	—	>4.9
Age 60+	>277	—	>5.5

Source: Kenneth H. Copper, M.D., M.P.H.: *Controlling Cholesterol*

Recommended Screening Tests

GRADE	TEST	WHO	WHEN	WHY
A+	Blood pressure measurement	Everyone	Every 1 to 2 years, beginning at age 3	To detect high blood pressure
A	Cholesterol test	Everyone	Every 3 to 5 years starting at age 21, or starting at age 2 for children in families in which heart attacks have occurred before age 50	To promote a healthier lifestyle
A	Mammography	Women at risk	Every 1 to 2 years beginning at age 50 **OR** According to risk as determined by Table 15.2 : Every year for women at high risk; every 3 years for women at moderate risk; every 5 years for woman at border-line risk; optional for women with low risk, but every 5 years is reasonable	To detect breast cancer
A	Pap smear	All women starting when regular sexual activity begins, or at least by age 21	Every year for 3 years; after 3 consecutive negative tests, every 3 years	To detect cervical cancer
A	Physician examination of the breast	Women	Same schedule as for mammography (See above)	To detect breast cancer
B	AIDS test	Persons who have had sex with many partners; have had sex with prostitutes; use intravenous drugs; have gonorrhea or syphilis; have had sex with anyone who has engaged in any of the above; anyone who received a blood transfusion or blood products between 1978 and 1985	Every 3 to 6 months for as long as the behavior creating the risk continues	To detect infection with the AIDS virus (human immunodeficiency virus, or HIV)
B	Gonorrhea, syphilis and chlamydia tests	Men and women with multiple sexual partners: pregnant women	At least every 6 months while risky behavior continues; early in pregnancy	To detect infection with gonorrhea, syphilis or chlamydia

Recommended Screening Tests

GRADE	TEST	WHO	WHEN	WHY
B	Tuberculin skin tests	Immigrants from areas where tuberculosis is common, or their children or grandchildren; persons living in crowded and impoverished conditions	Every 2 years	To detect exposure to tuberculosis
C	Breast self-examination	Women age 21 and over	Monthly	To detect any changes or lumps that could indicate cancer of the breast
C	Dental examination	Everyone age 4 and older	Every 1 to 2 years	To detect diseases of the teeth, gums and oral cavity
C	Hearing and vision tests	Children and older adults	Twice between ages 2 and 6 and every 2 to 3 years after age 65	To detect impaired hearing and vision and, in children, strabismus (crossed eyes)
C	Occult blood in the stool	Persons 50 years of age and older	Every 1 to 2 years	To detect colon cancer
C	Ophthalmoscopy or tonometry for glaucoma	Older persons, especially those with a family history of glaucoma	Annually after age 40 for those with a family history of glaucoma; every 3 years after age 44 for those with no family history of glaucoma	To detect glaucoma
C	Physical examination	Everyone	Five visits from birth to 18 months; two visits between ages 2 and 6; once every 10 years thereafter	To detect developmental abnormalities in children, and skin cancer, heart valve problems and abdominal aortic aneurysms in adults
C	Rectal examination of the prostate	Men over 40	Every 2 to 3 years, *if* seeing the doctor anyway	To detect prostate enlargement and prostate cancer
C	Sigmoidoscopy	Everyone over 50 years of age	Every 3 to 5 years	To detect cancer of the colon and abnormalities that increase the chance of cancer
C	Testicular self-examination	Men between the ages of 15 and 50	Monthly	To detect abnormalities that could indicate cancer of the testicles

cise and diet, as described in Chapters 6 and 7, are the mainstays of treatment for high cholesterol.

Cholesterol testing's virtue is that of being a strong motivator. Faced with the bad news of a poor test result, many people begin exercising and improving their diet. And getting their cholesterol "score" from time to time may motivate them to continue. By encouraging these lifestyle changes, the cholesterol test may produce benefits that justify its use. I hope so, because that is why it has been recommended for persons other than middle-aged men.

MAMMOGRAPHY

WHO: Women at risk
WHEN: Every one to two years beginning at age 50 *OR* by using Table 15.2 to determine individual risk, beginning at age 40: Every year for women at high risk; every three years for women at moderate risk; every five years for women at borderline risk; optional for women at low risk, but every five years is reasonable in this group
WHY: To detect breast cancer early enough to cure it

Mammography, or X-ray of the breast, can reveal cancers that are too small to be felt as lumps, and that are not likely to have spread. The X-ray—which may be either a conventional X-ray or a special type known as a xeromammogram—is interpreted by a radiologist.

Various types of equipment can be used to X-ray the breasts; most radiologists who specialize in mammography use an X-ray unit designed for that purpose. Depending on the type of machine, the woman will either lie down on a table or sit or stand in front of the machine. The mammography technician positions the breast on a flat surface that contains the X-ray plate, and then the breast is flattened out with a special device. This allows the X-rays to penetrate the tissues and produce as precise a picture as possible, but it may cause some discomfort. (Discomfort can be lessened by scheduling the test during the first half of the menstrual cycle, when the breasts are least apt to be swollen and tender.)

A typical mammographic study consists of two views of each breast, one from above and one from the side. All told, the test takes from 10 to 15 minutes. Then it is usually a few days before the radiologist reports the results to the referring physician.

Because radiation itself can cause cancer, in the late 1970s there was grave concern that mammography might be doing more harm than good. The techniques used today deliver such low doses of radiation that the risk of developing breast cancer from mammograms is much lower, although still present.

Certain X-ray findings, such as minute flecks of calcium known as microcalcifications or masses with irregular borders, are often linked with cancer; a well-outlined discrete spot is more apt to be a benign lesion, such as a cyst. However, the diagnosis often is not clear, even to a trained eye, and mammograms are very hard to interpret in the dense, glandular breasts of young women.

The main drawback to mammography is that almost any kind of finding is likely to lead to a surgical biopsy, "just to be sure." Because most of these findings are not cancerous, many women undergo biopsies unnecessarily.

Another option is to wait three to six months and have a repeat mammogram. The best information we have suggests that a few months' delay does not greatly increase risk if the finding should prove to be cancer. However, the wait may be hard on the woman's peace of mind, and physicians may not want to wait, for fear of being sued should the lesion turn out to be cancer six months later. As a result, even though waiting may be logical, it requires a woman who can deal with concern, and she may have to do this without her physician's active support.

While most authorities suggest that mammography should be done annually, there is controversy as to when it should begin. Some recommend starting at age 40, while others believe that there is little benefit to starting before age 50. And some suggest a "baseline" mammogram between ages 35 and 40 so it can be compared to other mammograms later on. I believe that current evidence favors starting at 50 if no other risk factors are considered (see below), but starting at age 40 may be reasonable. I strongly oppose mammograms before age 40 for any reason; there is every reason to believe they will do more harm than good. And there is no scientific basis for doing a "baseline" at any age.

These recommendations consider only one risk factor for breast cancer, which is age. A schedule based on determining your individual risk, that takes into consideration all of your risk factors, is the best way to increase the probability that findings are important and decrease the risk of unnecessary X-ray exposure and biopsies. This is sure to become the standard approach in the future. Currently, there is only one such schedule, and it is based on the work of physicians and scientists at Group Health of Puget Sound, Inc., in Seattle (Table 15.2). Although this is not as simple as the annual schedules recommended by most health organizations, I prefer it, because I believe that determining individual risk is the best way to gain the benefits and avoid the problems of mammography.

Pap Smear

WHO: All women, starting when regular sexual activity begins or at least by age 21

WHEN: Every year for three years; after three consecutive negative tests, every three years

WHY: To detect cervical cancer

During an examination of the pelvic organs, the doctor or nurse-practitioner takes a sample of cells from the vagina and cervix (the narrow base of the uterus that extends into the vagina). The woman lies on her back on the examining table with her feet supported in stirrups, and the vagina is held open with an instrument called a speculum. The examiner inserts a swab or a spatula and rubs or gently scrapes some cells from the cervix and the wall of the vagina. The procedure, which takes just a few minutes, may cause some slight discomfort,

---

Table 15.2
Estimating Breast-Cancer Risk

High Risk	Previous breast cancer or Mother with breast cancer or Age 50 plus any two variable risk factors
Moderate Risk	Below age 50 plus any two variable risk factors or Age 50 or older plus any one variable risk factor
Borderline Risk	Under age 50 plus any one variable risk factor
Low Risk	Any age; no variable risk factors

Variable Risk Factors

Previous other cancer
Other close relative with breast cancer
First menstrual period at age 10 or earlier
No pregnancies
First live birth at age 30 or older
Menopause at age 55 or older
Previous benign breast disease (not connected with lactation)

Source: Adapted from Carter et al. A clinically effective breast cancer screening program can be cost effective, too. *Preventive Medicine*, 1987; 16:19–34.

---

particularly when the speculum is inserted and the sample is taken.

The samples are spread on a microscopic slide and sent to a laboratory, where a pathologist or a trained technician (a cytologist) examines them under a microscope. The cells will be classed as benign, precancerous (showing certain abnormal cell changes), or malignant (cancerous). Results are usually available in a week or two.

When cancer is present, a Pap smear will reveal it in 60 percent to 80 percent of the cases. However, the presence of abnormal cells is not proof of cervical cancer or even of a precancerous condition; even a finding of "malignant" will turn out to be normal in some cases. A woman whose Pap smear is abnormal should have further tests to determine the significance of this finding.

Some experts believe that Pap smears should stop after age 65 if the woman has been regularly tested before that age and all tests have been negative. By stopping at 65, a woman probably loses little in benefit, but continuing is not much of a burden. It's your choice.

PHYSICIAN EXAMINATION OF BREASTS

WHO: Women
WHEN: When mammography is done
WHY: To detect breast cancer

Comprehensive studies of breast-cancer screening have shown that physician examination and mammography contribute to the early detection of breast cancer and a decrease in breast-cancer deaths. Each approach discovers some cancers not found by the other. While the evidence is not strong enough to recommend physician examination of the breast alone, it should be done when mammography is done. As a practical matter, it will also be done at younger ages when pelvic examinations and Pap smears are done; there seems little reason to discourage this practice at present.

While the woman lies on her back, the examiner (a physician or nurse-practitioner) uses the flat surface of the fingers to feel the breasts and the underarm area for lumps or irregularities. The examiner also inspects the breasts for visible changes in contour or texture, signs of dimpling or puckering, or discharge from the nipple.

Scheduling the exam in the first few days of the menstrual cycle, when the breasts are less likely to be swollen, makes them easier to examine.

B

AIDS TEST

WHO: Men or women who:
- Have had sex with many partners.
- Have had sex with prostitutes.
- Use intravenous drugs.
- Have gonorrhea or syphilis.
- Have had sex with anyone who has engaged in any of the above.
- Anyone who received a blood transfusion or blood products between 1978 and 1985.

WHEN: Every three to six months for as long as the behavior creating the risk continues
WHY: To detect infection with the AIDS virus (human immunodeficiency virus, or HIV)

Current tests for AIDS, made on a sample of blood, are not able to identify the virus that causes AIDS. Rather, they look for antibodies made by the body in response to the infection. The standard screening test is the enzyme-linked immunosorbent assay, or ELISA. When an ELISA is positive, the finding is always confirmed with a more accurate but more expensive test known as the Western Blot.

Typically, the ELISA test turns positive within one to three months of infection with the AIDS virus. Unfortunately, it is possible to be infected with the virus for long periods without the test turning positive. In a study of very-high-risk groups, 7 percent to 15 percent of persons with negative tests were infected with the virus.

Nevertheless, these tests are worthwhile in high-risk groups, such as persons who have had sex with many partners and intravenous drug users. Their value in populations that are not at high risk is less certain. A study conducted by the Congressional Office of Technology Assessment found that when HIV antibody tests are performed under ideal conditions, fully one-third of the positive results in a low-risk group, such as blood donors from rural Illinois, could be expected to be false positives. Worse yet, if the test conditions resembled those that actually prevail in U.S. laboratories, almost nine out of 10 positive tests in this low-risk group would be false positives. Presumably many of these false positives would be corrected by the more expensive and difficult Western Blot test. Still, so many false positives is a very strong argument against testing low-risk groups.

AIDS testing is further complicated by a number of other issues. Testing needs to be accompanied by counseling about AIDS prevention as well as interpretation of results. Keeping results confidential is necessary and may require special arrangements, but notifying sexual partners is essential when results are positive.

GONORRHEA, SYPHILIS AND CHLAMYDIA TESTS

WHO: Men and women with multiple sexual partners and pregnant women

WHEN: At least every six months while risky behavior continues

WHY: To detect infection with gonorrhea, syphilis or chlamydia

Persons at high risk for sexually transmitted diseases are those with many sexual partners. For such persons, periodic testing makes sense. Two points should be emphasized:

1. Frequent testing is no substitute for reducing risk by changing sexual practices.
2. Persons with positive tests are obligated to notify their sexual partners so that the partners can take steps to protect themselves from these diseases.

Gonorrhea is extremely common in the United States, and the incidence seems to be growing. It is found in all parts of the country and all social classes. It is also found in all age groups, although about 90 percent of the cases occur in teenagers and young adults.

Both men and women may be carriers of gonorrhea without having any symptoms, but this is more common in women. Even in men and women who go on to develop symptoms, there is often a long period in which the infection is present without causing problems.

Two techniques are used to diagnose gonorrhea, a laboratory stain and culture. A sample of genital secretions is collected by a doctor or other health professional. For women, the sample is obtained in much the same way as the sample for a Pap smear (see above), by swabbing the cervix. For men, a thin, cotton-tipped swab is inserted into the urethra to pick up a sample of any discharge. Part of the specimen is spread on a slide, stained and

examined under a microscope; part is put onto a culture plate and incubated to give the bacteria a chance to grow. Samples may also be obtained from the anus or throat.

Just about everyone who is infected with syphilis will show the signs and symptoms of primary syphilis (usually a painless sore called a *chancre*) or secondary syphilis (a variety of skin rashes). Unfortunately, this does not remove the need for screening of persons without symptoms for at least two reasons:

1. The chancre may be overlooked or ignored because it is painless and not obvious, or the skin rashes may be misdiagnosed because they vary and can resemble other problems.
2. There are long symptom-free periods between the initial infection and the appearance of the chancre (10 to 60 days), and between the healing of the chancre and the onset of skin rashes (about six weeks). Finally, after the skin rashes of secondary syphilis, the disease tends to enter a latent stage, in which the infection is still active but there are no symptoms. This stage may last for years or even for life. Despite the lack of symptoms, persons with latent syphilis can infect other people and run the constant risk of developing the severe and often fatal consequences of tertiary (advanced) syphilis.

The tests most often used in screening for syphilis, the VDRL and RPR tests, detect the presence of antibodies to the organism that causes syphilis (*Treponema pallidum*). These tests are fairly easy to do, although their sensitivity depends upon the stage of disease. For example, the VDRL test is positive in about 75 percent of persons with primary syphilis, just about 100 percent in secondary syphilis, about 95 percent in early latent syphilis, and about 70 percent in late latent syphilis or tertiary syphilis. These tests also produce a high number of false positives; a positive result is always confirmed by a more specific test, such as the FDA-ABS test. The FDA-ABS test is more sensitive and

Screening and Pregnancy

Pregnancy changes all the bets with respect to screening, because the fetus is at risk for serious problems caused by conditions that can be detected in the mother. Routine prenatal care should include tests for anemia, blood type, Rh(D) antibody, syphilis, gonorrhea, chlamydia, hepatitis B, diabetes and urinary-tract infection. Some of these tests should be performed as early in pregnancy as possible, so don't delay the start of prenatal care.

specific than the VDRL test, but it is also more difficult and costly to perform.

There is controversy with regard to routine testing for syphilis in pregnant women, marriage-license applicants, blood donors, military recruits and patients examined in physicians' offices or admitted to hospitals. It seems clear that, in the absence of such risk factors as many sexual partners, most of these people are at low risk. This means that most positives will be false positives, and that the number of true positives will be quite small. It seems that only in the case of pregnant women, where the determination must be made early to protect the baby's health, are these disadvantages outweighed by other considerations. Otherwise, it seems wiser to identify those at high risk, in whom testing is likely to give accurate and useful results.

Although not as well known as syphilis or gonorrhea, chlamydia is more common. An estimated 3 million to 4 million cases are diagnosed each year. Chlamydia causes about half of all infections of the urethra and epididymis (the structure attached to the testis that stores sperm) in men and about half of all pelvic inflammatory disease in women. Chlamydia infections are most common in young adults with multiple sexual partners.

Pregnant women with chlamydia can pass the disease on to their unborn children. This may result in serious eye infections and pneumonia in the newborn child.

The test for chlamydia is a culture similar to the one that tests for gonorrhea. It also is useful only when the risk is high—in individuals with many sexual partners and pregnant women.

TUBERCULIN SKIN TESTS

WHO: Immigrants from areas where tuberculosis is common, such as Southeast Asia, or their children or grandchildren; persons living or working in crowded and impoverished conditions
WHEN: Every two years
WHY: To detect exposure to tuberculosis

Tuberculosis (TB) can be a ravaging infection. Usually it attacks the lungs. Someone who has been infected with or vaccinated against the bacterium that causes TB becomes sensitized to the germ. When a small amount of a sterile extract of the dead bacteria is injected into the skin, an allergy-like reaction takes place.

The skin test is quick and at most only slightly painful. The extract is injected into the skin with a thin needle, or with a disk whose tiny prongs puncture the skin. Two to four days later, if the person has been exposed to the TB germ, the skin at the test site will grow red, swollen and perhaps blistered. It may itch, and if the reaction is very strong, it may be painful.

The person may return to have the health professional "read" the results or may be taught how to do it at home. A positive response is characterized by swelling, hardness and size. (Redness doesn't count.) A swelling larger than 10 millimeters across (slightly less than 1/2 inch) is considered positive, less than 5 millimeters is negative, and in-between is borderline, meaning that the test may have to be repeated.

A positive test does not mean that the person is ill with TB. It can signal an earlier infection that is dormant, or infection with a related but harmless bacterium. However, it does mean that further tests, including a chest X-ray and perhaps a sputum culture, may be prudent.

Breast Self-Examination

Women age 21 and older should examine their breasts every month, usually following the menstrual period, to detect any changes or lumps that could indicate cancer of the breast. Although most breast lumps are not cancer, women should report any suspicious changes to their physician.

The following steps outline the correct self-examination procedure. Keep this page in a convenient place for monthly reference.

Performing this test each month will familiarize you with the feel of your breasts, so that you can spot changes.

1. Stand in front of the mirror, and look at each breast to see if there is a lump, a depression, or a difference in texture.

2. Get to know how your breasts look, and be especially alert for any changes in the nipples' appearance.

3. Raise both arms and check for any swelling or dimpling in the skin of your breasts.

4. Lie down with a pillow under your right shoulder and put your right arm behind your head.

5. With the fingers of your left hand, repeatedly press or squeeze your right breast gently and circularly from the outside to the center.

6. Squeeze your nipple to see if there is any discharge. Repeat step 4, reversing right and left for your left breast.

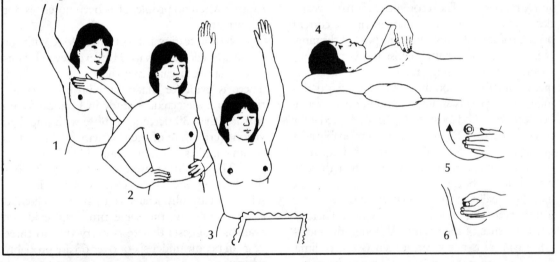

BREAST SELF-EXAMINATION

WHO: Women age 21 and over
WHEN: Monthly
WHY: To detect any changes or lumps that could indicate cancer of the breast

The controversy over breast self-examination (BSE) involves familiar elements. Those on the "pro" side say that, once learned, self-examination can be done often and without cost to the patient; also, the procedure itself does no harm. Those on the "con" side point out that there have been no scientific studies showing the test's usefulness. It is hard to get women to practice BSE, and it does cost money to provide training. Without training, the examination is likely to be inaccurate and, even with training, BSE may simply increase anxiety without improving a woman's health. Of six nonscientific studies that looked at the experience of different groups with BSE, four found value and two did not.

Again, unfortunately, this situation cannot be resolved on the basis of scientific data. Each woman must choose for herself. The promise of BSE seems great enough that we have chosen to provide instruction on the technique.

DENTAL EXAMINATION

WHO: Everyone age four and older
WHEN: Every one to two years
WHY: To detect diseases of the teeth, gums and oral cavity, including cancer

The value of fluoride treatments, flossing, brushing, sealants and professional cleaning in preventing dental problems is well established. In contrast, the value of screening (visual examination and X-rays) is not. The recommendation of a yearly dental examination is based largely on the current practice of annual visits for the purpose of cleaning. It is only logical for the dentist to examine your mouth during cleaning. However, the ideal frequency for these procedures has not been determined; one year is simply the traditional interval between visits, and most studies have adopted it for this reason alone. Every two years is probably adequate, especially for adults. Although frequently recommended, there is no evidence that there is benefit to a shorter interval such as every six months. Finally, the recommendation of every one to two years does not extend to X-rays. There is scant evidence of their value. Although the radiation involved is not great, it seems wise to limit these X-rays to about once every three to five years.

HEARING AND VISION TESTING

WHO: Children and older adults
WHEN: Twice between ages two and six and every two to three years after age 65
WHY: To detect impaired hearing and vision and, in children, strabismus (crossed eyes)

Hearing and vision screening programs always run into the same problem: How often does a significant hearing or vision problem develop unnoticed? Research has not settled this question, but most physicians believe that this sometimes occurs early and late in life, but almost never in between.

Hearing tests range from the simple test that every physician performs while examining infants and young children to complex tests requiring sophisticated instruments (audiometry). These tests may detect simple problems, such as impacted ear wax and, rarely, conditions that require immediate action, such as tumors of the ear (acoustic neuroma). Most often they detect such problems as the natural loss of hearing that occurs with age. The issue then is not to cure, but rather to decide when and how to improve hearing. Usually nothing is done until the hearing loss has become severe enough to outweigh the inconvenience of living with a hearing aid and its somewhat unnatural sounds. Thus, screening (testing when no problem has been noted) is not important.

Vision testing is most often done with the familiar Snellen eye chart. However, even infants a few days old can have their vision checked. There is evidence that vision problems sometimes go undetected. A study in London found that less than 30 percent of those with impaired vision were aware of the problem. Whether this finding applies to other groups is not known.

There is little reason to discourage the routine hearing and vision tests that are done in schools or by physicians as a part of well-child examinations. At the same time, the evidence available suggests that tests every two to three years in people under six or over 65 are probably adequate.

OCCULT BLOOD IN THE STOOL

WHO: Persons 50 years of age and older
WHEN: Every one to two years
WHY: To detect colon cancer

Using a test kit at home, the person obtains a series of stool samples, which are then treated chemically to determine if they contain hidden, or occult, blood.

There are several types of kits on the market. Some supply small sticks to be used for collecting the stool samples, chemically treated paper to spread them on and a developing solution that causes a color change if blood is present. Some require the samples to be sent back to the physician's office. One test kit uses chemically treated toilet paper; another uses a special test pad that is dropped into the toilet bowl after a bowel movement.

A major drawback to these simple screening devices is that some foods, medicines and problems other than cancer will give positive results. To decrease the chance of misleading positive results, it is necessary to watch one's diet for two days beforehand and, because the samples are generally collected from three consecutive bowel movements, for several additional days. The diet should contain fruits, vegetables and high-fiber breads and cereals, but should exclude several types of food, including red meats, turnips, radishes and horseradish, which can cause false-positive color changes on the tests. The individual should also avoid aspirin and other anti-inflammatory medications (ibuprofen, etc.), which can irritate the stomach and cause bleeding. The test results can also be thrown off by blood from hemorrhoids or menstruation.

Even when preparation for the test is excellent, the problem of false positives remains. Only 5 percent to 10 percent of positives in persons over age 50 will be true positives. And, of course, this problem is worse when the chance of colon cancer is low. Colon cancer is unusual before age 50, but occult blood tests are often done on people under this age.

Given these difficulties, it is not surprising that occult blood testing programs produce many false positives—between two percent and five percent of *all* those tested (not just those with positive tests). Although a positive result on any one of the samples should be discussed with the doctor, most do not signal cancer. Persons with several positive occult tests may be good candidates for sigmoidoscopy (see below), but the usual finding is apt to be no more than polyps or unsuspected hemorrhoids.

OPHTHALMOSCOPY OR TONOMETRY FOR GLAUCOMA

WHO: Older persons, especially those with a family history of glaucoma

WHEN: Annually after age 40 for those with a family history of glaucoma; every three years after age 44 for those with no family history of glaucoma

WHY: To detect glaucoma

At first glance, glaucoma seems to be an ideal candidate for detection by screening. Glaucoma appears to do most of its damage by raising the pressure inside the eye, and this pressure can be measured by one of several tests usually referred to as tonometry. Indeed, tonometry had routinely been recommended for the detection of glaucoma, especially in those with a family history of the problem.

Recently, this recommendation has been criticized for a number of reasons. First, as usual, the benefit of using tonometry for glaucoma screening has never been scientifically established. Second, it has long been known that technical problems with different types of tonometry might cause high-pressure readings to be missed; also, one type of glaucoma, so-called low-pressure glaucoma, does its damage without causing high-pressure readings. More importantly, newer studies suggest that treating high pressure might not be as critical as previously believed. These studies found that high-pressure readings were not a very accurate predictor of damage to the eye, especially in older adults, and that lowering pressure with treatment did not necessarily prevent damage.

Despite these problems, most physicians, including ophthalmologists (specialists in eye treatment and surgery) firmly believe that early cases of glaucoma should be treated in an attempt to prevent damage. As a result, emphasis has switched from detecting high pressure with tonometry to detecting the early stages of glaucoma with ophthalmoscopy (examining the inside of the eyeball with an ophthalmoscope).

In ophthalmoscopy, the patient sits in a darkened room, the pupil is dilated with the special eye drops and the inside of the eye is examined with the magnifying lenses of the hand-held ophthalmoscope. Of special interest is whether or not the optic nerve or the blood vessels of the eye show any signs of change that point to early glaucoma.

There are no scientific studies to help us resolve the dilemma of glaucoma screening, nor are there any in progress or even planned. Based on the best information we have, ophthalmoscopy may be the best approach, because it can detect problems other than glaucoma, but its advantages are unproven. Furthermore, it must be admitted that the age at which testing should begin and its frequency are unknown, making these recommendations educated guesses at best.

PHYSICAL EXAMINATION

WHO: Everyone
WHEN: Five visits from birth to 18 months; two visits between ages two and six; once every 10 years thereafter
WHY: To detect developmental abnormalities in children and skin cancer, heart valve problems and abdominal aortic aneurysms in adults

The term physical examination, or "physical," commonly refers to a process involving many tests and X-rays as well as a physical inspection of the body. Here it is used to mean just the actual examination—the looking, hearing and poking that the physician does with instruments no more complex than the stethoscope and ophthalmoscope, the familiar tools used to listen to the heart and lungs and look into the eyes and ears. Although many problems could be found during such an examination, there is almost no evidence to support the routine examination of your body.

The schedule suggested here is based on the following assumptions:

- The significant problems that may be detected by physical examination are developmental abnormalities, such as cleft palate in children and skin cancer, heart valve problems and aortic aneurysms (a bulging in the largest artery in the body) in adults.

Annual Physical, Complete Physical, Executive Physical: Trouble by Any Name

Why not have it all—physical examination, 40 or so laboratory tests, electrocardiogram, X-rays and more—every once in a while? There's a very good reason: Most of the tests are more likely to cause harm than be of help. Inappropriate procedures not only point to problems when there are none, they often miss problems that are there. And the more tests you do, the more problems you cause.

Moreover, an executive physical can't give you a "clean bill of health." In fact, a study of senior executives who died before retiring found that more than half had undergone complete physicals in the year before their death, and the problem that caused their death had not been detected. Why pay $500 to $2,500 for something that hurts more than it helps?

- Physical examinations can be part of visits to the doctor for other reasons, such as immunizations in children. (All but one of the recommended visits in children has to be made for an immunization anyway.)
- False positives are not as great a problem in examinations as they are in laboratory tests and X-rays. Occasionally, an uncommon problem will be detected, and this will be useful.

Although visiting the physician once a decade for a physical examination does not seem excessive, most of the benefit will probably be found before age six and after age 65.

RECTAL EXAMINATION OF THE PROSTATE

WHO: Men over 40
WHEN: Every two to three years, *if* seeing the doctor anyway

WHY: To detect prostate enlargement and prostate cancer

The prostate is a small gland that produces much of the fluid in semen. Because it lies next to the rectum, it is easy for a physician to check its condition by feeling it through the rectal wall.

The patient typically lies on his side with his knees drawn toward his chest. The doctor inserts a well-lubricated, gloved finger into the man's rectum and palpates the prostate gland. If the prostate is enlarged or if the side of the gland that faces the rectum contains possibly cancerous nodules or other irregularities, the physician will be able to feel them.

Prostate cancer is very slow growing, and studies at Stanford University show that it does not invade surrounding tissues until it is 3 to 4 cubic centimeters in size. Unfortunately, by the time cancer can be felt, it is apt to be fairly large. It is not easy to design studies to determine the benefits of rectal examination in men without symptoms, and so it is not surprising that there is little evidence that this common procedure is worthwhile.

If you are seeing a doctor for some other reason, it is probably wise to have this exam, but it's not worth scheduling a special visit.

SIGMOIDOSCOPY

WHO: Everyone over 50 years of age
WHEN: Every three to five years
WHY: To detect cancer of the colon and abnormalities that increase the chance of cancer

Using a flexible fiberoptic scope, the doctor looks at the lining of the rectum, which constitutes the last five to six inches of the large intestine, and, just above it, the stretch of colon known as the sigmoid colon. The physician can also remove tissue (biopsy) or abnormalities such as polyps with the scope.

The bowel needs to be emptied before the exam. Some doctors prescribe only a tap water or bottle enema an hour beforehand; others recommend a clear liquid diet for a day or two ahead, plus an enema the night before and another an hour or so before; yet others recommend something in between. The more elaborate the routine, the more likely the exam will be satisfactory because the bowel is empty, but the greater the inconvenience to the patient.

The patient lies on his or her side, with knees drawn up toward the chest, or he or she may rest on elbows and knees with the buttocks raised. The sigmoidoscope is inserted and gradually advanced through the rectum into the lower colon. The patient may feel some brief cramping and the urge to defecate. Sometimes puffs of air are blown in to help clear a path; a suction device may be used to remove stool, mucus or blood and improve the view.

Once the scope has been advanced as far as possible, it is slowly withdrawn while the doctor carefully inspects the lining of the bowel. The two-foot-long flexible sigmoidoscope contains a powerful light source and fibers that make it possible to see around bends.

The procedure lasts five to 10 minutes, or slightly longer if biopsies are taken or polyps removed. Typically the patient rests on the table for a few minutes afterwards. The physician can usually discuss some of the findings right away, although it will take a few days to get results from any laboratory tests.

Despite the instrument's length, its flexibility usually makes the exam more comfortable than one with its predecessor, the shorter but rigid sigmoidoscope. The test is low risk, with few serious complications. However, use of the fiberoptic scope requires some training and, because it is fairly new, it is not yet available everywhere. The test is also expensive, usually in the range of $50 to $200.

We don't yet know precisely when and if sigmoidoscopy should be done. Neither do we understand the balance between benefit, risk and cost. We can be fairly certain that the test should not be done before the age of 50, because colon cancer is uncommon before this age. The recommendation of every three to five years after age 50 is based on the experience of some screening programs. One study suggested that people who were

Testicular Self-Examination

Your best hope for early detection of testicular cancer is a simple three-minute monthly self-examination. The best time is after a warm bath or shower, when the scrotal skin is most relaxed.

Roll each testicle gently between the thumb and fingers of both hands. If you find any hard lumps or nodules, you should see your doctor promptly. They may not be malignant, but only your doctor can make the diagnosis.

Following a thorough physical examination, your doctor may perform certain X-ray studies to make the most accurate diagnosis possible.

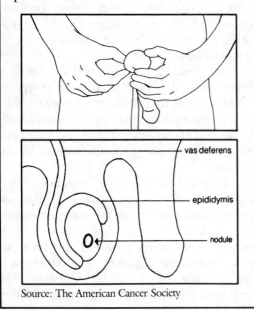

Source: The American Cancer Society

TESTICULAR SELF-EXAMINATION

WHO: Men between the ages of 15 and 50
WHEN: Monthly
WHY: To detect abnormalities that could indicate cancer of the testicles

Although testicular cancer does not pose the same threat to the nation's health as breast cancer does (5,000 vs. 145,000 new cases annually), the situation with respect to testicular self-examination (TSE) is much the same as that with breast self-examination (BSE). On the one hand, the test can be done frequently without cost once the technique is learned, and the examination itself causes no harm. On the other hand, we have no scientific evidence of its worth and there is concern that the test could cause more harm than good through creating anxiety and false positives. Again, there are no scientific trials of TSE that can help men decide what is best for them. One clear difference between TSE and BSE, but not a happy one, is that there are not even any research findings that would give us some indication as to what might happen if TSE were widely practiced.

So, as with BSE, information on the technique is offered so that men too can make a choice.

D

BLOOD CELL COUNTS

(including hematocrit, hemoglobin and complete blood count)

BLOOD CHEMISTRIES

(tests for liver and kidney function, gout, etc.)

BLOOD GLUCOSE

URINALYSIS

These tests have been grouped together for several reasons:

1. They are easy to do. Blood for a complete blood count and all of the blood chemistries, including blood glucose, can be obtained with a single needle stick. This hurts a little and sometimes people faint, but it hardly qualifies as major trauma.

completely normal on the first exam (no polyps, etc.) did not benefit from repeat examinations, while those who had any type of abnormality, even hemorrhoids, should have some repeat exams. There is a scientific trial under way now that will help resolve many of the questions concerning sigmoidoscopy. In the meantime, we are left with a recommendation whose wide range (three to five years) reflects uncertainty as to the test's value.

Figure 15.1
A Typical Report of a Complete Blood Count

Tests	Result	Reference Range*	Units
CBC			
RBC VALUES			
ERYTHROCYTE COUNT	4.63	4.00–5.60	mil./mm^3
HEMOGLOBIN	13.6	12.8–17.2	gm/dl
HEMATOCRIT	42.0	38.0–50.0	%
MCV	90.6	81.0–98.0	micron^3
MCH	29.4	23.0–34.6	picogm
MCHC	32.4	31.0–37.0	%
WBC TOTAL AND DIFF			
WBC TOTAL	7.79	4.00–10.60	1,000/mm^3
WBC PERCENT COUNTS			
NEUTROPHILS	65.8	50.0–75.0	%
LYMPHOCYTES	25.2	20.0–45.0	%
ATYPICAL LYMPHS	1.5	0.0–5.0	%
MONOCYTES	6.5	0.0–9.0	%
EOSINOPHILS	0.6	0.0–5.0	%
BASOPHILS	0.4	0.0–1.0	%
WBC DIFF ABSOLUTES			
NEUTROPHILS	5.13	2.00–7.00	1,000/mm^3
LYMPHOCYTES	1.96	1.10–2.90	1,000/mm^3
ATYPICAL LYMPHS	0.11	0.00–0.25	1,000/mm^3
MONOCYTES	0.51	0.10–0.80	1,000/mm^3
EOSINOPHILS	0.05	0.00–0.40	1,000/mm^3
BASOPHILS	0.03	0.00–0.12	1,000/mm^3
ADDITIONAL FINDINGS			
PLATELETS	ADEQUATE		

*This is the 'normal' range.

The procedure requires little in the way of equipment and can be done almost anywhere. Obtaining a specimen for urinalysis requires a disposable cup and a little maneuvering in the bathroom, but involves no discomfort.

2. Costs are not very high. While the tests are not cheap, they are not big-ticket items either.

3. They are the most frequently performed laboratory tests. Probably because they are easy to do and not very expensive, they tend to be a part of almost every "checkup."

4. **They fail as screening tests for the same reasons.** In short, a positive test in a person without symptoms doesn't mean much.

BLOOD CELL COUNTS

These tests are concerned with the cells in the blood. There are a number of different tests, and they may be combined into a complete blood count (CBC). A CBC usually consists of these tests:

• White-blood-cell count with differential. This is a measurement of the total number of white cells (leukocytes) per cubic millimeter

Figure 15.2
A Typical Blood-Chemistry Panel

	Results	Reference Range*	Units
CHEMISTRY-24			
CALCIUM	9.1	8.5–10.3	mg/dl
IONIZED CA, CALCULATED	2.1	1.8–2.3	meq/l
PHOSPHOROUS	3.0	2.1–4.5	mg/dl
GLUCOSE	80	70–118	mg/dl
URIC ACID	6.4	3.8–8.8	mg/dl
UREA NITROGEN (BUN)	9	8–22	mg/dl
CREATININE	1.1	0.7–1.4	mg/dl
CREATININE/BUN RATIO	0.12	0.03–0.12	
TOTAL PROTEIN	6.5	6.2–8.1	gm/dl
ALBUMIN	4.1	3.8–5.3	gm/dl
GLOBULIN	2.4	1.9–3.1	gm/dl
A/G RATIO	1.7	1.2–2.3	
TOTAL BILIRUBIN	0.7	0.2–1.2	mg/dl
ALT (SGPT)	21	0–35	IU/l
ALP (ALK. P'TASE)	86	30–125	IU/l
LD (LDH)	159	95–214	IU/l
AST (SGOT)	26	9–53	IU/l
GGT	52	0–52	IU/l
SODIUM	145	136–149	meq/l
POTASSIUM	3.8	3.2–5.5	meq/l
CHLORIDE	104	97–111	meq/l
CARBON DIOXIDE	27	20–33	meq/l
TRIGLYCERIDES	106	25–175	mg/dl
CHOLESTEROL	191	135–240	mg/dl

*This is the 'normal' range.

Table 15.3
The Quick Explanation

Test	Body Function or Disease
Calcium and phosphorus	Bone metabolism
Glucose	Diabetes
Uric acid	Gout
Urea nitrogen (BUN) and creatinine	Kidney function
Total protein, albumin and globulin	Infection and nutrition
Total bilirubin, ALT, ALP, LD, AST, GGT	Liver function
Sodium, potassium, chloride, carbon dioxide	Electrolytes
Triglycerides and cholesterol	Fat metabolism

Table 15.4

Introduction to a Sample Twelve-Factor Biochemical Profile

Test and Abnormal Values	Illustrative Associated Conditions
Calcium	
Increased	Metabolic disease (for example, hyperparathyroidism), malignancy, sarcoidosis, other bone disease (for example, Paget's disease)
Decreased	Hypoparathyroidism, malabsorption, renal failure, osteomalacia, pancreatitis
Glucose	
Increased	Diabetes mellitus, glucagonoma, mineralocorticoid excess (many causes), hyperthyroidism
Urea nitrogen	
Increased	Primary renal disease (for example, medullary cystic kidney, hereditary nephritis), secondary renal disease (infectious, immunologic, vascular, metabolic or obstructive), prerenal azotemia
Sodium	
Increased	Mineralocorticoid excess (many causes), heat stroke, diabetes insipidus, cerebral tumor or thromboembolism
Decreased	Volume depletion (many causes), mineralocorticoid deficiency (many causes), antidiuretic hormone excess (many causes)
Potassium	
Increased	Renal failure, metabolic acidosis (many causes), mineralocorticoid deficiency or renal unresponsive states (several causes)
Decreased	Mineralocorticoid excess (many causes)
Uric acid	
Increased	Gout, renal failure (many causes), myeloproliferative disorders, leukemia
Total Protein	
Increased	Systemic infection (for example, tuberculosis), systemic inflammation (for example, collagen vascular disease), malignancy (for example, lymphoma, myeloma), liver disease (many causes in addition to those above)
Albumin	
Decreased	Malnutrition, nephrotic syndrome (many causes), protein-losing enteropathies (many causes), severe liver disease (many causes)
Cholesterol	
Increased	Primary (for example, familial) and secondary hypercholesterolemia (for example, hypothyroidism, nephrotic syndrome, hepatitis)
Decreased	Hyperthyroidism, malabsorption, liver disease (many causes)
AST	
Increased	Hepatocellular inflammation (many causes), cardiac inflammation (for example, infarction, myocarditis, pericarditis), skeletal muscle inflammation (for example, viral infection, polymyositis)
LD	
Increased	Hemolysis, thromboembolism, systemic infection or inflammation, malignancy
ALT	
Increased	Liver disease (many causes), bone disease (many causes)

(mm^3) of blood, and a percentage for each of the different types of white blood cells.

- Red-blood-cell count. The total number of red blood cells (erythrocytes) per mm^3 is measured.
- Hematocrit. This test gives the percentage of blood that is red blood cells.
- Hemoglobin. The amount of hemoglobin in the blood is expressed as grams per 100 milliliters or deciliter (dl). Hemoglobin is a substance contained in red blood cells.
- Red-cell indices. These describe various aspects of the red blood cells and are derived from the hemoglobin, red-cell count and a measure of red-blood-cell size.

Hematocrits or hemoglobins are often done by themselves as screening tests for anemia. The other tests are rarely done other than as a part of a CBC. Abnormal white-cell counts and/or differentials may be seen in many diseases, including infections and leukemias.

A CBC may be done with as little as one milliliter (about one-fifth of a teaspoon) of blood obtained from a vein. The blood is then analyzed by machine. The white-blood-cell differential requires that a technician examine the blood under a microscope. If only a hematocrit or hemoglobin is to be done, other methods can be used. These require a little more than a drop of blood, which may be obtained by pricking the finger with a lancet or needle. (A typical CBC report is shown in Figure 15.1.)

Blood Chemistries

New technology allows one machine to perform a host of blood chemistries on a single blood sample. As a result, these tests are often referred to as panels or profiles. They may be referred to by a name that suggests their intended use, such as liver profile, or simply by the number of tests and the name of the machine, perhaps Chemistry 24 or SMAC 23. (A typical blood-chemistry panel is shown in Figure 15.2.)

A superficial (and inaccurate) understanding of the tests in a panel is often given to patients in the form of the following table of relationships between tests and body function or diseases as shown in Table 15.3.

Unfortunately, as any physician knows, each of these tests may be influenced by any of a number of conditions. To give you an idea of this, Table 15.4 is reproduced from a very brief introduction to these tests as offered to medical students. Even without an explanation of the medical terms, it is clear that many different conditions affect each of these tests.

The fact that any "abnormal" value on these tests may mean any number of things limits their usefulness, but the major problem with using these tests in screening is that an abnormal result probably means nothing. By definition, five percent of people without any disease will have an abnormal result on each of these tests. With 15 such tests, the chances are very good that one is going to have an abnormal result even when there is no problem.

Blood Glucose

Sometimes referred to as blood sugar, the blood glucose level is greatly influenced by the timing and content of meals. Thus, a *random glucose* test must have wide limits for normality, because it will be high soon after a heavy meal and much lower if it has been a long time since any food was eaten. To get around this problem, doctors often ask for a *fasting glucose*, which is done in the morning before any food is eaten. A *one-* or *two-hour postprandial glucose*, which is done one or two hours after eating a standard meal, was used in the past but proved to be so variable that it is now regarded as useless. *Glucose tolerance tests* involve making several determinations at various times after a standard amount of glucose is ingested.

Most glucose tests are done as a part of blood-chemistry panels and are usually random, although they may be classified as fasting if done before breakfast. A glucose test requires only a small amount of blood and, as noted, is most often done as a part of a blood-chemistry panel even if the other tests in the panel are not needed.

Urinalysis

Urinalysis usually consists of tests for the

presence of blood, protein, glucose and bilirubin in the urine, as well as a microscopic examination of the urine sediment for blood cells, bacteria and crystals. Tests for nitrite, ketones, urobilinogen, white blood cells and pH are often included in a urinalysis because they are very easily added. Many conditions may cause a positive on one or more of these tests, but the main reasons for testing are as follows:

1. The presence of nitrite, blood, protein, white blood cells and a high pH are associated with infections in the urinary tract, almost always of the bladder (cystitis).
2. The presence of blood also may be associated with uncommon kidney problems (nephritis or cancer in the urinary tract).
3. The presence of glucose or ketones may be associated with diabetes.
4. Bilirubin is associated with obstruction of the flow of bile from the liver; this may occur with gallstones and certain liver problems.
5. Urobilinogen is normally found in the urine; its absence may signal blockage to the flow of bile from the liver, and an increase may occur with some problems with red blood cells.
6. White cells, bacteria and red blood cells in the sediment are associated with urinary tract infections.
7. Crystals in the sediment may be associated with inherited diseases and/or kidney stones.

A urine specimen is collected in a disposable cup. Usually all the tests except for the examination of the sediment are performed using a plastic strip that carries up to nine different reagents. The plastic strip is dipped in the urine, and each reagent changes color according to the presence or absence of the chemical for which it is testing. The colors are then compared to standard charts, and an estimate of the substance can be made. To examine the sediment, the urine is spun in a centrifuge so that particles such as crystals and cells collect at the bottom. These are then spread on a glass slide and examined under a microscope.

ROUTINE TESTS, ROUTINE NONSENSE

If these tests are fairly easy, not too expensive and they detect so many things, why aren't they recommended?

Put simply, without symptoms, a positive result on these tests just doesn't mean very much. These tests are far from perfect. Most often when an unexpected abnormality is found, either the result is false positive or it indicates a condition for which no treatment will be required. In fact, in a recent study of what to do with these abnormalities, it was found that the best thing to do was to ignore the finding. The second-best thing was to repeat the test and hope that the abnormality went away, and the worst thing to do was to check out the finding with other tests. In short, these tests have all the problems in interpretation mentioned in Chapter 4.

Blood glucose determinations deserve special discussion, because they are so often promoted to detect diabetes. As noted recently by the U.S. Preventive Services Task Force (see end of this chapter), there is still no reason to believe that detecting a high blood-glucose level in an otherwise healthy person leads to any action that benefits him or her. See Chapter 21, Diabetes, for a more complete discussion of this problem.

F

CAROTID SONOGRAM
CHEST X-RAY
ELECTROCARDIOGRAM, RESTING
EXERCISE STRESS TEST
PULMONARY (LUNG) FUNCTION TESTS

These tests clearly do more harm than good as screening procedures. Fortunately, three of them (chest X-ray, resting electrocardiogram and pulmonary function tests) are widely recognized in the medical community as having no value as screening tests. Unfortunately, they are still often done as a part of a "complete" or "executive" physical.

Many physicians still believe that exercise stress testing has value in screening for heart disease in people without symptoms. Many would accept carotid sonograms, because screening is a fairly new use of this test, and they haven't seen the data pointing to its lack of value. While the continued use of chest X-rays, resting electrocardiograms and pulmonary function tests is to be deplored, the greatest threat to your health comes from carotid sonograms and exercise stress tests.

CAROTID SONOGRAM

The brain receives most of its blood via the carotid arteries. Blockage of these arteries can lead to stroke and other neurologic problems. Blockage and narrowing of the carotid arteries can be detected with a carotid sonogram, a test that uses sound waves to examine the flow of blood within the arteries. It was hoped that detecting and then surgically removing blockages would prevent such problems as stroke. (This surgery is called carotid endarterectomy.) It is now widely accepted that carotid endarterectomy in people without symptoms of blocked blood flow (see Chapter 20) has no benefit. Tragically, carotid endarterectomies are still done for this and other unacceptable reasons. A well-known study by UCLA and the Rand Corporation indicated that only about one-third of carotid endarterectomies were done for acceptable reasons. This is no small problem, because from two percent to five percent of patients who have this operation will have a major complication, perhaps a stroke, heart attack or death.

Four large studies of carotid blockage and carotid endarterectomy are currently under way; the results of these studies may change our view of screening for carotid blockages, but this is unlikely. At present, there is no reason to believe that surgery in persons without symptoms is of benefit.

Therefore, there is no reason to have a carotid sonogram unless there are symptoms.

CHEST X-RAY

The chest X-ray provides a look at the lungs, heart, large arteries, part of the diaphragm, ribs, collarbone, breasts and upper spine. It has been widely and wrongly used as a screening test.

A chest X-ray is taken by a technician and interpreted by a physician, usually a radiologist. The patient stands in front of a film holder, with the X-ray tube positioned several feet away. Usually two views are made, one from back to front, the other from the side. For the seconds while the X-ray is being taken, the person is asked to take a deep breath and hold it. The entire procedure takes about five minutes; results are available, if not right away, then by the next day.

When tuberculosis was widespread, there may have been a good reason for screening with chest X-rays, but this benefit was never proven. It may have a role for groups at high risk for tuberculosis today, but a tuberculin skin test is usually preferred. The chest X-ray is worthless as a screening test for lung cancer, because by the time the cancer shows up on an X-ray it is too late to affect survival. Like any X-ray, this one delivers a potentially harmful dose of radiation.

Although chest X-rays are often performed routinely on admission to the hospital or in preparation for surgery, several studies show that they simply do not provide important information often enough to justify their cost and risk.

ELECTROCARDIOGRAM (ECG), RESTING

Each day the heart beats about 100,000 times, and each of these beats comprises a complex set of electrical events. This electrical activity can be recorded as an electrocardiogram (ECG or EKG), and the patterns can be studied for signs of abnormality.

The ECG machine detects electrical impulses generated by the heart via wires connected to electrodes, small metal discs known as "leads." The test is usually performed by a technician, who rolls the ECG machine alongside the table where the person lies. The technician places the leads at specific sites on the chest, arms and legs; a paste is applied to the skin beneath each lead to improve electrical conduction. If the chest is hairy, small patches may be shaved. (The lead does not emit any electricity, so it cannot convey an electric shock.) The procedure is not uncomfortable, and it takes about 10 minutes.

The ECG machine presents the heart's electrical impulses as wavy tracings on graph paper. The rhythms and forms of the heartbeats can be categorized into patterns that indicate how the heart is functioning.

The ECG can show evidence of heart attacks both old and new, and of other types of heart disease, too. Unfortunately, the ECG also will miss a good amount of heart disease. Because of the large number of false negatives, the ECG is not useful in screening people who do not have symptoms of heart disease.

The ECG is recommended neither for screening nor as a routine test prior to hospital admission or surgery, although it may be considered for certain patients, including those with heart disease, diabetes and high blood pressure.

EXERCISE STRESS TEST

The exercise stress test is an ECG made while a person exercises. Physical stress increases the heart's demand for oxygen, and may help to reveal a problem in the coronary arteries, such as narrowing or blockage.

The exercise usually consists of walking on a treadmill or pedaling a stationary bicycle. The person begins slowly, but as the test proceeds, the speed and slant of the treadmill will be stepped up, or the resistance of the bike's pedals will be increased.

The ECG is recorded and blood pressure is monitored while the person walks or pedals. The test continues until he or she reaches a maximum heart rate (maximal testing) or a fixed percentage of that rate (submaximal testing). The test may be stopped short if the person develops chest pain, extreme shortness of breath, fatigue or ECG abnormalities.

Because there is a risk, albeit small, that the exercise might trigger a heart attack or abnormal heartbeat (arrhythmia), the test should never be done unless emergency equipment and someone trained in cardiopulmonary resuscitation are at hand. Submaximal testing is much less likely than maximal testing to cause a problem.

Although this test may be a useful diagnostic tool for persons who have unexplained chest pain, it cannot be recommended for screening.

In persons without symptoms, the exercise stress test leads to many false positives. Over 80 percent of positives in men will be false positives; in women the percentage is even higher! At the same time, the test will be negative in about half the people who have heart disease. Persons falsely positive may go on to have further diagnostic procedures, usually coronary arteriography, which carry a risk of major complications.

Stress testing's popularity comes from its image as a safer, easier, less costly alternative to coronary arteriography. In coronary arteriography a contrast material is injected into the arteries of the heart through a catheter that has been threaded up through an artery of the arm or groin. The coronary arteries are then X-rayed. Although coronary arteriography, also known as cardiac catheterization, is an accurate diagnostic tool, it carries its own risk of death, heart attack, stroke and other major complications (see below). Substituting stress testing for arteriography avoids this risk, but stress testing's inaccuracy makes this meaningless.

Perhaps the most disturbing aspect of exercise stress testing is that physicians and patients often fail to think clearly about what they will do with the results. Usually the results have no real impact even if they are accepted as valid. Faced with a positive result, there are only two choices:

1. Change risk factors, an approach in which the exercise stress test plays no role
2. Proceed with coronary arteriography and then with surgery if it is indicated by the results. Coronary arteriography and surgery is a fairly bold and infrequent choice

The Risk and Cost of Exercise Stress Testing

Many physicians have suggested that everyone over 35 years of age take an exercise stress test to detect coronary artery disease before undertaking any major increase in regular physical activity. What would happen if this recommendation were followed?

Researchers at the University of Pennsylvania developed a model for investigating what would happen if all 20 million joggers in the United States over the age of 45 had an exercise stress test and their results were followed up, when indicated, with coronary arteriography and coronary artery bypass grafting. They conservatively estimated the total cost of the program to be well over $9 billion (1985 dollars). More worrisome, more than 8,000 people would have major complications, and almost 2,000 would die from diagnostic testing and therapy. About half of the major complications and deaths would occur in persons *without* any disease. The cost for each person surviving surgery would be about $170,000. Would those surviving surgery benefit? No one knows.

in a patient without symptoms. The following discussion shows why.

There are really only three ways to treat atherosclerosis, the basic problem in coronary artery disease:

1. Improve lifestyle;
2. Treat high cholesterol and/or high blood pressure with drugs;
3. Perform surgery (coronary artery bypass grafting) to remove blockages. (An alternative to coronary artery bypass grafting, called percutaneous transluminal angioplasty, may be available to some patients, as discussed in Chapter 18.)

You do not need results from exercise stress testing to make decisions about the first two approaches. You already know what to do about such lifestyle risk factors as smoking, diet and exercise. Neither a positive nor a negative result on an exercise stress test would affect their importance, especially considering the inaccuracy of the test. When it becomes necessary to consider drugs for high cholesterol or high blood pressure in addition to changing lifestyle, the important tests are the cholesterol and blood pressure readings. Again, the results of an exercise stress test would not affect these decisions one way or the other.

That leaves the question of surgery. First, surgery can't be considered until a coronary arteriogram is done. If you are going to consider this alternative, then you must be willing to undergo coronary arteriography and accept its risks. These risks are approximately 1.4 deaths and 8.7 major complications (heart attacks, strokes) per 1,000 arteriograms.

Most surgery is done to relieve symptoms. But someone being screened does not have symptoms, so most of the experience with surgery is irrelevant. Surgery is being considered for a rather unusual reason: to prolong life rather than to ease symptoms. Surgery for certain types of blockages, mostly those in the two largest coronary arteries, does increase life expectancy, although modestly. The chances of finding such a blockage in a person with no symptoms is probably small, although there is no information available that would allow precise determination of the probability.

One way to get around all of the drawbacks might be to restrict screening to those with two or more risk factors. This would increase the likelihood of a positive result being a true positive. Unfortunately, the increased accuracy would only be modest (perhaps only 60 percent of the positives would be false positives), and it would not change the issues discussed above.

It has also been suggested that exercise stress tests be done on people above the age of 40 who are planning to begin an exercise program (see box). Again, this does nothing to alter the basic problems: The test's results are unreliable and do not affect decision making. After all, the people who will benefit most from exercise are those who have coronary artery disease. The safety of exercise depends on how you do it, not on whether or not you have had an exercise stress test.

Submaximal stress testing—testing up to a fixed percentage of someone's estimated maximum rate—can be useful as a motivating tool, by demonstrating the person's level of endurance. Someone who is confronted with the fact that his or her endurance is mediocre may be driven to improve it. However, there are easier and less costly methods that can provide the same information, such as the 1.5-mile walk/run test popularized by Dr. Kenneth Cooper in *The Aerobics Program for Total Well-Being* and other books.

PULMONARY FUNCTION TESTS

Pulmonary function tests (PFTs) have been included in physical examinations as both a general measure of health and a screening test for emphysema. While studies have shown that certain PFTs can accurately predict longevity, other studies have found that they have no value as screening tests.

When used in screening, PFTs are usually performed by having you breathe into a tube that is connected to a device that measures the amount and speed of air that you exhale. These devices are usually rather compact and may even be hand-held. More sophisticated PFTs use much more elaborate devices that collect air in bags; these tests may also involve inhaling certain mixtures of gases and taking blood samples for measuring the concentration of gases in the blood. These more elaborate tests are hardly ever done as screening procedures.

PFTs fail to be useful in screening because of limitations in the tests ability to detect emphysema and because there is nothing that stops the progression of emphysema other than stopping smoking. Clearly, smokers can be advised to stop without having them undergo PFTs. And, because PFTs do not detect the early damage of smoking, "normal" PFTs may give a false sense of security to smokers. In summary, PFTs do give some indication of lung function, but they do not lead to better treatment of emphysema or other diseases.

THE LOWDOWN ON SCREENING

So now you know the truth about screening tests. Only one, blood pressure, is worthwhile for all of the people all of the time. The value of some others depends on personal risk factors, such as your age and family history. Still others are of no proven merit.

When faced with decisions about screening tests, remember that a worthwhile test must yield reliable information that can lead to better treatment. Never submit to any screening test unless you are sure that its benefits outweigh its risks. If your physician or someone else pressures you to have a test not recommended in this chapter, simply say that you prefer to follow the recommendations of the U.S. Preventive Services Task Force as explained in its report, *Guide to Clinical Preventive Services*. The *Guide* is recognized as the best information on screening and is preferred over the recommendations of medical specialty groups, voluntary health organizations, even the National Institutes of Health. The information in *LifePlan* goes beyond that of the *Guide* in some areas and vice versa, but the recommendations in these books are compatible.

RESOURCES

Guide to Clinical Preventive Services: An Assessment of the Effectiveness of 169 Interventions. Report of the U.S. Preventive Services Task Force. Baltimore, MD: Williams and Wilkins, 1989.

IMMUNIZATIONS: Protection From Infections

*J*n November 1988, the traditional cross-town rivalry between the football teams of the University of Southern California and the University of California, Los Angeles, had reached fever pitch. The two teams were nationally ranked second and sixth, respectively, and both quarterbacks were contenders for the Heisman trophy. Midweek came the astounding news: USC's star quarterback, Rodney Peete, was flat on his back—and not with flu, as first thought, but with the measles.

By week's end some 40 other students at USC had come down with this highly contagious disease, and hundreds—including the players on both football teams—had lined up to get measles shots. There was even talk of canceling the game.

The afternoon of the game, UCLA fans showed up wearing medical masks and waving placards that taunted the "University of Something Contagious." But just before kickoff, Peete, who had missed practice all week, was named to start. And despite any lingering weakness or doubts, he threw for one touchdown and ran for another, leading USC's Trojans to a decisive 31–22 victory.

As for the UCLA fans, at least they got to watch the game. Later that same year, all fans were barred from a basketball game at Siena College in Loudonsville, New York, because of an outbreak of measles on campus.

BENEFITS, RISKS AND DOUBTS

The USC and Siena episodes were just two in a string of measles outbreaks at colleges and high schools in recent years. Before a vaccine was licensed in 1963, measles struck hundreds of thousands of Americans each year, mostly children under five. Improved vaccines debuted in 1965 and 1966, and the number of cases fell markedly over the next two decades. But then it began to rise again.

According to the Centers for Disease Control, the reasons for the increase are twofold. In some people, perhaps 5 percent, the vaccine does not "take." And not all children are being vaccinated.

To some extent, the vaccine programs designed to wipe out many infectious diseases have been victims of their own success. As the likelihood of infection drops, parents of young children underestimate the very real dangers posed by these diseases. Some have been frightened off by the small but real possibility of serious side effects, particularly from the pertussis vaccine. And programs to immunize adults against influenza are still tarred by the fiasco of the "swine flu" vaccine program. Figures from the Centers for Disease Control show that the percentage of two-year-olds fully immunized dropped between 1980 and 1985.

Historically, infectious diseases have been the bane of the human race. In the industrialized world their toll has been greatly reduced by many advances, including improved nutrition, sanitation and housing and, more recently, immunizations and antibiotics. In the past 25 years, global immunization programs sponsored by the United Nations have wiped out smallpox and made major inroads against measles, diphtheria, whooping cough, tetanus, polio and tuberculosis. Still, infectious diseases continue to kill some 14 million Third World children under five each year.

It is often impossible to avoid the bacteria and viruses that cause infectious illnesses, because they can be spread by contact with people or animals, or by airborne droplets. That's why immunization provides a practical means of protection. No immunization is 100 percent effective or safe. However, professionals and lay people alike almost always judge the benefits to outweigh the risks.

To encourage widespread vaccination and continued vaccine development, the government passed the National Vaccine Compensation Act. This 1988 law set up a trust fund, financed by a surcharge on each of the two major vaccines (DPT and MMR), to compensate children who suffer adverse reactions as well as their families. Parents who accept payment must agree to forgo further lawsuits. The fund is designed to compensate as many as 150 children a year, twice the number estimated to be affected.

If you have questions about a certain immunization, your physician or health department should be willing to explain in detail its risks, benefits and current recommendations. If you are not satisfied with the explanation, you can turn to any of the groups listed at the end of this chapter.

HOW VACCINES WORK

Immunization stimulates the body's immune defenses against specific, harmful germs, such as bacteria and viruses. This is done by introducing into the body a small dose of a germ that has been killed, weakened or otherwise altered. Although no longer able to cause serious illness, these substances can provoke the immune system to make antibodies and immune cells that will recognize and attack the germ.

Some vaccines contain just part of the germ. Still others substitute a related germ that causes a milder infection; for example, people were injected with the cowpox virus to protect against the much-deadlier smallpox. In some diseases, illness is caused not by the bacteria themselves, but by harmful toxins they secrete; in these cases, the vaccine may be a weakened form of the toxin, known as a toxoid. Sometimes chemicals that enhance the immune response are added to the mixture.

Vaccines that stimulate the body's own defense system are said to cause *active* immunization. It is also possible to be immunized *passively*, by receiving an injection of immune globulin ("gamma globulin"). This contains antibodies derived from the blood serum of donors who have a high degree of immunity to a certain disease. People with contaminated wounds may be given tetanus immune globulin; travelers to countries where hepatitis is widespread may receive gamma globulin. Infants, too, are often immunized passively when they receive antibodies from their mothers, either through the placenta or in breast milk.

Some immunizations, such as that for smallpox, produce lifelong immunity with a single injection. (Smallpox has achieved a unique distinction; it is the *only* disease ever to be eliminated.) Others need a series of shots to establish protection. In some diseases, including tetanus, immunity wanes over time and needs to be restored with "booster" shots. With a disease like influenza, immunization needs to be repeated each year, because the flu viruses that are going around change from one flu season to the next.

Vaccinations are not just for kids. Some of the immunizations of childhood—notably tetanus and diphtheria—need to be boosted throughout life. And other diseases, such as flu and pneumonia, become more serious concerns as age or certain chronic conditions weaken the ability to fight off infection. Some adults were never properly vaccinated when they were children—against rubella, for example. And some adults need to be protected against diseases they run into in the course of their work (hepatitis for health care workers, for instance) or travels.

CHILDHOOD IMMUNIZATION: THREE SHOTS AND ONE ORAL VACCINE

The DPT Shot

The DPT shot is a single injection that promotes immunity against three diseases—diphtheria, pertussis (whooping cough) and tetanus. The combination injection works as well as three separate shots and hurts less. The DPT shot is given four times during the first 18 months of life.

Diphtheria

Diphtheria is a serious, rapidly developing and painful infection that targets the throat and nose. (It can also develop in the skin or open wounds.) As the diphtheria bacteria multiply, they produce a toxin that kills nearby cells, creating a characteristic grayish film. The throat swells, making it hard to swallow or breathe. The toxin also travels through the bloodstream and injures the heart, kidneys and nerves. Even with treatment, diphtheria is fatal in about 10 percent of the cases. About 20 percent of patients become paralyzed; 50 percent suffer heart damage.

The diphtheria vaccine is a toxoid, made from an inactivated version of the deadly toxin. Reactions to the immunization are rare—usually nothing more than a slight swelling at the injection site—and immunity lasts for many years. Boosters use a somewhat weaker toxoid (signified by "d" on Table 16.1) than that used for primary immunization ("D").

Pertussis

Pertussis, or whooping cough, is a sometimes deadly and highly infectious disease of infancy and early childhood. It is characterized by severe and prolonged bouts of coughing. Robbed of air, the child breathes in violently, making the sound described as a whoop. The disease tends to last six to eight weeks.

Until the 1950s, whooping cough struck 100,000 American children each year. Between 4,000 and 5,000 died; many others suffered long-term nervous system injury. Widespread use of the pertussis vaccine reduced the number of cases to fewer than 3,000 a year, and the number of deaths to fewer than 20.

However, in recent years DPT shots have sparked controversy because of the side effects produced by the "P" component, which is made of the whole, killed pertussis bacterium. Minor reactions—fever, pain and fretfulness—are common. Nearly a third of the children who get the shot grow drowsy, and a fifth show some loss of appetite. More severe reactions, though less common, also occur. One child in 300 will develop a high fever (over 105 degrees Fahrenheit); one in 1,600 will experience a seizure or short period of collapse. Almost always, these reactions have no long-term effects; in a recent study of children who had suffered convulsions or lapses of alertness within 24 hours of vaccination (there were 18 such reactions in nearly 16,000 shots), all had recovered within 48 hours. Nearly a decade later, none of them showed any lasting damage.

In rare instances, the pertussis vaccine has been linked with brain damage or death. The Centers for Disease Control estimates that about 50 children suffer permanent brain damage each year in the United States, while the American Academy of Pediatrics estimates there are 70 to 75 severe reactions each year. The risk appears to be very low, about one or two in 100,000.

Table 16.1
The Immunization Schedule

Children

2 months	DPT (diphtheria, pertussis, tetanus)	and	Oral polio virus (OPV)
4 months	DPT	and	OPV
6 months	DPT	and	OPV (in certain areas only)
15 months	Measles, mumps, rubella (MMR)		
18 months	DPT	and	OPV
2 years	HbCV (Hemophilus conjugated vaccine)		
4–6 years	Td (Tetanus, adult diphtheria)	and	OPV
10–12 years	Rubella (only for girls who did not receive rubella vaccine, or with rubella hemagglutination test result that is negative or less than 1:16)		
14–16 years	Td		

Adults

Every 10 years	Td
Over 65 years*	Influenza yearly Pneumococcal pneumonia once

Special Situations

Chronic illness	Influenza yearly Pneumococcal pneumonia once
High risk for hepatitis B	Hepatitis B
Rabies exposure	Rabies (vaccine and antiserum)
Lack of immunity to measles, mumps or rubella	Measles, mumps or rubella

*Age 75 or 80 may be preferred. See page 267.

In Sweden, where pertussis vaccination was halted in 1979 on the grounds that it was too dangerous, the number of cases has increased yearly. In the United States, the number of cases reported to the Centers for Disease Control more than doubled between 1980 and 1985, from 1,730 to 3,589, simply because fewer parents had their children vaccinated.

Research to develop less toxic pertussis vaccines is under way. Vaccines made from one or more pieces of the pertussis bacterium, rather than the whole organism, have been developed by the Japanese and tested by American and Swedish scientists in Sweden. These have proved to cause fewer side effects, but to protect against disease somewhat less effectively. Current studies are looking at the value of making them more effective by giving booster shots.

Meanwhile, parents must weigh the risks of the current vaccine against those posed by the disease. It is my opinion that parents should go ahead with pertussis vaccination after discussing it with their own physician, but they should also keep abreast of reports on safety and efficacy.

Children who react to the first pertussis shot with more than minor side effects—temperature over 104 degrees Fahrenheit, convulsions, extreme drowsiness and loss of consciousness—should not have further shots. Rather, they should receive the DT immunization without the P.

Tetanus

Tetanus is caused when a deadly toxin produced by the tetanus germ attacks the nerves that control the voluntary muscles, and the muscles spasm. It usually affects the muscles of the neck and jaw, hence the name "lockjaw."

The tetanus bacterium and its spores are found everywhere—in dust, soil, pastures, and human and animal waste. They enter the body through wounds; because they grow only in the absence of air, the danger of tetanus infection is greatest with deep puncture wounds, such as those from gunshots, nails or knives, which can carry the bacteria beneath the skin. Even with the best of care, tetanus is still fatal in up to 40 percent of the cases.

Like the diphtheria vaccine, the tetanus vaccine is an inactivated version of a deadly toxin. Of all the vaccines available, tetanus is one of the best. It is nearly 100 percent effective, and any reactions are mild and brief. (That is, unless the vaccination is repeated too often; then, as some unhappy military recruits have discovered, the local reaction can be very painful.)

Once the initial series of shots is complete, immunity is renewed with a booster shot every 10 years. Also, a booster is often given when a person suffers a dirty wound and it's been more than five years since the last tetanus shot. Protection may be supplemented with tetanus immune globulin, especially if the basic series of shots is not complete (see Figure 16.1).

The MMR Shot

Like DPT, MMR is a three-in-one immunization. Given once around the age of 15 months, it protects against measles, mumps and rubella (German measles).

Measles

A classic childhood infection, measles is by no means a mild disease to be dismissed as a rite of passage. Before an effective vaccine was introduced in the mid-1960s, measles caused 400 deaths a year. More often, it produced severe complications, such as infection of the brain (measles encephalitis), often with permanent brain damage. Other complications include pneumonia, convulsions and blindness.

Caused by a virus, measles is highly contagious. It is spread by droplets from the nose, mouth or throat and by direct contact with items freshly soiled by nose and throat secretions. It can be transmitted for a period lasting from three to six days before the telltale rash appears until several days after it goes away.

Measles begins with fever, weakness, a dry, "brassy" cough, and eyes that are itchy, red and sensitive to light. Three to five days later, a pink, blotchy, mildly itchy, flat rash appears. It shows up first around the face, then gradually spreads to the trunk, arms and legs. It usually lasts for four to seven days.

Figure 16.1
Tetanus Shots

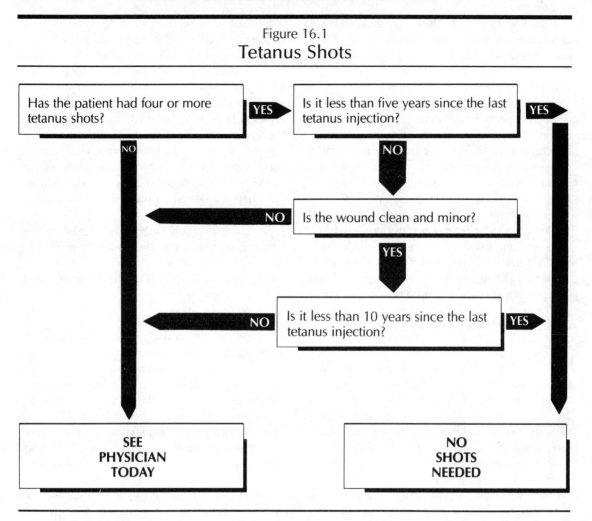

The measles vaccine in use today, introduced in 1966, is made of a weakened live measles virus. Reactions are mild—fever, slight irritability or rash.

The vaccine is usually given at age 15 months, although younger children may be vaccinated during epidemics. The incubation period for measles is 10 days, but protective antibodies develop within seven days of vaccination. This makes it possible to protect a child by getting him or her immunized immediately after exposure to the measles. However, it is more common to protect children who have been exposed by giving them measles immune globulin.

People who were immunized with the vaccines used between 1963 and 1967 may still be open to infection. Revaccination with the current vaccine is possible, but often produces adverse reactions. Consult your doctor if you received your MMR shot between 1963 and 1967.

Mumps

Mumps is caused when a virus infects the salivary glands. The major salivary glands are located just below and in front of the ear. When infected, they often swell up, producing the hallmark "chipmunk cheeks." Other salivary glands under the jaw and tongue can also be infected. The person may find it painful to chew or swallow and may also experience fever, headache, earache or weakness. About one-third of the people who get mumps don't have any swelling, so many people have mumps without knowing it.

Although highly contagious, mumps is usually a mild illness in children, with symptoms fading in about a week. In rare cases, it can lead to infection of the brain or pancreas, kidney disease, deafness, or damage to the testicles or ovaries. Adults are more likely than children to have problems with mumps.

The mumps vaccine is made from a live, weakened virus. After it was introduced in 1967, cases of mumps decreased steadily through 1985. In 1986 and 1987 the number of cases skyrocketed, largely due to outbreaks in high schools and colleges. But after states stepped up enforcement of school immunization laws, the numbers began to drop again in 1988.

Rubella

Also known as German measles or three-day measles, rubella is a mild, moderately contagious viral infection spread by droplets from the mouth or throat. It often produces a rash that starts on the face and spreads to the trunk, arms and legs; it can cause a mild fever and sometimes joint pain.

Many people have rubella and never know it; in itself, this disease is little cause for concern. The problem lies in the rubella virus's ability to cause birth defects: When a woman contracts German measles during the first three months of pregnancy, she runs a high chance of either miscarrying or giving birth to a baby with abnormalities, including cataracts, heart disease, deafness or mental retardation. During the last rubella epidemic in this country, in 1964, more than 20,000 babies were born with such defects.

To prevent a repeat of this misfortune, an immunization program was undertaken when a vaccine became available in 1969. This program aimed to immunize all children over the age of one year and was unique because for the first time, people were exposed to vaccination and its potential complications to protect not themselves, but others.

We are not yet certain how long the immunization's protection will last; we could be producing a generation of young women who will be susceptible to infection when they reach childbearing age. Other countries have adopted a policy of immunizing young teenage girls, who are closer to their reproductive years; however, side effects of the vaccination—mainly joint pains that can last as long as two years—are more common at this age. It is also possible that a teenager could be pregnant at the time of vaccination; however, no birth defects have ever been reported following vaccination.

There is a test (rubella hemagglutination) that tells whether someone is adequately immune to rubella. This test can be used to determine if teenagers or adult women need to be immunized.

Polio

As recently as the 1950s, polio was a fearsome scourge. Each summer the polio virus killed more than 1,000 Americans and, by invading and killing nerve cells, crippled tens of thousands of others. Many more people developed the infection but were not paralyzed. They suffered only a brief, feverish illness accompanied by headache, sore throat, vomiting and stiffness of the neck and back. Many thousands more remained apparently healthy carriers of the virus.

In 1955, Dr. Jonas Salk introduced the inactivated polio virus vaccine, which was given by injection, and the number of polio cases began to fall dramatically. In 1961, Dr. Albert Sabin developed a live polio vaccine to be taken by mouth. The oral polio vaccine, as this is known, offered even better protection against the virus, was less costly and was easier to administer. It largely replaced the injected vaccine.

Together, these vaccines virtually wiped out infection by wild polio viruses in this country; the last known case was reported in 1979. However, five to 10 cases still occur each year as a result of the oral vaccine itself, either in vaccinated children or, more often, in persons who come into contact with them. Although this number is small given the fact that some 3 million children receive the vaccine each year, these infections have triggered lawsuits as well as the newly legislated compensation fund.

The American Academy of Pediatrics now regards the injected vaccine as an acceptable alternative, particularly for families with members who have conditions that suppress their immune response and thus make them susceptible to illness. The injected vaccines carry a very small risk of serious muscle infections or nerve damage. Researchers are experimenting with ways to obtain maximum benefits by using both types of vaccine, starting with one or more doses of injected polio vaccine and then boosting with at least one dose of the oral vaccine.

Hib Vaccine/Bacterial Meningitis

Meningitis is an inflammation of the membranes around the brain and spinal cord. It begins with a high fever and irritability, and it often looks like influenza or a bad cold for a couple of days. Young children may complain of a stiff neck, or the "soft spot" on a baby's skull may bulge.

The leading cause of bacterial meningitis among American children is *Hemophilus influenza* type b, or Hib. Each year about one of every 200 children under five (at least 20,000 in the United States) becomes infected with this bacterium, and half of these children develop meningitis. (The infection often spreads rapidly through day-care centers.) In 10 percent of the cases it is fatal; 25 percent to 30 percent suffer serious and permanent nervous system disorders—partial paralysis, blindness, deafness and mild to severe mental retardation. Children who are spared meningitis can develop other types of infections—pneumonia, infectious arthritis, blood infection, and a serious form of croup called epiglottitis, in which swelling in the throat can lead to suffocation.

Since 1982, several types of Hib vaccine have been licensed. The most recent, released in 1987, is the Hib conjugate vaccine, or HbCV. It is made from just a part of the bacterium—the purified outer coat, or capsule, which has been chemically bonded (conjugated) to a diphtheria toxoid to make it better able to stimulate immune responses.

HbCV is approved for use in children from 18 to 60 months of age. (By age five most children develop natural immunity to Hib.) A single injection protects, and side effects are limited to some redness and tenderness at the injection site. Because the vaccine has no live components, there is no risk of spreading the infection.

The conjugate vaccine is now being tested —and appears to work—in younger children, too. Children under one year of age are at highest risk of Hib infection, but earlier versions of the vaccine didn't work in them, because their immature immune systems respond differently.

Chicken Pox

Chicken pox, which is caused by a type of herpes virus (herpes zoster, which is also known as varicella), is the last major childhood disease without a vaccine. Of the more than 3 million Americans it strikes each year, most are children. Usually it causes nothing more serious than fever and a tormenting itch.

Adults who get chicken pox often become seriously ill. Many develop viral pneumonia. Chicken pox can cause pregnant women to miscarry; in rare cases a fetus can become infected and suffer brain damage. Moreover, the herpes zoster virus, which lies dormant in nerves for years, can become reactivated later in life, causing the painful nerve inflammation and blister-like rash known as shingles.

In the early 1970s, Japanese scientists developed a vaccine using live attenuated viruses. This still-experimental vaccine is being tried in children whose immune systems are crippled by cancer therapy or AIDS and has proven safe and effective. And it does not cause shingles as was feared. The U.S. Food and Drug Administration has not yet approved it for general use, however, in part because scientists have no way of knowing if the immunity will last into adulthood, when the disease would pose a serious danger.

ADULT IMMUNIZATION
Td/Tetanus and Diphtheria

Each year a handful of American adults catch diphtheria and about 75 develop tetanus. What's more, surveys indicate that large numbers are not protected. Assuming you have already received the primary series of tetanus and diphtheria toxoids, you need a booster every 10 years. Boosting is simple, safe and highly effective, and should be routine. To help people remember, the American College of Physicians suggests scheduling boosters on mid-decade birthdays (35, 45, 55 and so on).

As with children, adults suffering a severe or dirty wound should get a booster if it's been more than five years since the last one.

The Td shot sometimes causes local redness or hardness, with or without tenderness. More severe reactions are rare, and the only contraindication is a history of severe allergic reactions.

Influenza

Although many common illnesses are mistakenly called "the flu," influenza is a specific viral infection of the respiratory tract—the nose, throat, airways and lungs. While its symptoms resemble those of other viruses, including the common cold, the flu is more likely to be severe and produce complications. The real flu usually starts with a headache, chills and dry cough; temperature shoots up and muscles ache. The fever begins to recede by the second or third day, and symptoms such as cough, chest pain and sore throat may be more prominent.

Most people recover fully within a week, although many feel unusually tired for some time. For some persons, especially those weakened by chronic illnesses such as heart or lung disease, flu can be deadly. The most common and serious complication is pneumonia. Each year flu claims more than 20,000 American lives; another 25,000 persons die of pneumococcal pneumonia.

Flu typically occurs in abrupt outbreaks, usually in the fall and winter. By the time the outbreak subsides, five or six weeks later, between 20 percent and 50 percent of the population will have been stricken.

Influenza is caused by three types of flu viruses: A, B and C. A and, to a lesser extent, B are able to change their genetic structure from one generation to the next. As the result of slight changes, every few years a flu virus will be "new" enough to escape the immune defenses already built up in a

population, and local epidemics ensue; a major genetic change can trigger a worldwide pandemic of the type that took more than 2 million lives in 1918.

The influenza vaccine, concocted anew each year to match the viruses currently making the rounds, is highly effective against the strains it contains; it reduces the incidence of illness and infection by up to 80 percent. And studies show that it can sharply curb flu-related deaths in older people. Nonetheless, only about 20 percent of high-risk people get the vaccine each year.

Flu Shots and Medicare

The number of persons receiving the flu vaccine is likely to rise if the shots are covered under Medicare. In 1988, the government approved a large Medicare project designed to demonstrate that increasing influenza immunization rates will reduce death, illness and health care costs among the aged and chronically ill. If the two-year study proves that providing flu vaccine is cost-effective, Medicare will begin paying for it in October 1990.

Made of inactivated (killed) virus, flu vaccine usually causes only mild side effects. Some people experience soreness and swelling at the injection site; 1 percent or 2 percent develop mild flu-like symptoms. (In 1976, the entire country was urged to get "swine flu" vaccine, because the swine flu virus was feared to resemble the one that caused the pandemic of 1918. A small number of cases of the paralytic Guillain-Barre syndrome occurred among persons receiving the vaccine. Fortunately, no other vaccine-related cases have since turned up.)

Because immunity is not long-lasting (and because of changes in the virus), high-risk people should get "flu shots" every year, preferably in the fall before the flu season starts. There may still be time to vaccinate high-risk people once a flu outbreak begins, although it takes a week or two for protection to develop. Sometimes an oral antiviral drug, amantadine, is given at the same time to tide these people over until they develop high enough antibody levels.

Most authorities recommend influenza immunization for anyone over the age of 65 as well as for persons with chronic diseases such as emphysema or heart disease. I don't like to recommend this immunization for people who are in excellent health just because they are over age 65. It seems likely that much of the benefit in the over-65 age group goes to those with chronic disease. I would prefer that the age be raised to 75 or 85 for persons in excellent health. Nevertheless, the shot schedule on page 261 reflects the standard recommendations.

Pneumococcal Pneumonia

Pneumonia is an infection of the lungs that makes it difficult to breathe. It can be caused by several types of germs. About half of the cases of human pneumonia are caused by bacteria, and most of these—an estimated 500,000 each year —are caused by round, bead-like microbes known as "pneumococci."

Pneumococcal pneumonia often follows influenza or other respiratory diseases. It can spread under crowded living conditions, and epidemics sometimes occur in schools and nursing homes. People with chronic illnesses are especially susceptible.

The disease often starts abruptly, with a severe shaking chill. This is followed by high fever, chest pains, headache and sometimes a rapid heart beat and shallow breathing. Many persons cough up blood-tinged sputum.

The pneumococcal pneumonia vaccine, which contains antigens from 23 types of pneumococci, produces long-lasting protection and should not be given more than once. Like the influenza vaccine, it can cause mild reactions at the injection site and, occasionally, low-grade fever. More severe reactions, including nervous system disorders, are rare.

Again, the standard recommendations for pneumococcal immunization include anyone over age 65 as well as anyone (including children) with a chronic illness. And again, I dislike recommending immunization for people in excellent health

just because they are over 65. I would prefer a higher age, say 75 to 80, for such people. Pneumococcal immunization does have the advantage over influenza immunization in that it is a one-time-only injection. The standard recommendations are listed in the shot schedule.

Hepatitis B

Hepatitis B, a debilitating and sometimes lethal liver infection, strikes some 300,000 Americans each year—up from 200,000 a decade ago—and kills about 200. Although most patients with acute hepatitis recover completely in a matter of weeks or months, each year between 4,000 and 6,000 Americans die from cirrhosis or liver cancer caused by the disease. Thousands of others have no symptoms but become life-long carriers, capable of spreading the infection to others. (There are now about 1.5 million carriers in the United States.)

The introduction of a good test for screening donor blood for the hepatitis B virus has greatly reduced the danger of infection through blood transfusions, but it has not eliminated it. Hepatitis still strikes some 36,000 transfusion recipients each year, but between 90 percent and 95 percent of these cases are due to a different hepatitis virus known as non-A, non-B; hepatitis B accounts for most of the rest.

Like the AIDS virus, the hepatitis B virus can be spread by contaminated blood, by sexual contact, and from mother to child around the time of birth. However, hepatitis is much more contagious than AIDS. Also, it is possible that it is spread through contaminated feces or body secretions. Persons at high risk include health care workers, especially those who come into contact with blood or instruments contaminated with blood; needle-sharing drug addicts; and persons with many sex partners. Others at risk are staff and residents of institutes for the mentally retarded, who frequently get hepatitis B; patients and staff of kidney dialysis units; and newborn infants of women who are infected or carriers.

The introduction of a good test for screening donor blood for the hepatitis B virus has greatly reduced the danger of infection through blood transfusions, but it has not eliminated it. Hepatitis still strikes some 36,000 transfusion recipients each year, but between 90 percent and 95 percent of these cases are due to a different hepatitis virus known as non-A, non-B; hepatitis B accounts for most of the rest.

The first hepatitis B vaccine, introduced in 1981, was made from blood plasma of hepatitis B carriers. (Unable to grow the hepatitis B virus in the laboratory, scientists learned how to obtain and purify the immunity-stimulating portion of the virus from the blood plasma of carriers.) In 1986, the government approved another vaccine, the first to be made through genetic engineering. Both vaccines have proven safe and effective, but they have been slow to catch on, even among at-risk health care workers, who should know better. Fewer than 40 percent of primary care physicians and other "front-line providers" have been vaccinated. Meanwhile, some 18,000 health care workers were newly infected in 1987 alone.

Rabies

Rabies, a deadly infection of the nervous system, is caused by a virus transmitted in the saliva of infected animals. The most common carriers are carnivorous wild animals, especially skunks, foxes and raccoons, as well as bats. Rabies has become rare in cats and dogs and is unusual in rodents, such as squirrels, chipmunks, mice and rats.

The bite of a rabies-infected animal does not always cause disease. Symptoms occur when the virus travels through the nervous system to the brain. They usually take about 30 to 50 days to develop, depending on the location and type of bite. Yet severe bites on the head can bring on symptoms in as little as 10 days.

The disease makes itself known with a feeling of depression, restlessness, abnormal sensations around the bite area, headache, fever, malaise, nausea, sore throat and loss of appetite. The person may also be highly sensitive to sound, light and changes in temperature. Other symptoms include muscle stiffness, dilated pupils and increased salivation.

As the disease progresses, bursts of irrational excitement and activity alternate with periods of alert calm. Violent convulsions are common. Severe and very painful throat spasms are triggered when the victim tries to swallow—or even sees—liquids. This gave rise to the disease's common name, hydrophobia, which means fear of water. Most patients die of cardiac or respiratory failure while in the excited state or from progressive paralysis. Although rabies had been thought to always be fatal, in recent years a few persons have recovered following supportive treatment that maintained their respiration and circulation.

The first line of defense against rabies is thorough cleaning of the wound. Whenever possible, the animal should be confined and observed for illness or killed and its brain examined for virus. Without proof that the animal is rabid, the decision to treat must be based on the details of the specific case—the species of animal, the extent of exposure, and the circumstances. (Rabid animals, their nervous systems damaged by infection, may attack for no reason.)

Both attenuated rabies vaccine and antirabies serum are available. Because of the long incubation period, it is possible to fend off disease by administering rabies vaccine *after* the bite. The antirabies serum, rabies immune globulin, can protect until the vaccine takes effect.

The vaccine used today is made from virus grown in cultured human cells; it does not cause allergic reactions like earlier vaccines grown in animal tissues, and it requires only five injections in the arm, compared to the 14 or more in the abdomen that once made rabies vaccination a dreaded procedure. Local reactions are common, but they are no reason to stop the series.

Persons such as veterinarians, who work regularly with animals, should receive rabies vaccine as a preventive measure. If bitten by a rabid animal, these people will still require vaccine, but fewer doses, and they will not need rabies immune globulin.

Measles

Young adults should be immunized unless they are known to be immune. The risk of infection is high for students living in crowded dormitories or military recruits.

Mumps

Most adults are likely to have had the mumps, but the vaccine is recommended for all adults, especially men, thought to be susceptible.

Rubella

Women of childbearing age need to be protected against rubella. Those who don't have a record showing they were vaccinated after their first birthday can have a lab test to find out if they are immune. Women who are not immune should be vaccinated, but should avoid becoming pregnant for at least three months.

INFECTIONS STILL POSE RISKS

Infectious diseases are not the widespread threat to health that they once were, but they still pose risks. Your personal risk depends on such factors as your age, sex, health status, occupation and previous immunity. Immunizations are an important defense against serious infections. Use the information in this chapter to update your immunizations and those of your children, if necessary. And remember that your immunization needs will change throughout life.

FOR MORE INFORMATION ON IMMUNIZATIONS

- American Academy of Pediatrics, Committee on Infectious Diseases, 141 Northwest Point Boulevard, Elk Grove Village, IL 60007.
- American College of Physicians, Committee on Immunization, 4200 Pine Street, Philadelphia, PA 19104.
- National Foundation for Infectious Diseases, P.O. Box 42022, Washington, DC 20015.
- Centers for Disease Control, Atlanta, GA 30333.

MEDICINES: Key Concepts

*I*f you want to know what a drug does, how to take it, how to store it, what its side effects may be and whether it will interact with food or other drugs, you can talk to your physician or pharmacist. You can also go to the library and read about the drug in the *Physicians' Desk Reference*, a thick book that contains all of the information that the U.S. Food and Drug Administration requires to be supplied with every package of every drug. The other books listed at the end of this chapter can supply this information as well.

But when it comes to the key concepts that you need for weighing a drug's benefits and risks, these resources often have little to offer. This chapter presents those concepts, so that you can make informed decisions about medication use.

This chapter does not contain all of the key concepts for all drugs, of course. It focuses on those situations in which your judgment of a drug's benefit and risk is most important. For example, the choice of medication in an allergy depends greatly on how much you are bothered by the allergy as well as how much you are bothered by the side effects of allergy medications. Likewise, the choice of a contraceptive method depends on personal feelings about pregnancy and the different types of contraceptive methods. On the other hand, if you have bacterial meningitis, a life-threatening disease that requires antiobiotic treatment, your physician will make the decision based on a number of factors, including the type of infection and your age.

In short, this chapter presents what physicians often refer to as "pearls"—small beads of knowledge that help guide decisions about benefit and risk.

ALLERGY

Four types of drugs are used to treat allergy:

- **Antihistamines** block the action of histamine, a body chemical that causes swelling, itching, sneezing, red and watery eyes and excessive mucus production in the nasal passages. Their main side effects are drowsiness and dryness of the mouth and nasal passages. Antihistamines available without prescription include pheniramine, chlorpheniramine, brompheniramine, pyrilamine, phenyltoloxamine, doxylamine, chlorcyclizine and triprolidine. Terfenadine (Seldane) is a fairly new antihistamine that is available by prescription only.

- **Decongestants,** by narrowing blood vessels, relieve swelling that has occurred as part of an allergic reaction. A common side effect is nervousness or "jumpiness," although decongestants sometimes cause drowsiness in children. At high doses, they may raise blood pressure. Popular decongestants available without prescription include phenylpropanolamine, phenylephrine, pseudoephedrine and ephedrine.

- **Corticosteroids** are powerful drugs that suppress the body's immune functions, including the allergic response. Short-term side effects include acne and mood changes, such as depression and manic behavior. Long-term use produces a variety of major problems, including cataracts, osteoporosis and peptic ulcers. Corticosteroids may be taken as pills (prednisone, prednisolone, methylprednisolone) or by injection (hydrocortisone, dexamethasone); these corticosteroids are available only by prescription.

- **Allergy shots** (hyposensitization) decrease the allergic response to one or more substances. Over time, tiny amounts of the offending substance are injected into the skin in gradually increasing amounts. Allergy shots appear to help about half of the people who try them. It may take months or years to see any benefit, and the shots must be continued indefinitely.

Key concepts:

- Remember that simply avoiding the substance causing the allergy may be the most important step in decreasing symptoms.

- None of these treatments will cure an allergy. Their purpose is to reduce symptoms; therefore, you must judge how effective they are. You must also balance their benefits against their side effects.

- Antihistamines and decongestants are the first line of defense, and often they are used together. Although Seldane causes less drowsiness, some physicians believe that it is somewhat less effective. Thus, there is little benefit in asking your physician to prescribe antihistamines and decongestants, because all that you need are available without prescription.

- Corticosteroids can be very helpful but must be used for a limited time. Therefore, they work best for people who have clearly defined seasonal allergies, such as someone who has a serious problem only in the spring or fall.

- Allergy shots are a last resort. They rarely remove the need for other drugs. The allergy testing used to select the type of shot is not precise, so most patients end up taking one of several standard types of shots.

ANXIETY

Anti-anxiety drugs may be referred to as "anxiolytics," but they are commonly known as tranquilizers. Tranquilizers are among the most frequently prescribed drugs and include such familiar names as Valium, Librium, Equanil, Miltown and Xanax. Tranquilizers slow mental activity and, in the process, help reduce feelings of agitation and restlessness. Some tranquilizers are effective as muscle relaxants, and Valium has a role in stopping seizures. Unfortunately, virtually all mental activity is slowed, so that drowsiness, forgetfulness and confusion are frequent side effects. Most tranquilizers can produce psychological and physical addiction.

Key concepts:

- Tranquilizers don't cure anything and do not solve problems.

Table 17.1
Expected Pregnancies

Pregnancy Rate (%) Among Married Women in the First Year of Contraceptive Use at Age*:

Method	15–19	20–24	25–29	30–44
Pill	2.3	1.5	1.2	0.8
Intrauterine device (IUD)	4.5	2.9	2.3	1.5
Condom	10.7	15.4	5.7	0.9
Diaphragm/spermicide	17.9	11.7	9.6	6.3
Rhythm	23.3	15.4	12.6	8.3

*Percentages shown are the lowest rates for each age group. From A. L. Shirm, J. Trussell, J. Menken and W. R. Grady, "Contraceptive Failure in the United States: The Impact of Social, Economic and Demographic Factors," *Family Planning Perspectives*, Volume 14, Table 2, p.68, 1982.

- It is a mistake to give tranquilizers to someone who is depressed. Be careful not to confuse so-called agitated depression (depression mixed with restlessness) with anxiety.
- Tranquilizers are especially likely to cause problems such as forgetfulness and confusion in older adults.
- Tranquilizers can be useful for a short period in persons who are very upset, but they have no place in treating chronic problems.
- A short period means short. Most often, this is a period of hours, or days at most. Use for longer than two weeks is seldom, if ever, appropriate.

CONTRACEPTION

The choice of contraceptive method is perhaps the best example of a decision in which your own judgment and values are paramount. Medical science cannot help you with the personal, moral and ethical issues involved. But medical science can help you understand the effectiveness of various contraceptive methods, as indicated in the tables below. Table 17.1 gives information on the effectiveness of various methods in preventing pregnancy. Generally, the risk of pregnancy for each method is somewhat lower after the first year of its use. Table 17.3 gives information on the risk of each method.

There are two sources of risk in contraception: risk from the method itself, and risk due to pregnancy when the method fails. While most pregnancies are normal and have a happy outcome, complications sometimes place a woman at risk and occasionally result in death. Some methods

Table 17.2
Cumulative Risk of Mortality Per 100,000 Women, Ages 15-44

No control	462
Abortion	41
Pill/non-smoker	251
Pill/smoker	977
IUD	45
Condom	23
Diaphragm/spermicide	53
Condom and abortion	1
Rhythm	68

Source: Howard W. Ory, "Mortality Associated with Fertility and Fertility Control: 1983." *Family Planning Perspectives*, Volume 15, Number 2, (March/April 1983), pp. 59–60. © The Alan Guttmacher Institute.

Table 17.3
Risks of Pregnancy and Contraceptive Methods by Age

Birth-related, Method-related and Total Deaths (per 100,000 women) Associated with Control of Fertility at Age:

Method of control and reason for death	15–19	20–24	25–29	30–34	35–39	40–44
No control, birth-related	7.0	7.4	9.1	14.8	25.7	28.2
Abortion, method-related	0.5	1.1	1.3	1.9	1.8	1.1
Pill/non-smoker	0.5	0.7	1.1	2.1	14.1	32.0
Birth-related	0.2	0.2	0.2	0.2	0.3	0.4
Method-related	0.3	0.5	0.9	1.9	13.8	31.6
Pill/smoker	2.4	3.6	6.8	13.7	51.4	117.6
Birth-related	0.2	0.2	0.2	0.2	0.3	0.4
Method-related	2.2	3.4	6.6	13.5	51.1	117.2
IUD only	1.3	1.1	1.3	1.3	1.9	2.1
Birth-related	0.5	0.3	0.3	0.3	0.5	0.7
Method-related	0.8	0.8	1.0	1.0	1.4	1.4
Condom, birth-related	1.1	1.6	0.7	0.2	0.3	0.4
Diaphragm/ spermicide, birth-related	1.9	1.2	1.2	1.3	2.2	2.8
Condom and abortion, method-related	0.1	0.1	0.1	—	—	—
Rhythm, birth-related	2.5	1.6	1.6	1.7	2.9	3.6

—, Less than 0.1.

Source: Howard W. Ory, "Mortality Associated with Fertility and Fertility Control: 1983." *Family Planning Perspectives*, Volume 15, Number 2, (March/April 1983) pp. 59–60. © The Alan Guttmacher Institute.

(condoms and rhythm) have virtually no risk in and of themselves, but the risk in their use comes from pregnancies associated with their failure; their failure rates are relatively high compared to other methods. On the other hand, a method such as the pill is quite effective in preventing pregnancy, but the method itself has more risk. Also, risks change with age. Table 17.2 gives a measure of the total risk if one method were to be used for all of the reproductive years.

Key concepts:

- Not using birth control is riskier than using any of the birth-control methods.

- Use of the pill by a smoker may seem to be an exception, but in that case the real issue is smoking, not contraception. All the other risks of smoking will remain unless the woman stops smoking. Choosing another birth control method misses the point.

- Consistent and proper use is the issue with condoms and diaphragms. The risk to the woman rises rapidly with inconsistent or improper use, because the risk of pregnancy rises rapidly.

- Intrauterine devices (IUDs) generally are not recommended for women who have never had children. This is because there is an increased risk of pelvic infection with IUD use that in turn leads to an increased risk of infertility. (If a pelvic infection has not occurred, removing the IUD usually restores normal fertility.)

- The pill has the greatest number of situations in which it should not be used because it is a medicine taken internally. There are at least 20 such situations, so a thorough discussion with your physician of your medical history is required before the pill is prescribed.

- Surgical sterilization (tubal ligation or vasectomy) is the most common contraceptive method used in the United States. It should be considered permanent sterilization, although reversal may be possible in 30 percent to 80 percent of cases. Even with careful counseling, 3 percent to 4 percent of patients regret their decision, and about 1 percent will request reversal of the procedure.

DEPRESSION

There are two main types of antidepressant drugs, tricyclics and monoamine oxidase inhibitors (MAOIs). Both appear to relieve depression by increasing the amount of certain chemicals in the brain called neurotransmitters. These chemicals are the means by which one brain cell stimulates another. Tricyclics (amitriptyline, amoxapine, desipromine, doxepin, imipramine) can produce drowsiness, dry mouth, blurred vision and difficulty urinating. MAOIs (isocarboxazid, phenelzine) have a long list of side effects, some of which (high blood pressure, headache and vomiting) occur when people taking the drug consume foods containing tyramine, such as cheese, meat and red wine.

Key concepts:

- Just about everyone is depressed at one time or another, and most depression passes within a few days or weeks. Drugs are not used for this kind of depression, because it usually takes from 10 to 14 days before any benefit is noticed, and it may be six to eight weeks before the drug's full effect is felt.

- On the other hand, chronic depression may go undetected or be mistaken for anxiety, senility or some other problem. Use of antidepressants in such cases may relieve symptoms thought to be due to other illnesses.

- Some tricyclics, such as amitriptyline, produce drowsiness and may be especially useful in people who have trouble sleeping. Others, such as imipramine, are stimulants and may help people who feel fatigued.

- MAOIs seem to work better than tricyclics in people who are anxious as well as depressed or in those who have phobias.

- While the above information is helpful in determining who might benefit from an antidepressant drug, only the person taking the drug can determine its benefit and decide if it is worth the risk involved.

KEEPING MEDICINES

When it comes to storing medications, there is one basic rule: Keep only those medicines that you are likely to need in the near future. Unless you have a chronic medical problem, these are likely to be a pain reliever, an antacid, hydrogen peroxide, sodium bicarbonate and, if you have small children, syrup of ipecac for inducing vomiting in case of poisoning.

Key concepts:

- Cool, dry and dark—that's the place to keep your medicines. Be aware of this when traveling, too—the temperature in a car's trunk or glove compartment can easily rise to 100 degrees Fahrenheit or more even when it is not very hot outside.

- Throw away any medicine that has passed its expiration date, any drug for which you don't know the expiration date, and any medicine without a label clearly stating what it is, what it's for and when to take it.

- Keeping an antibiotic around is a bad bet, even one that is properly labeled and has not expired, unless it was prescribed for a recurrent or continuing problem. Otherwise, the chances are very small that you will have a problem for which exactly the same prescription will be given, but you may eventually be tempted to treat yourself. And taking antibiotics on your own is usually a mistake.

MENOPAUSE

Many of the symptoms of the menopause (hot flashes, sweating, vaginal dryness and mood changes) are caused by the drop in estrogen that occurs at this time. Taking synthetic estrogens (estradiol, ethinyl estradiol) or conjugated estrogen (naturally occurring estrogen obtained from the urine of pregnant mares) will relieve these symptoms. And it now appears that taking estrogen may prevent one of the major problems with the menopause, the risk of osteoporosis. Unfortunately, long-term use of estrogen appears to increase the risk of endometrial cancer (cancer of the lining of the uterus). There are also concerns about increased risk of breast cancer, heart disease and stroke. Estrogens may cause fluid retention, nausea, vomiting, breast tenderness, headache, dizziness and depression.

Key concepts:

- If symptoms such as hot flashes are your only concern, then estrogen use can be limited to a period of two to four years, because these symptoms usually disappear during this time. The risk in using estrogen for a limited time appears to be fairly small.

- If vaginal dryness is the only concern, creams containing estrogen are usually effective. The amount of estrogen absorbed into the blood from such creams is not great, so the impact on other symptoms is very small—but so are the risks.

- It is thought that the risk of uterine cancer is decreased by combining estrogen with a synthetic progesterone (progestin), such as medroxyprogesterone, megestrol or norgestrel (progesterone is another female hormone that decreases during menopause). Taking estrogens intermittently (25 days of estrogen followed by five days off) may also reduce the risk.

- Concerns about heart disease and stroke are based on studies involving certain kinds of estrogen-progesterone pills used for contraception; no such risk has been linked with estrogen use in menopause. Indeed, some experts believe that estrogen use restores the protection against cardiovascular disease that women enjoy in the years before menopause and might even reduce that risk by up to 50 percent. But just to keep things complex, there is some evidence that the use of progestin with estrogen blocks the protection against cardiovascular disease.

- Whether estrogen increases the risk of breast cancer is controversial. A recent study from Sweden found that long-term use of synthetic estrogens resulted in an increase in the risk of breast cancer, especially when combined with progestin. Other studies have pointed to a decreased risk of breast cancer for combined estrogen-progestin pills.

- Many physicians summarize the risk questions as follows: The risks of breast cancer and cardiovascular disease are a toss-up; the increased risk of uterine cancer is real but is decreased by combining estrogen with progestin or by using estrogen intermittently.

- All other concerns aside, the use of estrogen will not prevent aging, although it may make you feel better while you age gracefully.

- Many physicians, myself included, believe that weight-bearing exercise and calcium supplements can help to prevent osteoporosis. This allows the dose of estrogen, if it is used, to be lowered and any risk reduced further. This is especially important, because anything done to prevent osteoporosis must be continued for the rest of a woman's life—on average, 30 years or more.

Obesity

Reduced appetite is a side effect of certain nervous system stimulants, such as amphetamines. Unfortunately, amphetamines are notorious for being abused, and their other side effects include agitation, sleeplessness, anxiety, shaking, sweating, palpitations, seizures, delusions and hallucinations.

Over-the-counter "diet pills" contain phenylpropanolamine, a decongestant commonly used in cold and allergy medications, and this is often combined with caffeine. Side effects of such pills include sleeplessness, palpitations and raised blood pressure; in large doses, their use may lead to a psychotic episode or stroke.

Key concepts:

- Amphetamines are out of the question. Even if they suppress appetite, their continued use leads to addiction, which is far more destructive than obesity.

- Diet pills available without prescription have been associated with increased weight loss, but only a small amount of weight is lost (a pound or two) within a fairly short period (four weeks). There is no information on what happens after that time. All other evidence suggests that diet pills play no useful role in controlling obesity and may cause harm by distracting you from the effective methods described in Chapter 8.

- The bottom line is simple: Drugs aren't the answer.

Pain

There are three categories of pain-relieving drugs (analgesics): non-steroidal anti-inflammatory drugs (NSAIDs), narcotics and acetaminophen. NSAIDs include aspirin, ibuprofen and many other well-known drugs (see Table 17.4).

Table 17.4
Non-Steroidal Anti-Inflammatory Drugs (NSAIDs)

Generic Name	Brand Name
Aspirin	Many
Diflunisal	Dolobid
Fenoprofen	Nalfon
Ibuprofen	Advil, Medipren, Midol 200, Motrin, Nuprin, Rufen, etc.
Indomethacin	Indocin
Meclofenamate	Meclomen
Mefenamic acid	Ponstel
Naproxen	Naprosyn, Anaprox
Phenylbutazone	Butazolidin
Piroxicam	Feldene
Sulindac	Clinoril
Tolmetin	Tolectin
Diclofenac	Voltaren

Their popularity is due to their usefulness in arthritis as well as in relieving the everyday aches and pains that we all suffer. As their name implies, NSAIDs not only relieve pain, but they also reduce the swelling, redness and heat of inflammation. They do this by blocking prostaglandins, chemicals that cause these symptoms. Although NSAIDs act on the brain to some extent, their primary action is at the site of pain. Narcotics act almost exclusively on the brain, where they block the transmission of pain signals and alter the perception of pain. Acetaminophen is a special case. Like NSAIDs, it blocks prostaglandins, but it works only in the brain and has no effect on inflammation.

The most worrisome side effect of NSAIDs is irritation of the stomach lining which can lead to ulcers. Acetaminophen is less likely to irritate the stomach, but prolonged use may damage the kidneys and, possibly, the liver. Use of narcotics is limited by their addictive potential. They may also cause drowsiness, nausea, vomiting and constipation. Overdoses of just about any analgesic can be serious and even fatal.

Key concepts:

- NSAIDs are powerful drugs that are more likely than acetaminophen to relieve pain. This is especially true when inflammation is a part of the problem, as it is in arthritis, bursitis and sprains. But aspirin must *never* be given to children or teenagers suspected of having a virus, and many physicians prefer not to use aspirin for any problem in children or teenagers. Although other NSAIDs have not been implicated in the problem associated with aspirin use in children (Reye's syndrome), it is best to avoid them. For this reason, acetaminophen is the best choice for reducing pain and lowering fever in children and teenagers.

- NSAIDs are more alike than different. You cannot find one that is very effective but has no risk of stomach irritation. On the other hand, any particular NSAID may be more effective in one person than another. Trial and error may be needed to find the best NSAID for a certain person.

- Fear of addiction should not exclude the use of narcotics, but effective pain relief can usually be obtained with one of the NSAIDs or acetaminophen. Narcotics are most useful for severe pain or when the side effects of NSAIDs limit their use.

Seniors and Drugs

Older bodies handle drugs differently than younger ones. While drug absorption does not change with age, drugs tend to remain in the body longer. For this reason, drug doses usually should be lower the older we get.

And the older we get, the more likely we are to use more than one drug at a time. This means that interactions between drugs, as well as mix-ups in their use, are more likely to occur.

Key concepts:

- Always look for chances to reduce the number of drugs being used. Often lifestyle changes can work as well as, or even better than, a drug. For example, by improving your sleep habits, you can eliminate the need for a sleeping pill (see page 279).

- Drugs that affect the central nervous system are most likely to cause mischief. Be especially careful with tranquilizers, antidepressants and sleep aids.

- If you have a chronic medical problem, be sure you know how it affects any medicine that you might take. Kidney or liver diseases are especially likely to affect drug therapy. For example, decreased kidney function requires reduction in the dosages of many drugs, including digitalis, verapamil and captopril.

Sleep Aids

When the drugs in sleeping pills are used for other purposes, drowsiness is an undesirable side effect; in a sleeping pill, it is the benefit. Virtually all tranquilizers have been used as sleeping pills. Those promoted as sleeping pills today are those in which drowsiness is a very strong side effect. Sleeping pills available without prescription are simply antihistamines, usually pyrilamine. Tranquilizers, which are available only by prescription, are far more powerful in putting you to sleep, but the sleep they induce is not the same as natural sleep. Some people feel less rested and others complain of

Why Do the Elderly Fall?

Falls are the sixth leading cause of death in elderly persons. In those over age 65 living in the community, 30 percent will be injured in falls each year. The rate rises to 40 percent in those over age 80. Falls are cited as a contributing factor in 40 percent of all nursing home admissions.

Falls are most often blamed on hazards in the environment, such as stairs and objects left on the floor, or illness. According to an excellent study reported in the *New England Journal of Medicine*, while these factors play a role, by far the most important risk factor for falls in the elderly is the use of sedatives.

Independent Risk Factors for Falls in the Elderly

Factor	Risk*
Use of sedatives	28.3
Mental impairment	5.0
Lower extremity disability	3.8
Palmomental reflex**	3.0
Foot problems	1.8
Number of abnormalities in balance and gait	
Up to 2	1.0
3 to 5	1.4
6 to 7	1.9

* Average risk = 1
** A sign of brain disease.

Falls occurred in 32 percent of elderly people with two independent risk factors and 60 percent of those with three risk factors and 78 percent with four or more risk factors.

Environmental hazards, dizziness, and acute illness were mentioned as contributing factors in 48 percent, 13 percent and 10 percent of falls respectively.

Interestingly, no independent association was found between falling and depression, alcohol consumption, postural hypotension or environmental hazards in the home.

a "hangover" effect the following day. Antihistamines are best thought of as "promoting" sleep by making you drowsy rather than actually putting you to sleep. Their chief side effects are a dry mouth, blurred vision and trouble passing urine.

Key concepts:

- Sleeping pills are a "Catch 22": They are useful only if getting to sleep is a rare problem. In other words, usually the benefits outweigh the risks only when the day's events have you so keyed up you can't sleep—*if* such days are infrequent.
- If you have a continuing problem getting to sleep, drugs aren't the answer; you need to change your sleeping habits. See the box at right for help.

KEY CONCEPTS, KEY QUESTIONS

In the years ahead, you will face a number of decisions regarding medication use for yourself and other family members, perhaps young children or aging parents. The key concepts relating to many of those decisions have been outlined here. In other cases, they have not.

Yet whenever you are faced with a decision about medication use, you can get the information you need by asking your doctor or pharmacist some key questions:

- What are the drug's benefits?
- What are its risks?
- What side effects should I watch for?
- Are there alternatives to drug therapy that I might try, such as lifestyle changes?

RESOURCES

Guide to Prescription and Over-the-Counter Drugs, a publication of the American Medical Association. New York: Random House, Inc., 1988.

The Essential Guide to Prescription Drugs, 1989, by James W. Long, M.D. New York: Harper and Row, 1989.

Sleeping Well

If you are having trouble sleeping, give the following program a try. It is the regimen that physicians prescribe most. If it doesn't work, see your doctor. But don't expect too much—remember that drugs are seldom the answer.

To help with your sleep:

- Avoid alcohol in anything but the smallest amounts. Just like other drugs, it disturbs rapid-eye-movement (REM) sleep, periods characterized by deep muscle relaxation and vivid dreams. Also, it may cause you to feel agitated and fatigued the next day.

- Establish a regular bedtime, but do not go to bed if you feel wide awake. Try to find a bedtime that you associate with sleepiness.

- Relax upon retiring. Read, watch television or listen to soothing music. (I find that trying to get through something I should read but don't want to makes me drowsy almost instantly.) It's best not to do these things in bed. That way, you will associate your bed with sleep only.

- Avoid caffeine in the two hours before bedtime. Remember that soft drinks and chocolate contain large amounts of caffeine, as do coffee and tea.

- Eat or don't eat, depending on what works for you. Eating seems to affect people differently. Foods such as milk, meat and lettuce contain a natural sleep inducer called L-tryptophane. However, a single glass of milk probably does not contain enough L-tryptophane to explain the effect of the traditional glass of warm milk at bedtime. Whatever the reason, a glass of milk or a snack seems to help many people fall asleep.

- Fix the dripping faucet. Do something about those little sounds or lights that annoy you in the night. Sleep masks, ear plugs, darker window shades and sound-proofing the bedroom sometimes help.

- If you are sleeping for a couple of hours during the day, it's only common sense that you will want to stay up later at night. You can either accept this routine or gradually reduce the length of your daytime naps.

- Exercise regularly. Exercise is conducive to sleep and especially to those deeper stages of sleep that are associated with restfulness. But avoid exercising within two hours of bedtime. This has been shown to interfere with sleep, with one very important exception. One of the most effective and healthful sleep inducers known is—you guessed it—sex.

People's Pharmacy 1988, by Joe Graedon and Teresa Graedon. New York: St. Martin's Press, Inc., 1988.

The Complete Guide to Prescription & Nonprescription Drugs (7th edition), by H. Winter Griffith, M.D. Los Angeles, CA: Price/Stern/Sloan, Inc., 1990.

Books Written for Professionals

Physicians' Desk Reference for Nonprescription Drugs (10th edition) Oradell, NJ: Medical Economics Company Inc., 1989.

The Handbook of Non-Prescription Drugs, 8th edition (1986). Available from the American Pharmaceutical Association, 2215 Constitution Avenue, N.W., Washington, DC 20037, (202) 628-4410.

SECTION V

DEFEATING MAJOR DISEASES

- ❑ Heart Disease
- ❑ Cancer
- ❑ Stroke
- ❑ Diabetes

HEART DISEASE

Some 100,000 times a day, your heart—a strong, fist-sized muscle —faithfully pumps blood that carries oxygen and nutrients to tissues throughout your body. It speeds up when you run and settles down when you rest. Although at times it may skip a beat, jump for joy or catch in your throat, for the most part you take its steadfast performance for granted. But as hundreds of thousands of Americans learn each year, a lot can happen to disturb the heart's rhythmic work.

TYPES OF HEART DISEASE

The country's number-one killer, heart disease, can strike different parts of the heart. Sometimes just the muscle is affected; such diseases, relatively rare, are known as cardiomyopathies. A second type of heart disease involves the valves that control the flow of blood through the heart; a prime example is rheumatic heart disease, in which the valves are damaged by rheumatic fever, an inflammatory condition that develops in the wake of a streptococcal infection, usually a strep throat. (The valve damage is not caused by the bacteria themselves; it is due to an abnormal immune response to infection.)

However, most of the time what we mean when we talk about heart disease—and what you will read in this chapter—is a disease that affects the arteries that supply blood to the heart. Because these arteries circle the heart like a crown, they are known as the coronary arteries, and the disease is called coronary heart disease (CHD). Because it usually results from blocked arteries (atherosclerosis), it is also known as atherosclerotic heart disease. Strictly speaking, arteriosclerosis (hardening of the arteries due to aging) is a rare cause of CHD. However, arteriosclerosis and atherosclerosis often occur together, so that CHD is sometimes referred to as arteriosclerotic coronary vascular disease. Additionally, because it involves the loss of blood supply (ischemia), it is sometimes called ischemic heart disease.

The Scope of Coronary Heart Disease

- Nearly 5 million Americans alive today have had heart attacks and/or angina (heart pain).
- 1.5 million Americans have heart attacks each year.
- More than 500,000 die each year from heart attacks—60 percent of them within the first hour.

An adequate supply of blood is critical to all body tissues, of course, but it is especially important for the constantly pumping heart. If heart muscle is deprived of its oxygen supply completely or for more than a few minutes, muscle cells die; this is a heart attack. (Another name for a heart attack is a myocardial infarction, or MI.) A less drastic cutoff of the blood supply, one that falls short of causing muscle to die, is known as ischemia. Ischemia in almost any tissue results in pain, the body's most direct way of letting us know something is wrong. Heart pain due to ischemia is known as angina pectoris, or simply angina. Heart attacks and angina are almost always caused by CHD.

Many physicians consider hypertensive heart disease (heart disease due to high blood pressure) to be separate from CHD. Certainly there are cases in which a person who dies with high blood pressure has an enlarged heart, a prominent sign of hypertensive heart disease, but no evidence of CHD. On the other hand, over 90 percent of persons with high blood pressure will have evidence of CHD at autopsy. Thus, a diagnosis of hypertensive heart disease usually means that the problems of high blood pressure were more severe than those of CHD. For the sake of simplicity, we will regard high blood pressure primarily as contributing to CHD rather than as causing a separate type of heart disease.

Sometimes heart attacks and atherosclerosis set the stage for yet another type of heart problem, congestive heart failure. Here the heart is unable to pump strongly and efficiently. As a result, the circulation slows down and blood backs up in the veins, causing tissues to grow congested and swollen. The muscle damage that leads to congestive heart failure is usually caused by heart attacks and atherosclerosis, but high blood pressure, congenital heart defects and rheumatic fever can also be the cause, as can high blood pressure in the lungs resulting from lung disease.

ATHEROSCLEROSIS: THE ROOT OF THE PROBLEM

The problem underlying most coronary heart disease is atherosclerosis. In this condition, the arteries' inner walls grow thick with gunk —fatty substances, cholesterol, waste products from cells, calcium and clotting material from the blood. Also, the smooth-muscle cells that make up the artery walls grow abnormally.

This complex buildup, known as plaque, causes the artery walls to bulge inward, narrowing the channel and endangering the blood flow in various ways. Sometimes the plaque itself obstructs the artery. In other cases, an artery wall becomes distended and weakened by plaque, and bleeds. The blood clot that forms rapidly blocks the already narrowed artery. Occasionally, a blood clot breaks off and travels to, lodges in and obstructs smaller vessels downstream; in medical terms, such a clot is an *embolus*.

Blood flow to the heart can also be cut off when an artery goes into spasm. This can happen with normal arteries as well as vessels that are atherosclerotic; the reasons are not well understood.

Heart Disease, the Number-One Killer in America

	Deaths
Heart attack	524,100
Rheumatic fever and rheumatic heart disease	6,400
Hypertensive heart disease	30,100
Congestive heart failure	38,000
Congenital heart defects	6,000

Source: U.S. Public Health Service

Figure 18.1

Risk Factors For Coronary Heart Disease
(rate per 1,000 men age 30–59 at entry)

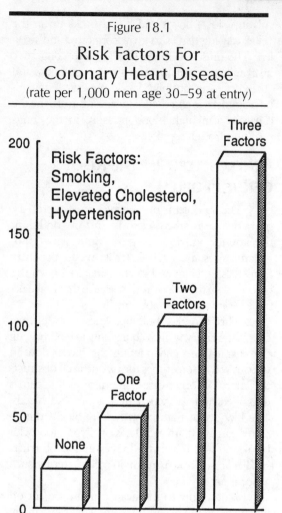

Source: *Health Consequences of Smoking, 1983*

WHAT CAUSES ATHEROSCLEROSIS?

The many studies that have looked into this question have identified a number of factors that go hand in hand with atherosclerosis. Exactly how such so-called risk factors do their dirty work is not clear, but this doesn't lessen their importance. You can do something about each one of them. They include:

- Cholesterol:
  High LDL-C or total cholesterol
  Low HDL-C (see below)
- Smoking
- High blood pressure
- Lack of exercise
- Obesity

A family history of heart attacks or sudden death before age 55 appears to be another risk factor. Although a large part of the risk that has been chalked up to heredity is probably due to a combination of the other risk factors, some risk is attached to a family history of CHD in and of itself. It is hard to know just how large this risk is. Even so, a family history of CHD should strengthen your commitment to change other risk factors, because you can't change your family history.

The more risk factors you have, the likelier you are to develop heart disease. Risk factors often interact, and they have a nasty tendency to gang up on you. Blood pressure tends to go up as fat goes up. People who seldom exercise are often overfat, and people who are overfat often have elevated LDL-C and decreased HDL-C. Worst of all, risk factors may not just add up to a big problem, they can multiply! That is, the risk of three or more factors together is greater than the sum of the risks for each of those factors separately (see Figure 18.1).

Cholesterol: Good and Bad

Cholesterol is a waxy substance that helps to make up all body cells as well as some hormones. Eighty percent of the cholesterol in the body is produced from saturated fats in the diet, found largely in animal products—meat, poultry, eggs and whole-milk dairy products, including cheese. The remaining 20 percent is absorbed directly from cholesterol-containing foods (all of animal origin). Research shows that a rise of two percent in total blood cholesterol raises the risk of heart disease one percent.

Cholesterol is carried through the bloodstream by substances known as lipoproteins (fat–protein combinations). Low-density lipoproteins, or LDL-C, are the major cholesterol carrier in the blood. High levels of LDL-C in the blood correspond with an increase in cholesterol deposits in artery walls. This has given LDL-C its reputation as the "bad" cholesterol.

In contrast, high-density lipoproteins, or HDL-C, are thought to carry cholesterol away from cells and back to the liver, where it is eliminated. Because high levels of HDL-C are associated with a decreased risk of coronary heart disease, HDL-C is known as the "good" cholesterol.

The contrasting behaviors of these two types of cholesterol help explain why a measurement of total cholesterol has not always been a very good predictor. The difference also goes a long way toward explaining why women have a decreased risk of heart attacks during their childbearing years. They usually have more HDL-C and less LDL-C than men. (It also seems to explain why dogs don't have much heart disease—they, too, have high levels of HDL-C.) However, because total cholesterol is easier to measure and consists mostly of LDL-C, most cholesterol testing consists of measuring total cholesterol or total cholesterol and HDL-C.

A total cholesterol level of 200 milligrams per deciliter of blood (mg/dl) or less has been called "desirable" (although 180 would be better), with levels between 200 and 240 considered "borderline" and 240 or above "undesirable." But HDL-C levels are important also. The Framingham Heart Study found that people with an HDL-C level of 35 are 50 percent more likely to develop heart disease than those with an HDL-C level of 45. Researchers at Johns Hopkins University Medical School discovered that, among 1,000 people with cholesterol levels below 200, almost a fourth had heart disease, and that these people typically had HDL-C levels below 35. In a Boston study of nearly 800 people with "desirable" cholesterol levels, 60 percent had heart disease; of this group, three quarters had HDL-C levels below 40. An HDL-C level of 45 or higher in men and 55 or above in women is desirable. A level in excess of 75 is associated with a very low risk of coronary heart disease; such a level is not uncommon among persons who exercise often.

Although there are some differences in how habits affect LDL-C and HDL-C, diet has more impact on LDL-C and exercise has more impact on HDL-C. As a rule, those things that make LDL-C

Stress and Heart Disease

Stress has long been considered a factor in heart disease, but exactly how it does its damage is still unknown. In the past, there has been much discussion and controversy concerning the connection between the "Type A" personality—impatient, hard-driving, intolerant—and coronary heart disease. It now seems clear that the Type A personality is not the whole story; it is just part of a complex interaction between mind and body. Although much remains to be learned, we know that (a) relaxation techniques lower blood pressure and (b) intensive practice to improve mind-body interactions is part of the lifestyle program that has successfully reversed the process of coronary heart disease. Thus, relaxation techniques are recommended for the control of high blood pressure and you are urged to explore the potential of mind-body interactions as discussed in Chapter 11.

go down make HDL-C go up. Beneficial effects on cholesterol are associated with:

- Regular exercise
- Not smoking
- A diet low in fat, especially saturated fat
- A diet high in fiber
- A diet high in fish oil
- Low body fat

High Blood Pressure

Like obesity, high blood pressure adds to the heart's workload; it stresses the arteries and worsens atherosclerosis. People with high blood pressure are three times as likely to develop CHD and six times as likely to develop congestive heart failure as persons with normal blood pressure.

Desirable blood pressure levels are associated with:

- Regular aerobic exercise
- Not smoking

- Low body fat
- A diet low in sodium (salt)
- A diet high in calcium
- A diet high in potassium
- Use of relaxation techniques

Smoking

Smoking raises your risk of heart disease no matter what else you do. Smokers have twice the risk of heart attack as non-smokers and when they do have heart attacks, smokers are more likely to die, and die suddenly. Even having an ideal weight and low blood pressure will not save you from the ravages of smoking. But quitting can undo them: After just six months, the ex-smoker's risk of dying from a heart attack plummets by about half; after three years, the ex-smoker's risk is almost the same as that of a person who has never smoked.

Lack of Exercise

An analysis of several dozen studies examining the relationship between physical activity and heart disease has documented a clear link between the two: A person who is sedentary has almost twice the risk of developing CHD as a person who regularly exercises for 20 minutes three times a week. More recently, researchers reported a study in which they used the treadmill exercise test to evaluate the fitness of more than 3,000 men. The men were divided into four equal groups, according to their fitness level. Over the next eight years, the death rate from heart disease was 8.5 times higher in the group who were least fit than in the group who were most fit; death rates for the men in the two middle groups were in between.

Obesity

Being overweight has several strikes against it. Most obviously, the excess poundage puts added strain on the heart. Obesity is closely linked to other risk factors, including high blood pressure and elevated cholesterol levels (higher LDL-C and lower HDL-C). It promotes diabetes, which also increases the risk of heart attack. But more than that, obesity itself is a risk factor, regardless of these other issues: The Framingham Heart Study has found that even those rare obese people who have normal levels of cholesterol and blood pressure are unduly prone to heart attacks. The risk of heart disease rises with weight, and fat that is carried around the middle—the waist and belly—seems most dangerous.

HOW CAN WE PREVENT HEART DISEASE?

Lifestyle changes that eliminate risk factors will go a long way toward preventing heart disease. The risk factors most often emphasized are high blood pressure and high cholesterol levels. This is understandable, because they are easily measured and have been the subject of much research. In my opinion, however, the key risk factors are the lifestyle issues. A person who exercises regularly, eats a diet low in saturated fats, controls weight and doesn't smoke will automatically lower his or her LDL-C, raise HDL-C and normalize blood pressure. Medicines have a place in halting the progress of atherosclerosis, but only after healthful lifestyle changes have been made. And Americans have made important changes in their lifestyles, as Table 18.1 shows.

In addition, the number of persons exercising regularly has increased greatly. In 1961, only 24 percent of American adults exercised regularly. If you saw a man running down the street, you looked to see who was chasing him! But by 1984, that number had risen to 59 percent. While this exercise is often not very vigorous—only about 7.5 percent of adults regularly exercise at 60 percent or more of their maximum capacity (see Chapter 6)—we now know that moderate exercise also helps reduce the risk of heart disease.

Importantly, such changes in lifestyle have been paralleled by major drops in death rates due to heart disease and stroke. From 1976 to 1986, deaths from coronary heart disease declined by more than 27 percent, and deaths from stroke declined by more than 40 percent. Medical care has played only a small role in these improvements. The major factor has been the public's awareness of the importance of lifestyle. Keep this in mind the next time you hear someone say that anti-smoking

Table 18.1
Change (per Person) in Use of Certain Products
from 1963 to 1987

Product	Percentage of Change
Tobacco products	−34%
Animal fats	−21%
Eggs	−19%
Coffee	−22%
Vegetable fats and oils	+43%
Fish	+20%
Poultry	+46%

Source: U.S. Department of Agriculture

or other health-information campaigns don't work.

It has been suggested that alcohol, in moderation, may help fend off deaths due to heart disease. A major research project known as the Honolulu Heart Study reported that people who have one or two drinks a day are less likely to die of heart disease than people who drink more or who don't drink at all. This may be because moderate alcohol use is associated with an increase in HDL-C and a decrease in LDL-C. The reason might also be something as straightforward as stress reduction: The person who sits down with a drink before dinner is taking time to relax, and the benefit might accrue even without alcohol. Whatever the reason, a small amount of alcohol is OK. But even though a little may be good, a lot is definitely *not* better (see Chapter 10).

Aspirin, too, has been proposed as a shield against heart attacks: This multi-purpose chemical discourages the buildup of blood clots in blocked arteries by decreasing the "stickiness" of platelets, cells that normally form clots by clumping together. In a five-year study of more than 22,000 healthy male physicians, those who took one aspirin tablet (325 milligrams) every other day had about half the heart attacks of those who did not. However, they also had more strokes due to bleeding, or hemorrhage. At present, it seems that the benefit of aspirin may outweigh the risk, but all of the information is not yet in. The rationale may be strongest for persons who have several risk factors—except

for high blood pressure, because of the apparent risk of hemorrhagic stroke. It is possible that a different dose, 75 to 100 milligrams taken daily, might prove safer.

PREVENTING AND TREATING ATHEROSCLEROSIS

The big news is that atherosclerosis can be stopped in its tracks and even reversed. This was first achieved in 1987, with the use of powerful cholesterol-lowering drugs. Even more remarkably, by 1988 researchers had shown that arteries could be unblocked with lifestyle changes alone.

In one study, a small group of patients with severe heart disease was "treated" with diet, exercise and stress-management techniques. Their diet was stringent—vegetarian and very low in fat. (Eight percent to 10 percent of total calories came from fat, compared to 37 percent in the average American diet and the 30 percent recommended by experts.) Their exercise was moderate—walking three times a week. To cope with stress they were taught yoga, meditation, relaxation exercises and other techniques. A year later most of these people had less blockage than they started out with (and none had more), while disease in an untreated control group of their peers had grown worse.

In a different study, milder lifestyle changes also halted the progression of atherosclerosis. A group of men with heart disease was given extensive nutritional counseling and advised to reduce

Where is Your Cholesterol Going?

Total Cholesterol Projections for Men, by Age

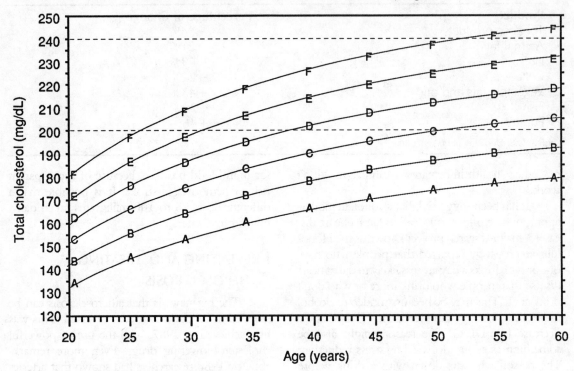

Age (years)

The Centers for Disease Control have recently developed graphs that show the relationship between age and total cholesterol levels (nomograms). These allow you to estimate what your total cholesterol level will be in the future.

Adapted from *Morbidity and Mortality Weekly Report*, May 26, 1989.

---

daily fat intake to about 27 percent of calories. Those who followed the advice to eat less fat, saturated fat and cholesterol did not form new coronary artery blockages in the months that followed.

CONTROLLING CHOLESTEROL

The first step is to get your cholesterol levels measured. (It's a simple blood test; see Chapter 15.) If your total cholesterol is under 200 mg/dl (180 mg/dl is better), and you follow a healthful lifestyle—exercising regularly, not smoking, eating a diet low in saturated fat, keeping your body fat

low, practicing healthy mind-body interactions— you probably are doing OK. Still, lowering your total cholesterol (and raising your HDL-C) through further lifestyle improvements will lower your risk even more.

If your total cholesterol is above 200 (or 180 if you are following my preferences), then you need to make some changes and decide whether you need your doctor's help. Traditionally, recommendations have been based on a person's cholesterol level and whether or not he or she already has CHD, symptoms of CHD, or other risk factors for CHD. In short, if you had a cholesterol level above

Where is Your Cholesterol Going?

Total Cholesterol Projections for Women, by Age

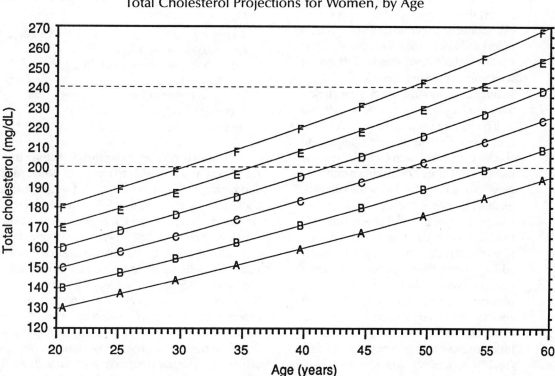

For example, if you are a 25-year-old man with a total cholesterol of 175, these nomograms would predict a cholesterol of over 200 by age 40. These nomograms are especially important for young adults who may be lulled into a false sense of security by a "low" total cholesterol level.

Adapted from *Morbidity and Mortality Weekly Report,* May 26, 1989.

240, or if you had CHD or its symptoms, or if you were at high risk because of several risk factors, a visit to the physician was recommended. This is an overly complex approach and results in inappropriate doctor visits for the following reasons:

- If you already have CHD, then you should be under a physician's care. Cholesterol testing should be part of this care and not regarded as a screening procedure to be interpreted on its own.
- The physician can only do two things with respect to cholesterol that you cannot do for yourself:

- Determine if there is an unusual cause for your cholesterol problem, such as a hereditary disease, hypothyroidism (underactive thyroid) or kidney disease.
- Prescribe drugs to lower cholesterol.
- Having several risk factors doesn't change the fact that lifestyle changes come first, although it should motivate you to make lifestyle changes as quickly and completely as possible.

In view of the above, we can simplify the next step for total cholesterols above 200:

1. If your total cholesterol is 240 or above,

contact your physician to obtain the tests needed to look for unusual causes for high total cholesterol. These include tests of HDL-C, triglycerides, lipoprotein electrophoresis, thyroid function (free T4 index) and kidney function (urinalysis). If your total cholesterol is under 240, get on with improving your lifestyle.

2. In three to six months, check your cholesterol level again. If it is below 240 and well on its way toward being under 200, continue with your lifestyle changes and check your cholesterol again in six months. If you are not making much progress, take a long, hard look at your program. Have you really made major changes in your lifestyle? If you conclude that you have not and are able and willing to try harder, then give it a go. Consider adding more fiber (psyllium or extra bran) or even niacin (see below) as supplements. Check your cholesterol again in another three to six months.

3. If, after six to 12 months, you are making little progress toward your goal of 200 (or 180 preferably), contact your physician to consider the use of cholesterol-lowering drugs. This is a last resort that is to be avoided, if possible.

Note that the above does not require HDL-C determinations unless the total cholesterol is above 240. This is a standard and acceptable approach. Nevertheless, a low HDL-C level is a risk factor for CHD independent of total cholesterol and is well worth considering, especially if total cholesterol is under 200 and there is a family history of CHD. I also think an HDL-C test is worthwhile if total cholesterol is under 200 and your lifestyle doesn't seem to fit the number. In other words, an acceptable total cholesterol in someone who smokes, doesn't exercise and/or is overweight may be hiding a low HDL-C level that indicates high risk. In short, it's wise to have an HDL-C measurement any time the total cholesterol seems too good to be true.

With or without further testing or drugs, the main concern is lifestyle. Here is where you can find the information in this book that you need to make changes that will improve your cholesterol levels and your chances:

Change	Chapter
Increase exercise and activity	6
Lower dietary fats, especially saturated fats	7
Increase dietary fiber	7
Decrease body fat	8
Stop smoking	9

These changes are powerful. Switching from the typical American diet to one that is lower in fat and higher in fiber can be expected to lower total cholesterol by 30 to 40 mg/dl or more if your total cholesterol is especially high to begin with. A diet very low in fat (less than 7 percent of calories from fat) will lower the total cholesterol level an additional 15 to 30 mg/dl. Smoking raises total cholesterol about 0.5 mg/dl for every cigarette smoked. So if you are a two-pack-a-day smoker, you can expect your cholesterol to decrease by about 25 mg/dl when you quit. HDL-C can be raised 5 to 20 mg/dl through a program of vigorous physical activity. Losing five pounds of body fat will usually raise HDL-C by 3 or 4 mg/dl. And stopping smoking will add another 3 to 5 mg/dl to the HDL-C level.

Some people will not meet their cholesterol goals through these changes, or they will not be completely successful in making the changes. The next step is to consider the use of supplements. Psyllium fiber is available in granular form (Metamucil, Effer-Sylium and many other brands); a tablespoonful three times a day has been shown to reduce total cholesterol.

Niacin (nicotinic acid), a B vitamin, is effective in reducing cholesterol and the risk of CHD when taken in large doses (1 or 2 grams three times a day with meals). However, its side effects, chiefly flushing and itching, make it unacceptable to many people. It also may activate peptic ulcers, cause liver problems or skin rashes, and raise your plasma-glucose level. If you decide to use niacin, a phone call to your physician to discuss its use might be wise. By the way, niacinamide (nicotinamide) does not have the cholesterol-lowering effect of niacin, even though it is sometimes sold as being essentially the same.

A recent study suggested that adding 200 micrograms (μg) of chromium per day to the diet will lower total cholesterol. Because 200 μg is the daily intake of chromium recommended by many authorities, this is not likely to be a dangerous supplement, but its effects on cholesterol need to be confirmed by other studies. The principal source of chromium as a supplement is brewer's yeast.

Fish oil capsules may reduce cholesterol modestly, but many capsules per day are required and the changes may not last. It's probably a better idea simply to eat more fish.

Finally, for a few people, lifestyle and supplements are not enough to bring cholesterol levels into the safe range. In these cases, drug therapy may be appropriate. Several types of drugs have proven effective in lowering blood cholesterol. Cholestyramine and colestipol are known as bile acid sequestrants; through a complex process they stimulate the removal of LDL-C from the bloodstream. Both have been shown to reduce not only LDL-C (by 15 percent to 30 percent), but also the risk of heart disease. However, they are not easy to use and have side effects, chiefly bloating and constipation or diarrhea, which cause many patients to stop using them. Gemfibrozil lowers cholesterol 5 percent to 15 percent and has been shown to reduce the damage of CHD. It is less likely to cause problems such as constipation, but its long-term safety is not clear. Lovastatin and probucol interfere with cholesterol synthesis in the liver and are effective in reducing LDL-C by 25 percent to 45 percent and 10 percent to 15 percent, respectively, but neither their effect on heart disease nor their long-term safety are yet known. And, unfortunately, probucol may lower HDL-C. Thus, lovastatin and probucol should only be used as a last resort in patients with severe problems.

None of these drugs is as safe and inexpensive as including 1-1/2 cups of oat bran in your diet each day, a habit that will lower LDL-C by 10 percent to 20 percent. Please be sure you have given lifestyle a chance before you consider drugs.

CONTROLLING HIGH BLOOD PRESSURE

More than 60 million Americans have high blood pressure—a systolic blood pressure of 140 millimeters of mercury (mm Hg) or above, and/or a diastolic blood pressure of 90 mm Hg or above. (High blood pressure and blood pressure measurement are described in Chapter 15.) It is more common among older persons and blacks.

High Blood Pressure

Range	Classification
Systolic Blood Pressure (when diastolic pressure is less than 90)	
Under 140	Normal blood pressure
140–159	Borderline isolated systolic hypertension
Over 160	Isolated systolic hypertension
Diastolic Blood Pressure	
Below 85	Normal blood pressure
85–89	High normal blood pressure
90–104	Mild hypertension
105–114	Moderate hypertension
Over 115	Severe hypertension
A Simplified Version Using Both Systolic and Diastolic Pressures	
120/80 or below	Normal blood pressure
140/90	Upper limits of normal
Above 140/90	Hypertension

Like atherosclerosis, high blood pressure can work its devilment for years without producing symptoms. It causes the heart to work harder, hardens the arteries, and damages the heart, brain and kidneys. Many people have high blood pressure and feel fine; the only way to tell if your blood pressure is out of line is to have it measured. This is a simple matter; you can even find reliable machines to do it at many pharmacies.

The higher the blood pressure, the more devastating its effects. In persons with moderate hypertension (diastolic blood pressure above 104 mm Hg), controlling blood pressure clearly decreases heart disease and subsequent deaths. In so-called mild hypertension (diastolic pressure between 90 and 104 mm Hg), lowering blood pressure has been shown to protect against stroke, congestive heart failure, and progression to more severe hypertension, as well as to cut overall mortality.

As with cholesterol, the basic means of controlling blood pressure is lifestyle. And, fortunately, many of the habits that have a good effect on cholesterol have a good effect on blood pressure, too. Exercising regularly, not smoking and lowering body fat are important both for high blood pressure and cholesterol. However, some parts of your diet that are important for blood pressure have no known effect on cholesterol. Diets that are low in sodium (salt), high in calcium or high in potassium are associated with lower blood pressure. Such diets are compatible with the low-fat, high-fiber diet recommended for controlling cholesterol. For instance, apples are an excellent source of both fiber and potassium. However, sometimes a little maneuvering is required. Dairy products are an excellent source of calcium, for example, but they often contain large amounts of saturated fat. Thus, it's necessary to obtain calcium from low-fat or skim dairy foods, or other sources, such as sardines, canned salmon and broccoli, or from calcium supplements. Here's where to find the information in this book that you need to control blood pressure:

Change	Chapter
Increase exercise	6
Stop smoking	9
Lower body fat	8
Eat more calcium	7
Eat more potassium	7
Eat less sodium (salt)	7
Practice relaxation techniques	11

When lifestyle changes alone fail to bring blood pressure under control, drugs are used. In addition to the traditional diuretics and beta-blockers, two new classes of drugs are calcium antagonists and angiotensin-converting enzyme inhibitors, or ACE inhibitors. Because all of these drugs have about the same ability to lower blood pressure, any one of them may be the first tried. If in a month or two blood pressure has not reached normal levels, the doctor may increase the dosage, add a second type of drug or switch to another class of drug altogether. Eventually, through trial and error, the most suitable combination of drugs is worked out for each person. (Different people may respond differently to a particular drug.) However, lifestyle remains most important. Without good habits, drug dosages will be much higher than they need to be (causing more side effects) or blood pressure will remain high despite high drug doses.

CAN WE DETECT CORONARY HEART DISEASE BEFORE IT CAUSES SYMPTOMS?

As a practical matter, the answer is no. As originally defined, CHD meant that a person had developed symptoms such as angina (heart pain) or a heart attack. These events set the victim apart from the vast majority of middle-aged or older Americans, who were likely to have some coronary atherosclerosis. A study of soldiers killed in the Korean War, whose average age was 22, showed that 77 percent already had atherosclerosis in their coronary vessels. And a large autopsy study of Americans of all ages killed in accidents showed that 75 percent had more than 25 percent blockage in at least one of the three main coronary arteries.

The advent of coronary arteriography, an X-ray procedure that shows the flow of blood in the coronary vessels, changed the definition of CHD. Today CHD means significant blockage—typically at least 50 percent—of one or more coronary arteries.

If you have not had a heart attack and don't have any symptoms, then coronary arteriography is the only way (short of autopsy) to diagnose CHD. Unfortunately, coronary arteriography itself carries a risk of disability and death. It is clearly unacceptable as a screening test.

The electrocardiographic stress test, which consists of taking an ongoing electrocardiogram during harder and harder exercise, has been proposed as a way to detect CHD before it shows symptoms. However, it, too, leaves a lot to be desired. Studies show that 60 percent to 80 percent of the people with "abnormal" stress tests do not have CHD on coronary angiography, while more than half of those with "normal" stress tests do. (See the discussion of stress tests in Chapter 15.)

WHAT ARE THE SYMPTOMS OF CORONARY HEART DISEASE?

Atherosclerosis develops for many years in silence. Only after an artery is about 70 percent blocked is the oxygen-starved heart likely to cause the pain known as angina. Angina is sometimes mild, sometimes severe. It is not always the first symptom of CHD. For many people, the first symptom is a full-blown heart attack.

The pain of a heart attack, like angina, is usually located in the center of the chest and may extend to the arms, jaw, neck or back, but it is likely to be much more severe. The pain is often described as a crushing feeling, like the pressure from a great weight on the chest or the squeezing of a severe spasm or cramp. It often causes dizziness, sweating, nausea or shortness of breath.

TREATING THE SYMPTOMS OF HEART DISEASE

A number of drugs work fairly well in relieving the symptoms of heart disease. Angina, for instance, can be relieved by drugs that improve the heart's oxygen supply, such as nitroglycerin, which relaxes the blood vessels so that the channels enlarge. Yet other drugs counter angina by reducing the heart's need for oxygen; some lower blood pressure, whereas others slow the heart rate.

Other drugs are quite helpful in offsetting certain abnormalities of the heartbeat (arrhythmias) and relieving the shortness of breath and ankle swelling that occur in congestive heart failure. In other words, medicines can relieve some of the symptoms of these diseases, sometimes dramatically. However, there is very little evidence that these drugs actually do much to change the course of the disease. They can make someone feel better, but they cannot cure the underlying problem.

In recent years doctors have attempted to stop heart attacks in progress with drugs that dissolve the blood clots that are blocking the oxygen supply to the heart. In the short term, the benefits of such drugs—which include streptokinase and tissue plasminogen activator, or t-PA—appear to outweigh the risks; by reopening choked arteries they can decrease the death rate in the first few days following a heart attack by 35 percent to 50 percent. Longer-term benefits are less clear, however; the drugs produce certain unwanted side effects, such as bleeding, and the drug-opened arteries tend to close again. And, of course, drugs have no effect on the underlying disease process.

A disappointment has been the coronary care unit (CCU). With its careful monitoring, expert personnel, drugs and high-tech equipment, the CCU once was expected to reduce deaths from heart attacks by as much as 50 percent. The most recent data show that the real number is closer to 5 percent. Several studies have shown CCUs to be no better than standard hospital wards in decreasing deaths in congestive heart failure, and one study shows that at least one group—older men with uncomplicated heart attacks—are better off *at home*.

This is understandable. The CCU is a dangerous place that exposes patients to a great deal of stress. It can effectively fight some of the complications of heart attacks, such as arrhythmias, but it is helpless against the disease itself. Worse yet, its victories are short-lived: Many of the people whose deaths are prevented in the CCU die before the year is out.

Types of Heart Disease

Coronary heart disease (CHD) is the most common type of heart disease and is responsible for almost all heart attacks and angina.

▶▶▶

Hypertensive heart disease, caused by high blood pressure, is characterized by an enlarged heart that cannot pump effectively. Although it is a separate form of heart disease, it is most often found together with CHD.

Valvular heart disease occurs when damaged or misshaped valves make the heart's pumping action ineffective. Most often it is present at birth or due to rheumatic fever.

Cardiac myopathies are uncommon diseases that affect only the heart muscle.

The Causes of Coronary Heart Disease

Atherosclerosis is by far the most common cause of CHD. The walls of affected arteries accumulate a variety of substances—fats, cholesterol, cellular debris, calcium and clotting material—from the blood. Also, smooth muscle cells in the artery walls grow abnormally. This buildup blocks the flow of blood to the heart.

▶▶▶

Arteriosclerosis is the hardening of the arteries that occurs with aging. Strictly speaking, arteriosclerosis without atherosclerosis is a rare cause of CHD; most often the two occur together in CHD.

Spasm of the coronary arteries may also block the flow of blood simply by constricting these vessels. It is an unusual cause of CHD. Why the spasm occurs is not known.

Risk Factors for Atherosclerosis

High LDL-C or total cholesterol, and low HDL-C are associated with an increased risk of CHD, especially in middle-aged men.

▶▶▶▶▶▶▶

High blood pressure probably does more damage by contributing to CHD than by causing hypertensive heart disease.

▶▶▶▶▶▶▶

Lack of exercise has been shown to increase the risk of heart attacks and death due to heart attacks.

High body fat is often associated with cholesterol problems, high blood pressure and lack of exercise, but also seems to increase the risk of CHD by itself.

Smoking causes more deaths through atherosclerosis than through lung cancer.

Controlling Risk Factors

Most Important
1. Aerobic exercise
2. Diet:
   Less fat, especially
      saturated fat
   More fiber
   More complex
      carbohydrates
   More calcium
   More potassium
3. No smoking
4. Relaxation, healthy
mind-body interaction

Optional Supplements
1. Psyllium preparations
2. Calcium
3. Niacin (nicotinic acid)
4. *Chromium
5. *Fish oil

The last resort: Drugs
1. Cholestyramine
2. Colestipol
3. Gemfibrizol
4. Lovastatin
5. Probucol

* The value of these supplements is
uncertain.

Is Coronary Heart Disease Present?

Screening
An exercise stress test is often advised as a screening test for CHD, but there are too many false positives (60 percent to 80 percent) to consider this a reliable test. Unfortunately, there is currently no acceptable screening test.

Symptoms
The major symptoms are angina (chest pain), shortness of breath, swelling of the ankles and heart attack.

Treating Heart Disease

Lifestyle changes are the first line of treatment for CHD!

Drugs can often relieve the symptoms of CHD, but they cannot cure the disease, and probably cannot change its course.

Surgery effectively relieves angina. In some patients, it increases life expectancy. However, it does not cure atherosclerosis, so problems may recur. It is not for all patients, has risks and is expensive.

SURGERY FOR HEART DISEASE

Another approach to the treatment of CHD—a last resort for a selected group—is surgery. There are two main types, balloon angioplasty (or PTCA, for percutaneous transluminal coronary angioplasty) and coronary artery bypass grafting (CABG). Both have become common in recent years: In 1988 more than 200,000 Americans had angioplasty and more than 300,000 had bypass surgery. Neither, however, is a panacea.

PTCA does not require that the chest be cut open or even that the patient be put to sleep. Rather, a balloon-tipped catheter is slipped through a small incision into a large artery, usually in the groin. The catheter is threaded up through the blood vessels until it reaches the heart. When its tip is positioned in an obstructed coronary artery, the balloon is inflated, widening the blocked channel so that more blood can flow through. For PTCA to have a good chance of success, the blockage must meet several criteria; it can help only about 10 percent of the candidates for heart surgery.

Though less drastic than open-heart surgery, PTCA is not without risk. The pressure from the balloon can irritate or even damage the artery wall; it can also break debris free from the plaque. About 4 percent of the time, the procedure itself triggers a heart attack; it can also cause other complications, such as prolonged angina or, rarely, a ruptured artery. The mortality rate is about 1 percent. Sometimes the attempt just doesn't work. For instance, the plaque may be too hardened or too maze-like to let the catheter through. And, unfortunately, a recent study suggests that channels widened by PTCA often narrow again in a fairly short time.

CABG exploits a simple concept: A vein or artery (an artery is best) from another part of the body (usually the leg or chest wall) is used to bypass a blocked section of a coronary artery. The operation itself is as delicate as the concept is simple: sewing a small and squiggly vessel into the artery of a living human heart so that it will carry blood around an obstruction. It requires a dedicated team of health professionals using complex machinery as well as a patient able to withstand several hours of major surgery.

Bypass surgery effectively relieves angina; about 70 percent of the patients have complete relief and another 20 percent experience partial relief. Some, probably most, of this relief comes from improved blood flow to the area of heart muscle that was starved for oxygen.

However, there are at least two other ways in which the surgery might relieve pain. First, the heart tissue causing the pain may die during the operation—creating, in effect, a heart attack; dead tissue causes no pain. Such a heart attack weakens the heart even though pain disappears. Second, it is known from earlier studies of angina that a sham operation in which the chest wall is opened but nothing is done to the heart will bring relief in about 40 percent of patients. This is the placebo effect, and it is very powerful. Indeed, a review of bypass surgery studies showed that pain relief is just about the same in patients who have open grafts permitting blood flow and patients whose grafts have closed down.

CABG's track record in improving life expectancy is less impressive. The best information suggests that it improves life expectancy only when performed for certain kinds of problems. Time is most likely to be gained when there is an almost complete obstruction of the most important coronary artery, the left main coronary artery, or there is significant blockage of all three of the heart's principal arteries. On average, such patients can expect to live six to 12 months longer than if they had been treated with drugs.

A recent review of one large medical center's experience with bypass surgery suggested that the procedure increased the life expectancy of all patients regardless of the type of blockage. However, this was not a scientific study and the increase was modest in most cases. Nevertheless, if confirmed by scientific studies, this finding would be most welcome.

Some of surgery's benefit may be due to better lifestyles adopted after surgery. This has been shown to be important in preventing more problems, and most surgical teams stress this to their patients.

As you would expect, the risk of surgery is related to the severity of the heart disease. It is also related to the skill of the operating team. The death rate when a competent surgical team operates on an "average" mix of patients should be less than 4 percent.

Between 5 percent and 10 percent of patients will suffer a heart attack during surgery or immediately after. About 5 percent will suffer other serious complications, such as severe bleeding and serious infection.

There are three generally accepted criteria for considering PTCA or CABG:

1. Disabling angina persists despite optimal medical therapy.
2. The obstruction is located where it can be approached surgically.
3. The heart is not already severely damaged.

Your doctors must decide on the last two factors, but you are the one who decides how severe the pain is. If pain is minor, but coronary arteriography has shown you have the type of lesions that are most successfully treated by surgery, you face a tough choice. Current statistics show that you may improve your life expectancy by having the operation, but just about all of the patients studied had a great deal of pain. (That's why they were operated on.) It is not clear that the results will be the same if you have little or no discomfort, because this may mean your disease is less severe. Claims are also being made that new drug therapies can improve the outcomes of patients not treated with surgery. In this situation it is best to obtain advice from more than one physician. At least one of your advisors should be an internist or cardiologist who is *not* part of the cardiac surgery team. And you and your advisors must remember that it is possible to *reverse* atherosclerosis through lifestyle changes with or without cholesterol-lowering drugs.

Surgery for heart disease includes heart transplants, but these are best regarded as a medical curiosity and last-chance procedure that has provided some very expensive headlines but no breakthrough in the treatment of heart disease.

WHAT SHOULD YOU DO ABOUT HEART DISEASE?

Heart disease *can* be prevented, and lifestyle is the key. Lifestyle is also the key to treatment. And it is the key whether or not you have symptoms or a diagnosis of heart disease. You already know what you want to do: Alter your lifestyle to keep your arteries as clean as possible.

During the average lifetime, the heart beats some 2.5 billion times. Pursuing a healthful lifestyle is your best insurance that your heart will be able to complete its fair share.

RESOURCES

The American Heart Association (AHA) publishes numerous brochures on heart disease. Call or write your local chapter or the AHA National Center, 7320 Greenville Avenue, Dallas, TX 75231. (214) 373-6300.

Or contact the National Heart, Lung and Blood Institute (NHLBI), 9000 Rockville Pike, Bethesda, MD 20892. (301) 496-4000.

CANCER

Cancer is not one disease but many, each with its own characteristics and quirks. With hundreds of different kinds of cancer, the chance of finding a single cure is just about nil.

The link between all of these diseases is cells out of control. Cancer cells grow without restraint, invade nearby tissues and spread to other parts of the body. These transformed cells are unable to function normally; most can do nothing but grow, but some may actually overproduce substances ordinarily found in the body. For example, cancers of the ovary sometimes produce sex hormones. Cancers may also produce toxins, which have been blamed for the anemia and weight loss that often accompany these illnesses. Still, most cancers do their greatest damage by invading and replacing normal tissue.

Medically, the term tumor simply means swelling. Most tumors are not cancerous; they do not spread and invade other tissues. Although these tumors are called benign, they can sometimes cause serious problems merely by creating pressure on other structures. This happens with benign tumors of the brain, for instance, because the skull cannot expand to relieve pressure. Benign tumors are more likely than malignant ones to produce normal tissue substances. For example, a thyroid tumor that produces thyroid hormones is much more likely to be benign than malignant.

The history of cancer patterns in this country can teach us some valuable lessons.

The age-adjusted cancer death rates for males and females shown in Figure 19.3 and Figure 19.4 can be divided into three groups:

1. Clearly going up: lung cancer, with women beginning to reap the "rewards" of equality in smoking.
2. Clearly going down: cancers of the stomach and uterus, for reasons that are not certain (see below).
3. Not clearly going anywhere: everything else. For example, the death rate for breast

Figure 19.1

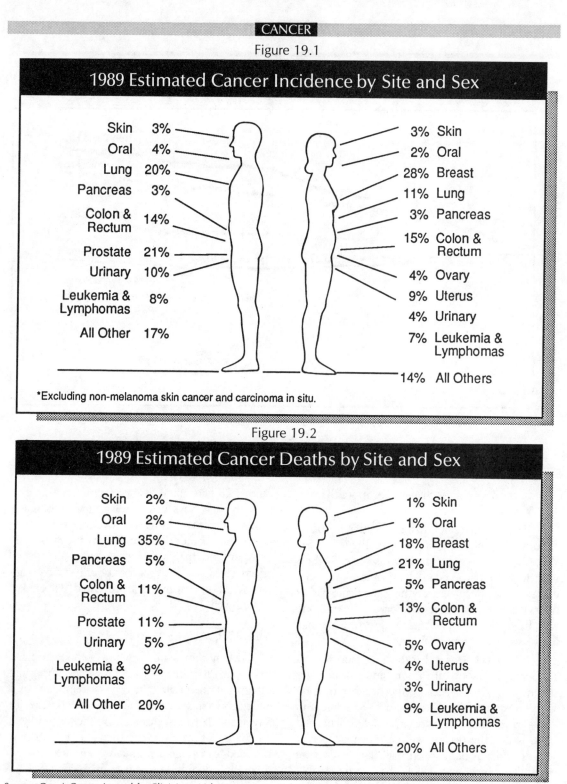

1989 Estimated Cancer Incidence by Site and Sex

Skin	3%	3%	Skin
Oral	4%	2%	Oral
Lung	20%	28%	Breast
Pancreas	3%	11%	Lung
Colon & Rectum	14%	3%	Pancreas
Prostate	21%	15%	Colon & Rectum
Urinary	10%	4%	Ovary
Leukemia & Lymphomas	8%	9%	Uterus
All Other	17%	4%	Urinary
		7%	Leukemia & Lymphomas
		14%	All Others

*Excluding non-melanoma skin cancer and carcinoma in situ.

Figure 19.2

1989 Estimated Cancer Deaths by Site and Sex

Skin	2%	1%	Skin
Oral	2%	1%	Oral
Lung	35%	18%	Breast
Pancreas	5%	21%	Lung
Colon & Rectum	11%	5%	Pancreas
Prostate	11%	13%	Colon & Rectum
Urinary	5%	5%	Ovary
Leukemia & Lymphomas	9%	4%	Uterus
All Other	20%	3%	Urinary
		9%	Leukemia & Lymphomas
		20%	All Others

Source: Ca - A Cancer Journal for Clinicians, Vol. 39, No.1 (Jan/Feb 1989) pp. 3-21, and The American Cancer Society.

Figure 19.5
Cancer Mortality

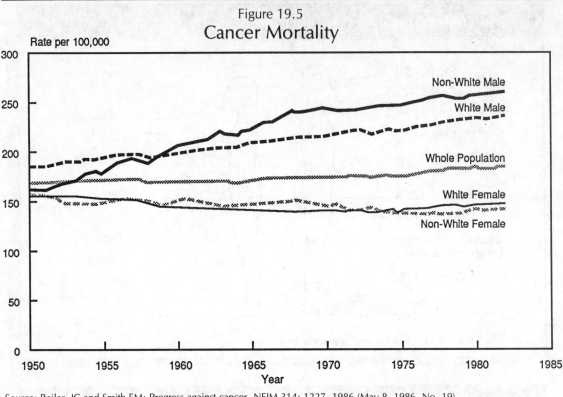

Rate per 100,000

Non-White Male
White Male
Whole Population
White Female
Non-White Female

Year

Source: Bailar, JC and Smith EM: Progress against cancer. NEJM 314: 1227, 1986 (May 8, 1986, No. 19)

cancer has been unchanged for more than 50 years.

The overall result is that the death rate due to all forms of cancer is going *up* (see Figure 19.5). Why? Because an epidemic of a disease caused by lifestyle and environment—lung cancer—far outdistances the effects of everything medicine has to offer. Pause a moment in memory of the millions who have died of a preventable disease while billions have been spent to find a "cure."

The good news is that the lung cancer death rate in men will soon turn around and start heading downward. This is because the number of men who smoke has fallen sharply, from 53 percent in 1964 to less than 33 percent in 1985. The bad news is that the decline will be much smaller in women and may not happen at all. The percentage of adult women who smoke has declined only modestly between 1965 and 1985, from 34 per-

cent to 28 percent. Worse yet, more teenage girls than teenage boys now smoke, and smoking is actually increasing in women over age 60.

This chapter discusses those cancers that are not rare and that may be prevented or treated effectively. These account for about half of all cancers. Most others cannot be prevented, detected or treated well.

WHAT CAUSES CANCER?

Many things are known to produce cancer, from acids to sunlight to X-rays. One important category is chemicals. The term "carcinogen" usually refers to such a chemical, but it may be used for any agent that causes cancer. By the same token, anything that causes cancer, such as radiation, may be called "carcinogenic." Finally, substances that by themselves do not cause cancer may act with other substances to do so. These are called "co-carcino-

Table 19.1
Environmental Causes of Cancer

Carcinogen	Cancer
Aromatic amines	Bladder
Arsenic (inorganic)	Lung, skin
Asbestos	Lung, pleura, peritoneum, pericardium
Benzene	Leukemia
bis-Chloromethyl ether	Lung
Chromium	Lung
Radiation	Almost all organs
Isopropyl alcohol production	Nasal sinuses
Mustard gas	Lung, larynx, nasal sinuses
Nickel dust	Lung, nasal sinuses
Polycyclic hydrocarbons	Lung, scrotum, skin
Radon	Lung
Sunlight (ultraviolet)	Skin, eye
Vinyl chloride	Liver
Wood dust	Nasal sinuses

gens."

About 20 chemicals are known to cause cancer in humans; Table 19.1 lists some of them and the human cancers with which they have been linked. Many other industrial chemicals, pesticides, food dyes and additives, and chemicals used in cosmetics have been shown to cause cancer in laboratory animals. How these relate to human cancer is a subject of great controversy. At present it can only be said that these findings cast an ominous shadow over the future, because these chemicals are in widespread use and the effects of carcinogens often are not seen for years after exposure begins.

Tobacco causes more cancer in Americans than all other carcinogens combined—not only lung cancer but also cancers of the mouth and throat, esophagus, pancreas, bladder and kidney. Tobacco smoke contains several carcinogens, but it is not certain which ones do the most harm. Long-term exposure to tobacco smoke in the air (passive smoking) has also been linked to an increased lung cancer risk. And so-called "smokeless tobacco" has been shown to increase the risk of oral cancers.

Table 19.2 lists drugs that may cause cancer; ironically, many of these drugs are used to fight cancer.

Viruses, which have long been known to cause certain cancers in animals, have been tied to a number of human cancers as well. For instance, the hepatitis B virus has been linked to liver cancer, the Epstein-Barr virus to some cases of Hodgkin's lymphoma, the retrovirus known as HTLV-1 to adult T-cell leukemia/lymphoma, and human papillomavirus to cancer of the cervix.

The theory that diet may influence cancer comes from studies showing that the incidence of stomach and intestinal cancers varies widely between countries where people eat very different diets—and cancer patterns change in populations that migrate from one country to another. For instance, Japanese who move to the United States lower their risk of stomach cancer but become more likely to develop colon cancer, which is more common among white Americans.

Despite a lot of research, no one diet has been shown to cause or prevent cancer. But there are some very promising leads. Diets low in fiber and high in calories and fat have been linked to

Table 19.2
Drugs That May Cause Cancer

Drug	Cancer
Alkylating agents (melphalan, cyclophosphamide, chlorambucil, nitrosoureas)	Leukemia, bladder
Androgenic steroids	Liver
Cyclosporine	Lymphoma
Diethylstilbestrol (prenatal exposure)	Vagina
Immunosuppressive drugs (azathioprine, cyclosporine)	Lymphoma
Phenacetin	Kidney, bladder
Synthetic estrogens	Uterus

cancers of the breast, uterus, prostate and colon; so has obesity. Diets that are high in fiber and rich in green vegetables and fruits, vitamins A, C and E (all antioxidants), and such minerals as calcium and selenium might reduce cancer deaths by more than one-third. (See Chapter 7 for help in meeting these dietary recommendations.)

Preservatives and food additives have come under scrutiny. However, only stomach cancer is clearly declining in both sexes. There is evidence that the food preservatives BHT and BHA, which are both antioxidants, have contributed to this decrease.

Radiation, from X-rays, the sun and such natural sources as radon gas, has long been known to cause cancer. Yet before 1950 some doctors used X-ray treatments to shrink the tonsils and adenoids, and to treat acne and ringworm of the scalp (tinea capitis). Today we see the effect: an increase in cancers of the head and neck. For example, the incidence of cancer of the thyroid gland may be 100 times greater than in persons never exposed to such radiation.

Undoubtedly those doctors believed that the amount of radiation used was too small to do harm. From the days of Madame Marie Curie (who discovered radium and died from cancer caused by radiation) to the present, there has been a continuing debate as to how much radiation can produce a malignancy. It now appears that even small amounts of radiation increase the risk of cancer, but the increase is slight and depends on the person's age. For example, mammography (X-ray examination to detect breast cancer) has been estimated to cause breast cancer in about one in 1,000 women who have the exam at age 20. However, this risk falls to about one in 2,500 at age 40, and one in 60,000 at age 50. (The effect of age is largely due to the fact that cancer may not appear until many years after the X-ray is done.) Because each X-ray adds to this risk, it is easy to see why there is a real difference in the risk of starting annual mammograms at age 30 or 40 and waiting until age 50.

Heredity influences cancer at several levels. In a few rare cancers, such as the eye cancer known as retinoblastoma, susceptibility is the work of a single flawed gene. Much more often, a person's susceptibility is shaped by a number of subtle genetic differences.

A tendency to develop some of the more common cancers—of the breast, colon and brain—appears to run in families. A woman whose mother or sister has had breast cancer, for example, is at increased risk of developing the disease. Cancer of the colon, often preceded by polyps, also shows a familial pattern—as was suggested in 1985, when both President Reagan and his brother were treated for the disease.

Identifying specific causes of cancer is tricky, because various causes may interact, thus multiplying the total effect. For example, heavy asbestos exposure doubles the chance of lung cancer, as does smoking. But when a smoker is also exposed to asbestos, the risk of cancer rises not four times, but more than 50 times.

Increasingly it appears that cancer development requires more than one factor—exposure to carcinogens along with genetic susceptibility. The strange case of Burkitt's lymphoma is a good illustration. This cancer is found almost exclusively in Africa. However, the virus that causes Burkitt's lymphoma appears to be the same virus that causes infectious mononucleosis, the Epstein-Barr virus. Why do Americans get mono while Africans get cancer? Clearly there's more at work than just the virus.

CAN WE PREVENT CANCER?

Yes! At least one-third of all cancer deaths can be prevented. And that's a conservative estimate. Two Nobel Prize winners contend that more than 75 percent can be prevented.

Cigarette smoking is responsible for more than 85 percent of lung cancer deaths among men and 75 percent among women. It also causes cancer of the lip, mouth, larynx, esophagus and bladder. *If stopping tobacco use were the only preventive measure taken, the number of cancer deaths would drop by about one-third.*

Heavy alcohol use is associated with increased rates of cancer of the liver, larynx, esophagus, stomach and bladder. Much liver cancer would be prevented if alcohol abuse were limited.

Prolonged exposure to the sun is associated with an increased risk of the most common and curable types of skin cancer, basal cell and squamous cell carcinomas. Recent studies show that sun exposure is also a major factor in the development of the deadly type of skin cancer known as melanoma. Unfortunately, limiting exposure to the sun may not be very practical for many persons, such as farm laborers who work outdoors. But especially if they are fair-skinned, these people should try to cover up, particularly between 10

a.m. and 3 p.m., when the sun's ultraviolet rays are the strongest. Sunscreens probably help, but they have not been proven to prevent skin cancer.

Unnecessary medical and dental X-rays add to the risk of cancer caused by radiation. About one-half of all the radiation to which Americans are exposed comes from these X-rays. Sometimes these X-rays are intended as screening procedures or ordered as "routine" upon entry into the hospital. Regardless of the excuse given, the use of X-rays for screening should be limited to mammograms (see Chapter 15). Other X-rays should be done only when the physician is certain that they are essential for investigating a specific medical problem. Even then, you should always request the use of a gonadal shield, a lead apron to protect the ovaries or testes. X-ray technicians often don't offer these shields even though they know they should. Finally, as a rule, X-ray examinations of stomach and intestines involve the most radiation. The recommendation for these examinations should be questioned and thoroughly discussed with your doctor.

Diets rich in antioxidants, such as vitamins A, C and E, offer promise in preventing cancer. Fortunately, the foods that contain antioxidants are also likely to benefit your heart and help you maintain a low body-fat level. (See Chapter 7 for more information on how to use nutrition to look better, help your heart and, perhaps, prevent cancer.)

It appears that the cancer risk in the environment is large and growing. Consider these realities:

- The risk of death due to lung cancer is greater in Los Angeles than in Chicago. Because the percentage of smokers is about the same in both cities, the most likely reason for the difference is Los Angeles's notorious air pollution.
- The concentration of asbestos is rapidly rising in our water sources, in the air and in the earth. Some of this contamination is due to industrial pollution, but a more widespread threat appears to be the asbestos from worn automobile brake linings.
- The ozone layer absorbs much of the sun's

ultraviolet radiation and prevents it from reaching the earth's surface. Fluorocarbons used in spray propellants, air conditioning units, refrigerators, and solvents have the capacity to destroy this protective layer. As it deteriorates, our radiation exposure increases.

- A large number of pesticides and other industrial chemicals appear to be capable of causing cancer. We do not yet know how much of a threat they pose.
- Radon is a naturally occurring radioactive gas that may accumulate in poorly ventilated spaces that come in contact with the ground, such as basements. It may also be dissolved in well water. It is estimated that more than 1 million American homes have radon concentrations that raise the risk of lung cancer due to radon 10 times or more. Radiation from radon may cause as many as 20,000 cases of lung cancer each year in the United States.

Ironically, as the amount of cancer rises, the percentage that is preventable will also rise. The first strategy in the war on cancer should be prevention.

CAN WE DETECT CANCER BEFORE IT CAUSES SYMPTOMS?

It often takes years for a single malignant cell to grow into a tumor large enough to cause symptoms. The goal of cancer screening tests is to detect cancer in this early stage, or even in a "precancerous" stage, when there is less chance that it has spread and more chance that it can be cured. A few tests meet this goal; they are discussed in Chapter 15. In short, mammography, physician examination for breast cancer and Pap smears for uterine cancer are recommended. A few others—breast self-examination, testicular self-examination, rectal examination for prostate cancer, sigmoidoscopy and testing for occult blood in the stool—may be considered, but are of no proven benefit. Others, such as chest X-ray for lung cancer, do more harm than good.

CAN WE TREAT CANCER?

Cancer treatment is clearly getting better, yet its effectiveness is a subject of constant debate. Is a treatment effective if it extends life for a year but the person still dies of the disease? Is that year worth living, considering the pain and disability the treatment frequently causes? These questions can be resolved only on a case-by-case basis. The answers depend more on the patient's own values than anything else. However, it must be remembered that cancers vary greatly in their prognosis. Most lung cancer patients will be dead within six to 12 months following the diagnosis, whereas most breast cancer patients will survive for more than five years. This is true regardless of the type of treatment or whether there is any treatment at all. The five-year survival rate for all cancers did not improve between the 1974–76 and 1979–84 periods, but there was improvement for some types (see Table 19.3).

With some exceptions, surgery to remove a cancer that has not spread is the only method that permits a cure. The likelihood that the cancer has spread prior to surgery depends on the characteristics of the particular cancer and just plain luck. For example, cancer of the lip grows slowly and is likely to be noticed and removed before it spreads. More than 95 percent of the people with this cancer will be cured. Just the opposite is true with cancer of the pancreas, a silent disease that produces symptoms only in its last stages. Fewer than 10 percent of those who have this cancer will be alive one year after its discovery.

The thought that surgery would be more successful if performed earlier is logical. Yet there is surprisingly little scientific evidence that we can discover cancers earlier than in the past or that we will be able to do so in the foreseeable future. The desire for successful treatments has led to an unfortunate emphasis on annual physicals and other ineffective procedures.

Treating cancer with radiation and/or drugs has produced cures in some types of cancers. Cancers of the lymph glands, including Hodgkin's disease, are treated effectively with radiation or drugs or a combination of the two. Perhaps the first

Table 19.3
Survival Trends in Cancer

Site	1960–63 Relative 5-year Survival Rate (Percent)		1970–73 Relative 5-year Survival Rate (Percent)		1974–76 Relative 5-year Survival Rate (Percent)		1979–84 Relative 5-year Survival Rate (Percent)	
	White	Black	White	Black	White	Black	White	Black
All Sites	39	27	43	31	50	38	50	31
Oral Cavity & Pharynx	45	–	43	–	54	35	54	31
Esophagus	4	1	4	4	5	4	7	5
Stomach	11	8	13	13	14	15	16	17
Colon	43	34	49	37	50	45	54	49
Rectum	38	27	45	30	48	40	52	34
Liver	2	–	3	–	4	1	3	5
Pancreas	1	1	2	2	3	2	3	5
Larynx	53	–	62	–	66	58	66	55
Lung & Bronchus	8	5	10	7	12	11	13	11
Melanoma	60	–	68	–	78	62	80	61
Breast (Female)	63	46	68	51	74	62	75	62
Uterine Cervix	58	47	64	61	69	61	67	59
Uterine Corpus	73	31	81	44	89	61	83	52
Ovary	32	32	36	32	36	41	37	36
Prostate	50	35	63	55	67	56	73	60
Testis	63	–	72	–	78	77	91	82
Bladder	53	24	61	36	73	47	77	57
Kidney & Renal Pelvis	37	38	46	44	51	49	51	53
Brain & Nervous System	18	19	20	19	22	27	23	31
Thyroid	83	–	86	–	92	88	93	95
Hodgkin's Disease	40	–	67	–	71	67	74	69
Non-Hodgkin's Lymphomas	31	–	41	–	47	47	49	49
Multiple Myeloma	12	–	19	–	24	28	24	29
Leukemia	14	–	22	–	34	30	32	27

cancer to be cured with drugs is a fairly rare tumor of the uterus, choriocarcinoma. In recent years, successful chemotherapy has been developed for a number of other cancers, most notably acute lymphocytic leukemia in children. Before drugs were available, most children with this disease succumbed within months. Now, more than 80 percent survive for more than five years and are considered cured.

These therapies are hazardous in themselves. Usually they cause at least some discomfort or disability, and the patient may even die of a complication of the therapy itself. Rather than cure, radia-tion and drugs usually bring temporary relief from the disease—a remission.

Remissions vary greatly depending on the type of cancer as well as the person. For example, remissions in breast cancer often last for years, whereas remissions in lung cancer are infrequent and usually short when they do occur.

WHAT SHOULD YOU DO ABOUT CANCER?

Prevent it. Prevention is your best bet by far. If you don't smoke and avoid the dangerous chem-

Figure 19.3
Cancer Death Rates in Women

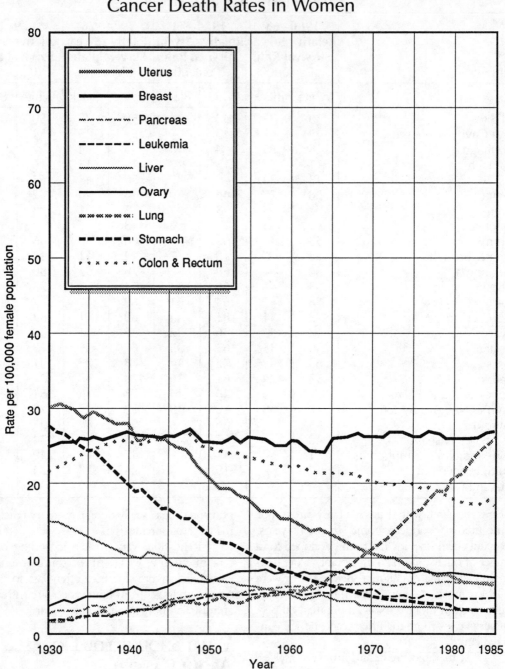

Sources of Data: U.S. National Center for Health Statistics and U.S. Bureau of the Census.
*Adjusted to the age distribution of the 1970 U.S. Census Population.

Figure 19.4
Cancer Death Rates in Men

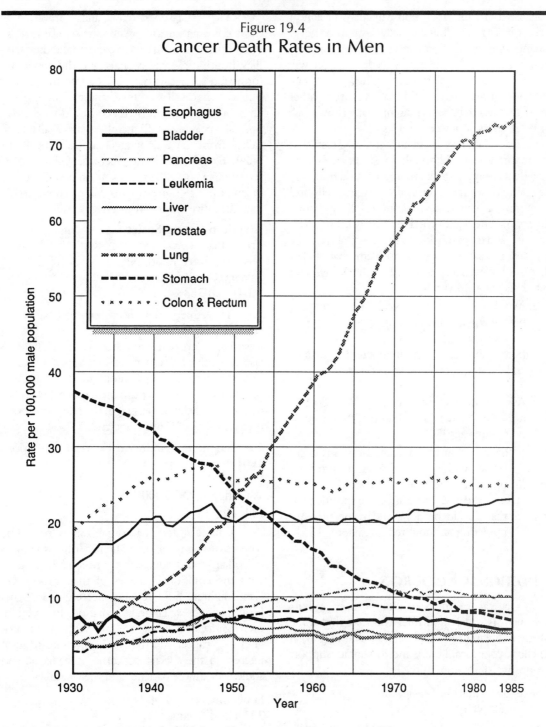

Rate per 100,000 male population

Year

Sources of Data: U.S. National Center for Health Statistics and U.S. Bureau of the Census.
*Adjusted to the age distribution of the 1970 U.S. Census Population.

icals listed in Table 19.1, you will cut your cancer risk in half. You will be virtually assured of never having lung cancer, liver cancer or several uncommon tumors, and your risk of bladder cancer will be reduced. If you stop smoking, you will not only cut your cancer risk, you will enjoy a score of other important health benefits ranging from a lower risk of heart attack to fewer wrinkles.

Be very choosy about any screening tests that involve radiation. Although most diagnostic X-rays deliver only a small amount of radiation, any excess increases the chance of damaging cells and triggering a malignancy. "Routine" X-rays done for annual physicals, dental examinations or work permits, and on admission to the hospital are to be avoided unless you have a problem that makes them necessary. Keep a record of the X-rays you get. This will help you to:

- Avoid "repeats" because you can't remember whether, when or where you had a certain type of X-ray.
- Better understand the number of X-rays and the amount of radiation you are receiving.
- Ask specific questions, such as, "Why do I need this X-ray when I had the same one six months ago?"

Whenever you do have an X-ray, insist on being provided with a gonadal shield to limit the amount of radiation to ovaries or testes.

Detect it early. There are some specific procedures that should be done and some that are worth considering, as indicated in Chapter 15.

ADDITIONAL RESOURCES

General information about cancer and its treatment is widely available. You may find some of the following resources helpful. You may wish to check your local library and to contact support groups in your community.

Cancer Information Service
1-800-4-CANCER

In Hawaii, on Oahu, call 524-1234 (call collect from neighboring islands).

The NCI-supported Cancer Information Service is a nationwide telephone service that answers questions from cancer patients and their families, health care professionals, and the public. Information specialists can provide information and publications on all aspects of cancer. They also may know about cancer-related services in local areas. Spanish-speaking staff members are available to callers from the following areas (daytime hours only): Florida, California, Georgia, Illinois, New Jersey (area code 201), New York, and Texas. By dialing the CIS number, you will be connected to the CIS office serving your area.

American Cancer Society
Tower Place
3340 Peachtree Road, NE
Atlanta, GA 30026
(404) 320-3333

The American Cancer Society (ACS) is a voluntary organization that offers a variety of services to cancer patients and their families. The ACS also is involved in cancer education and research. You can get additional information about ACS programs and services from the national headquarters or a local chapter (listed in the telephone book under American Cancer Society).

Candlelighters Childhood Center Foundation
1901 Pennsylvania Ave., NW
Suite 1001
Washington, DC 20006
(202) 659-5136

Candlelighters is an organization formed by parents of young cancer patients. It helps families of pediatric and adolescent cancer patients cope with the emotional stresses of their experience. Candlelighters hold regular meetings to discuss problems and exchange information. In addition, the organization works to gain support for programs of cancer research and to stimulate local interest in the special concerns of pediatric and adolescent cancer patients and their families.

Leukemia Society of America
733 Third Avenue
New York, NY 10017
(212) 679-1939

The Leukemia Society of America (LSA) is a voluntary health organization that offers patients with leukemia and related disorders financial assistance, transportation, and consultation services for referrals. You can get additional information about LSA programs and services from the national headquarters, or a local chapter (listed in the telephone book).

American Red Cross
17th and D Streets, NW
Washington, DC 20006
(202) 737-8300

The American Red Cross is a network of local chapters that provides health education materials and programs, including courses designed to give individuals the skills needed to care for ill family members.

Make Today Count
P.O. Box 222
Osage Beach, MO 65065
(314) 348-1619

Make Today Count is an organization that helps patients and families cope with cancer and other serious diseases and improve their quality of life.

STROKE

*W*e are all familiar with the devastation—the aging parent groping for words that won't come, the retired neighbor whose foot drags and arm hangs useless, the young mother who collapses while weeding her flower bed. Each of them, it turns out, has had a stroke. Each is one of the more than 400,000 Americans a year who experience an interruption in the brain's vital blood supply.

Strokes are especially frightening, because they can occur quickly and randomly, and none of us can guarantee that we are beyond their reach. Still, it is possible to take out insurance against strokes, because most result from atherosclerosis, the artery-clogging process that also underlies most heart disease, or high blood pressure. This insurance consists of exercise, a healthful diet, fat control, no smoking and drinking alcohol in moderation.

What Happens in a Stroke?

The delicate tissues of the brain require a constant supply of oxygen and nutrients, which are transported by the blood. When blood flow is cut off even briefly, brain cells die. The outcome of such a cut-off depends on which area of the brain is affected, as well as how long the stroke lasts. Some stroke victims suffer no more than slurred speech. Others become crippled, and yet others will never again be able to care for themselves. (Stroke is responsible for a large number of nursing-home admissions; the annual bill for hospital and nursing-home services for stroke patients comes to almost $10 billion.)

About one-third of all strokes are fatal; only heart disease and cancer cause more deaths. The good news is that the number of stroke deaths in the United States has been declining sharply. It fell more than 40 percent between 1976 and 1986 (Figure 20.1). This remarkable trend is the result of healthful living and better control of high blood pressure.

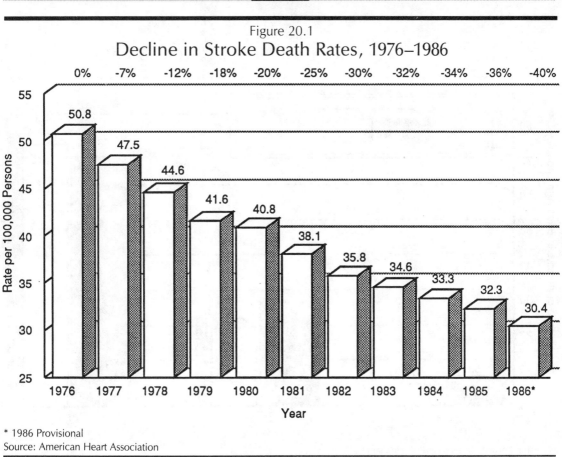

Figure 20.1
Decline in Stroke Death Rates, 1976–1986

* 1986 Provisional
Source: American Heart Association

TYPES OF STROKE

There are four main types of stroke. Two occur when a clot obstructs a blood vessel; two occur when a blood vessel bursts.

Strokes due to clotting are by far the most common, accounting for about 75 percent of the total. The damaging clots typically result from atherosclerosis. Most often the clot builds on the thickened wall of a diseased artery in the brain; the medical name for this clot is *thrombus*, and this type of stroke is known as *cerebral thrombosis*. Less often the clot will have formed elsewhere in the body —usually in the heart—and have been carried by the blood into the brain. Such traveling clots are known as *emboli*, and this type of stroke is called a *cerebral embolism*. Usually emboli form only when there has been some previous damage to the heart,

perhaps from a heart attack or rheumatic heart disease, or when there is a certain type of irregular heartbeat known as atrial fibrillation.

Hemorrhagic strokes occur when a blood vessel ruptures, either deep within the brain (a cerebral hemorrhage) or on the surface of the brain (a subarachnoid hemorrhage). Some hemorrhages occur when an aneurysm ruptures. An aneurysm is a weakened section of artery that balloons out into a little pouch. About 10 percent of Americans are born with aneurysms, but most never rupture. Not only does a hemorrhage interrupt the brain's blood supply, but the escaping blood floods, compresses and damages surrounding brain tissue. Hemorrhagic strokes are more lethal than strokes due to clotting—half of the victims die. But those who survive recover more completely.

Figure 20.2
Age/Sex Distribution of Stroke Events

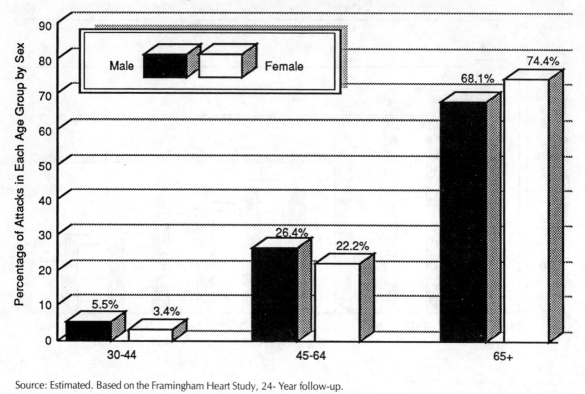

Source: Estimated. Based on the Framingham Heart Study, 24- Year follow-up.

WHO HAS STROKES?

Strokes are much more common in older people. The risk of having a stroke doubles each decade over the age of 50; more than two-thirds of all strokes occur in people over 65. For persons between 65 and 74, the risk of having a stroke is about 1 percent a year, unless they are veterans of a "little stroke," or transient ischemic attack (TIA), described below; then their risk rises to between five percent and eight percent a year. One younger group at high risk for stroke consists of women who take oral contraceptives and smoke. Strokes are more common in men than in women, and much more common in blacks than in whites, in part because more blacks have high blood pressure.

WHAT ARE THE SYMPTOMS OF STROKE?

Because different areas of the brain rule different senses and activities, strokes can produce an almost unlimited number of problems. Strokes can interfere with memory, reasoning and judgment. They can numb the senses, distort the personality and affect behavior. Often strokes impair the ability to speak, or to make sense of what is heard or read. Most strokes affect muscle control, producing weakness (paresis) or paralysis.

Most strokes are said to be "localized"—that is, they affect just part of the body. Because of the way the brain is built, this usually means that the stroke affects one side of the body—the side opposite the site of the brain damage. For example, a person who experiences a stroke on the right side of the brain might develop weakness in the left arm and leg. He or she may also have trouble with spatial perceptions, and may behave impulsively. Someone with left-brain damage, in contrast, will experience paralysis on the right side of the body, may have difficulty speaking, and is more likely to be cautious, anxious and disorganized. A stroke so massive as to affect both sides of the brain and body is usually fatal.

Some stroke victims experience a condition known as hemispheric neglect. Damage to one half, or hemisphere, of the brain cuts off input from half of the body. They may be unable to see things in the left (or right) field of vision, and they may simply ignore anything on that side—even their own arms and legs.

Many stroke patients lose some control over their emotions and may cry or laugh at the wrong times, moan or lash out in anger. In addition, about half of all stroke victims develop serious depression sometime in the following year. This reaction, characterized by anxiety, sleep disturbances and loss of energy, weight and appetite, appears to be caused at least in part by damage to the brain (perhaps because of a decrease in an important brain chemical). It is not simply an emotional response to misfortune.

Another common problem is aphasia, or trouble with words. The person may have problems speaking, understanding what is being said or read, and remembering names. But the fact that a person's speech is jumbled doesn't necessarily mean that he or she isn't thinking clearly. Some people know what they want to say but cannot find the words. A related problem is called dysarthria: Because the stroke has damaged the part of the brain that controls the muscles used in talking, the person's speech may be slurred or distorted, and hard to understand. (Chewing and swallowing may also be a problem.)

By damaging the brain centers that control thinking, judgment and memory, strokes can cause dementia, or a decline in mental ability. It is not unusual for a series of small strokes to progressively damage the brain. Known as multi-infarct dementia, this condition is second only to Alzheimer's disease as a cause of mental deterioration in older people. Whereas Alzheimer's disease usually develops gradually, the damage from multi-infarct dementia is more likely to appear as several abrupt changes.

THE TIA, OR MINISTROKE

Some people experience a fleeting interruption in blood supply to the brain. Known as a transient ischemic attack, or TIA, such a "ministroke" produces symptoms similar to those of a full-fledged stroke—weakness or loss of feeling in an arm and/or leg and/or the face, loss of sight in one eye, difficulty speaking or understanding speech. Sometimes the person feels dizzy or has double vision. The major difference is that the TIA and its symptoms are quickly over; most last just a few minutes, although by definition a TIA can go on for as long as 24 hours.

TIAs are the subject of much controversy today. The debate stems from the notion that because more than a third of the people who experience TIAs later go on to have strokes, TIAs should be searched out and treated vigorously. Unfortunately, it appears that we are only modestly effective at best in preventing strokes in persons suffering from TIAs. Moreover, symptoms such as dizziness are so general that the diagnosis of TIA is often uncertain. Dizziness is almost never a signal of TIA in persons under 40, and it is rarely so even in the aged. However, any episode that involves difficulty speaking or weakness in one part of the body should be brought to a physician's attention.

CAN WE DETECT A STROKE BEFORE IT CAUSES SYMPTOMS?

There is no test that can signal an impending stroke. Only when a TIA precedes a stroke is any warning given—but it's an imperfect warning at best. Ninety percent of all strokes are *not* heralded by a TIA. Should a TIA occur, it may be days, weeks or even months before a stroke develops.

Abnormal Heart Rhythms and Stroke

The million or so Americans who suffer from a type of abnormal heartbeat known as atrial fibrillation are especially susceptible to stroke; their risk is five times higher than that of the average person. The problem arises because the two small upper chambers of the heart, the atria, flutter instead of beating effectively. Blood is not fully pumped out with every heartbeat, so it tends to stagnate and form clots. Recent research suggests that it is not unusual for people with atrial fibrillation to have so-called "silent" strokes—strokes that occur without the person being aware of any symptoms. They are usually small and occur in areas of the brain that involve memory and complex thought. Studies are under way to identify subgroups of people with atrial fibrillation who have the highest risk of stroke.

Indeed, nearly two-thirds of the people who experience TIAs don't ever have a stroke.

CAN WE TREAT STROKES?

The acute phase of a stroke lasts from minutes to hours (or, rarely, days) and then typically ends of its own accord. While a stroke is in progress, the patient may be given drugs—anticlotting drugs for a thrombotic stroke or drugs to lower blood pressure or encourage clotting for a hemorrhagic stroke. However, it is vital to know what kind of stroke it is, so the medication doesn't do more harm than good. Special X-rays called computerized axial tomography (CAT scans) can often show where there is blockage or if there is bleeding.

Occasionally a hemorrhagic stroke can be headed off with emergency surgery. In 1988, Senator Joseph Biden of Delaware suffered a bleeding aneurysm; luckily for him, the bleeding was light, and it was located in an area of the brain where surgeons could reach it and "clip" it off. More often, surgery is no solution; the hemorrhage is too abrupt or too massive, or the bleeding site can't be reached. An added problem is that when surgery can be attempted, the blood vessels frequently react with little understood but often-fatal spasms.

In the two or three days following a severe stroke, brain tissue may swell, producing further damage. Some patients rally and improve; others worsen or slip into a coma. It is a period of anxious watching and waiting. Doctors will make frequent checks on the patient's reflexes, mobility and feeling, but only time can tell how extensive the damage will be.

Fortunately, stroke symptoms tend to improve with time. Many patients recover quickly, reaching their full potential within weeks. (The most complete and quickest recoveries occur in persons whose stroke symptoms last less than an hour.) For others, recovery is a long, drawn-out process; some never fully regain their former abilities. However, even seriously paralyzed stroke patients can make remarkable progress.

To maximize recovery and prevent the muscle deterioration that sets in when a person is immobile, rehabilitation and physical therapy should begin as soon as the patient is out of danger. Physical and occupational therapists, social workers, speech-language specialists, and other experts can help the patient re-learn how to walk or sit, improve balance, or speak clearly—whatever it takes to let the person lead as independent and productive a life as possible. Stroke victims usually continue this therapy after they leave the hospital; some enroll in programs at rehabilitation institutes.

Families, too, can benefit from counseling. Family support and encouragement are essential to the patient's recovery, but family members need to understand what the patient is going through. They need to learn how to tap into community resources. And they have to help the patient work out ways to compensate for his or her impairments, obtain self-help devices or make adjustments around the house. Stroke Clubs, sponsored by area hospitals and local chapters of national health organizations, are a good source of information, encouragement and recreation for both patients and their families.

CAN WE PREVENT STROKES?

Because stroke damage can be so swift, devastating and hard to reverse, prevention is paramount. Some of the risk factors for stroke—age, sex, race and a family history of stroke (especially having a mother who died of stroke)—cannot be altered. But the most important risk factors are things we can control. As you will see, these are largely the same as the risk factors for heart disease, discussed more fully in Chapter 18.

- **High blood pressure** tops the list of risk factors for strokes of all kinds. The higher your blood pressure, the greater your risk. (High blood pressure is discussed in Chapter 18.) It is just as dangerous for women as for men, and for seniors as for younger people. High blood pressure can often be controlled by *exercise* and *fat loss*. *Moderating salt intake* is also important.
- **Heart disease** of just about any kind doubles your risk of stroke, regardless of your blood pressure. You can cut your risk of coronary heart disease by *lowering your cholesterol level*—once again, the magic words are *exercise* and *fat loss*, along with eating a *low-fat diet*—and *not smoking*.
- **Cigarette smoking** increases the chances of stroke, even in people with no other risk factors. The risk goes up with the number of cigarettes smoked and falls off when a person quits. (In the Framingham Heart Study, the risk returned to normal after five years of not smoking.) Studies in volunteers show that smoking cuts down on blood flow to the brain—which can't do anyone any good. The obvious conclusion: *Don't smoke.*
- **Smoking and oral contraceptives** interact to markedly increase the chances of having a stroke. Studies have shown that the risk is four to 13 times higher in women who take birth control pills and smoke than in women who do neither.
- **Obesity** clearly contributes to high blood pressure. Poundage and pressure often rise

Cholesterol and Stroke

Can cholesterol ever be too low? Several large studies have recently uncovered an unexpected link. The combination of high blood pressure with a very low cholesterol level—below 160 mg/dl—appears to be linked to an increased risk of stroke due to hemorrhage. Because cholesterol is an essential component of cell membranes, it has been suggested that too little cholesterol may weaken artery walls, making them more likely to rupture, especially under high pressure. However, other scientists contend that the low cholesterol levels don't contribute to strokes. Instead, they are a marker of whatever is really at fault. (I think the latter is more likely.) Whatever the case, few Americans have cause to worry. The average cholesterol level in this country is 210 mg/dl. Striving for lower cholesterol levels remains essential —while maintaining low blood pressure is as important as ever.

together. Obesity also plays a role in diabetes. Getting rid of excess fat will reverse both of these damaging conditions. *Exercise* and *eat wisely*.
- **Physical inactivity,** it has been suggested, may be linked to stroke. The Framingham Heart Study found that stroke appeared to be higher in persons with sedentary jobs, although the numbers didn't meet the scientists' criteria for being "statistically significant." What is clear, however, is that physical activity helps fight most of the risk factors for stroke—high blood pressure, heart disease, high cholesterol, diabetes and obesity. The solution? *Get moving*.
- **Alcohol** appears to have a mixed effect on strokes. According to a large California study, light drinking (no more than two drinks a day) is associated with a decreased risk of strokes due to blood clots, whereas

Stroke in the Streets

To all the woes that drugs can beget, add another. There are now several well-documented cases of healthy young men with no known risk factors suffering strokes within minutes of taking "crack," a highly potent, smokable form of cocaine. These strokes resulted from a blocked blood supply, not a hemorrhage. Exactly how crack works its damage is not clear, but cocaine is known to narrow arteries and may trigger a sharp rise in blood pressure.

heavy drinking (three or more drinks a day) almost quadrupled the risk of hemorrhagic stroke. (Heavy drinking also raises blood pressure.) So, if you drink, *drink in moderation*.

- **TIAs.** More than a third of all people who experience TIAs go on to have strokes. Drugs that interfere with blood clotting, such as heparin and aspirin, have been used in an attempt to decrease this chance. Aspirin appears to have some benefit, and patients who have experienced TIAs or non-disabling strokes are often told to take an aspirin a day. However, aspirin also presents a drawback. In a Harvard study of 22,000 American physicians, taking an aspirin every other day did decrease the doctors' risk of having a heart attack (by almost half), but it also slightly increased their risk of hemorrhagic stroke.

- **Diabetes,** a disorder of body chemistry that results in high levels of sugar (glucose) in the blood, is a key risk factor for stroke, especially in women. (Diabetes is discussed fully in Chapter 21.) The risk is compounded for those many diabetics who also suffer from high blood pressure. Moreover, recent research suggests that having a high plasma-glucose level increases the damage wrought by stroke, and

that stroke patients with high plasma-glucose levels have a poorer prognosis than those with normal blood sugar. Like so many other diseases, diabetes often responds to weight loss achieved through *a healthful diet* and *exercise*.

- **A high red blood cell count** can hoist the risk of stroke by increasing the thickness of the blood and thus the chances that it will clot. This condition can be treated with blood thinners.

- **Multiple risk factors.** Certain risk factors, when combined, spell extra trouble. Researchers have identified a treacherous five-part combination: high blood pressure, high cholesterol, abnormal plasma glucose (indicating diabetes), cigarette smoking and enlargement of the left side of the heart (left ventricular hypertrophy). About one-third of all strokes occur in people who fit this description.

Surgery, too, has been used to prevent stroke by removing deposits clogging arteries in the neck (the carotid arteries) in persons who have had TIAs or who have shown evidence (via a test known as a carotid sonogram) of reduced blood flow in these arteries. Although this surgery, known as carotid endarterectomy, is performed on many thousands of Americans each year, it has been vastly overrated as well as overperformed. A study by UCLA and the Rand Corporation found that only about one-third of all carotid endarterectomies are performed for acceptable reasons. In addition, only a small percentage of strokes are due to deposits that can be reached by surgery.

Not only have the benefits of this surgery never been proven in careful studies, the operation is dangerous: Close to three percent of the patients die, and in another six percent, the operation triggers a stroke. Large studies are under way to see if it is possible to identify certain groups who might possibly benefit from this procedure. Arguing against such a benefit are studies in which brain scans (using positron emission tomography) have shown that despite significantly blocked carotid arteries, many persons have normal blood flow and blood pressure within the brain.

Clearly, the best—really the only—anti-stroke prescription is a healthful lifestyle.

FOR MORE INFORMATION

American Heart Association (AHA) publications, available from local chapters, include "Recovering from a Stroke," "Strokes: A Guide for the Family," "Up and Around: A Booklet to Aid the Stroke Patient in Activities of Daily Living," and an excellent discussion of physical and behavioral changes written by Roy S. Fowler, Jr., and W. E. Fordyce, "Stroke: Why Do They Behave That Way?" AHA chapters gather information about local sources of stroke treatment and rehabilitation, financial assistance and equipment. They also sponsor Stroke Clubs.

"Stroke: Hope Through Research" and "Aphasia: Hope Through Research" are available from the National Institute of Neurological Disorders and Stroke, National Institute of Health, Bethesda, MD 20892. (301) 496-5751.

The National Easter Seal Society concerns itself with treatment and rehabilitation for persons with physical disabilities and speech and language problems. It also sponsors Stroke Clubs. The address is 70 East Lake Street, Chicago, IL 60601. (312) 726-6200.

Information on federal benefits and rehabilitation services can be obtained from the Clearinghouse on the Handicapped, Switzer Building, Room 3132, 330 C Street, S.W., Washington, DC 20202.

DIABETES

The first time Lillian Rogers showed up in my office, she was a sick woman. She had the symptoms, blood tests and medicines to prove it. She had been told she had diabetes. And she had friends with diabetes—one had even had a foot amputated. At 63, this heavyset housewife had resigned herself to ill health and fading horizons. In fact, she and her husband (newly retired from the National Park Service) had moved into our community to live near their daughter in their twilight years. She had come to me to get her prescriptions renewed.

Mrs. Rogers told me she was feeling pretty bad. She was tired, she was often nauseated, and sometimes she had diarrhea. Every so often she would have a shaky, dizzy, quivery spell. Actually, the woman was worried that she would soon be dead.

I had my doubts. The medications could have been causing some of her symptoms, so we stopped them. Her plasma glucose rose, but not dangerously. As you might guess, I started her on a low-fat diet. And she took up walking for exercise. She lost a couple of pounds, and her plasma glucose fell a few points. Then she lost a few more pounds. Her plasma glucose fell some more. And her energy and her spirits rose.

In a matter of months, Mrs. Rogers was a totally different person. Her plasma-glucose level was normal; her weight was the lowest it had been in 15 years. Her notions about disabling illness and early death were replaced by vigor and enthusiasm. She and her husband bought a large travel trailer and headed west for a tour of the national parks so dear to their hearts. When she touched base with me after their first six-month circuit, she was feeling great and her plasma glucose was fine. I haven't seen her again, but I suspect she's still on the road.

DIABETES AND DIABESITY

Like millions of other Americans, Mrs. Rogers suffered from a condition that has been dubbed "diabesity." Although I am not a fan of medical jargon, this is one term for which I would make an exception. Diabesity describes a common state in which obesity is closely linked with high plasma glucose. If high plasma glucose is not controlled, it can damage many parts of the body. But diabesity almost always responds to changes in lifestyle —loss of fat through diet and exercise.

Diabesity is the most common of the disturbing and complex diseases of body chemistry known as diabetes. Diabetes mellitus, or "sugar diabetes," is not one disease but several. One, insulin-dependent diabetes mellitus (IDDM), is a severe disease that is impossible to prevent and hard to control; treatment requires daily injections of insulin as well as a controlled diet, exercise and careful monitoring of glucose levels in the urine or blood. It usually begins in childhood and used to be called juvenile-onset diabetes. A second form, non-insulin-dependent diabetes mellitus (NIDDM), often is directly related to obesity and inactivity—in a word, diabesity—and does not require insulin. It usually occurs in middle age or later and formerly was called adult-onset diabetes. A third type, gestational diabetes, appears during pregnancy.

Diabetes of all types is characterized by a disturbance in the body's ability to use food as fuel. It involves a number of chemical abnormalities that damage blood vessels and nerves over time. The long-term outcome can be kidney failure, heart disease or stroke. Diabetes causes more than 37,000 deaths a year; indirectly, it is responsible for another 100,000. Each year it produces 8,000 new cases of end-stage kidney disease and necessitates some 30,000 amputations. It is the leading cause of adult blindness. Diabetes during pregnancy sharply increases the risk of birth problems and birth defects. Most of this damage is done by IDDM, even though it accounts for only 5 percent to 10 percent of all diabetes.

THE SCOPE OF DIABETES

Lots of numbers get thrown around regarding diabetes, but they can be misleading. Estimates based on data from the National Health and Nutrition Examination Survey, published in 1985, state that about 6 million Americans have diabetes. An-

Blood Sugar by Any Other Name

When doctors talk to patients about diabetes, they often refer to "blood sugar." Yet when they talk among themselves or write about diabetes, they usually use the term "plasma glucose" or "serum glucose."

The reasons for the different terms are fairly simple. Glucose is the type of sugar found in the blood, so saying glucose instead of sugar is just being more precise. When glucose is measured in the laboratory, it is done after the red blood cells have been removed from the blood sample by one of two methods, spinning or clotting. When red blood cells are removed by spinning, the remaining fluid is referred to as plasma. When they are removed by clotting, the fluid that is left is called serum. Thus, serum glucose or plasma glucose is a more accurate term than blood glucose, which implies that the test was done on whole blood. Plasma and serum concentrations of glucose are identical and run 10 percent to 15 percent higher than whole-blood determinations. Whole-blood determinations are hardly ever done nowadays. Most tests for diabetes routinely use plasma glucose.

other 5 million are said to have "undiagnosed diabetes." The number of persons with IDDM is estimated to be between 300,000 and 600,000.

The significance of these figures is debatable. First of all, many people are labeled "diabetic" on the basis of a single blood test. Even though most people whose tests show mild abnormalities will not develop true diabetes, all too often they are given the diagnosis of "chemical diabetes" and started on drugs when what they need is to exercise and eat sensibly.

Chemical diabetes is touted as "asymptomatic diabetes," diabetes that hasn't yet produced symptoms. Chemical diabetes is something of a Frankenstein's monster, concocted of half good intentions and half ignorance. Unlike the original, this monster won instant acceptance and endless promotion by those who portrayed it as a rampant killer that can be controlled if detected and treated in time.

The argument for promoting the concept of chemical diabetes (and screening programs to detect it) is simple: An abnormal plasma-glucose level means diabetes, even if it is not causing any symptoms. Early treatment might prevent some of the complications, such as blindness and kidney disease. Even if treatment doesn't help, at least it won't hurt; it involves drugs that are safe and can be taken by mouth (and therefore do not hurt, as insulin injections do).

The problems with this argument are many. To begin with, the significance of an abnormal plasma-glucose test is often not clear. Plasma-glucose levels change throughout the day, rising quickly after a meal and then falling as the body, with the help of insulin, burns glucose or stores it. What's more, plasma-glucose levels naturally rise with age. Plasma-glucose tests, especially types used in the past, often showed these normal changes as "abnormal" results. This led to many people, especially older ones, being wrongly diagnosed as diabetic. A related problem has to do with finding "undiagnosed" diabetics. Unfortunately, there is no evidence that treating someone before symptoms appear helps to head off any damaging complications. Finally, there is ample evidence that oral anti-diabetes drugs (oral hypoglycemic agents) can be hazardous. All have side effects, some of them serious. One of these drugs, phenformin, was removed from the market after it was shown to cause a serious and sometimes fatal reaction called lactic acidosis.

The punch line to all this is that almost all of those millions of Americans with "undetected diabetes" have a condition that: 1) causes no symptoms; 2) is defined on the basis of a laboratory test; and 3) has a treatment with no known benefits but real hazards.

What Is Diabetes?

In diabetes the body's food-processing system is out of whack. Normally the body converts sugars and starches (carbohydrates) into a form of sugar called glucose, which it can burn for heat and energy. What it doesn't need right away is stored in the liver or muscles as glycogen, or as fat. In diabetes, however, the body is unable to use or store glucose properly. This results in a high level of glucose in the blood; the excess spills over into the urine and is excreted.

A big part of the trouble lies with insulin, a hormone produced in the pancreas. Insulin is needed to convert plasma glucose into energy. In some cases, the pancreas doesn't produce enough insulin. This is the problem in IDDM. In other cases, insulin is present but for some reason does not work well. This is called insulin resistance; it is the main problem in NIDDM. Insulin resistance is related to too much body fat and not enough exercise. Thus, NIDDM most often is the same as diabesity. Whatever the reason—lack of insulin or insulin resistance—too much glucose builds up in the blood.

What Causes Diabetes?

What causes diabetes is not yet known. IDDM is suspected to involve an abnormal immune-system response, in which the body's defenses mistakenly attack the insulin-producing cells of the pancreas. Studies also suggest that at least some cases of IDDM may be related to a virus. A hereditary component seems very likely as well. The current theory is that the virus triggers the abnormal immune response in persons who have inherited a tendency to develop IDDM.

NIDDM, in contrast, is closely linked to obesity. Excess fat is known to impair the body's ability to use insulin; in other words, it creates insulin resistance. However, losing fat helps to restore insulin's effectiveness. Most of the people who develop NIDDM—about 80 percent—are overweight. What's more, their chance of developing the disease climbs with weight. Recent studies show that risk is greatest for people who carry their excess fat in the waist and belly rather than in the buttocks, thighs and arms.

Gestational diabetes appears during pregnancy. It is thought to occur in about three percent of all pregnancies, and it sharply increases the risk of congenital malformations, birth problems (the babies are often very large), and death and illness in the newborn. Although most patients have no symptoms, the condition can be detected by routine testing of pregnant women for elevated plasma glucose. (The basic treatment is diet.) Although this kind of diabetes often disappears after the baby's birth, many of these women will develop NIDDM later in life.

WHO WILL GET DIABETES?

The typical diabetic is middle-aged and overfat—and the incidence goes up as age and fat increase. In this country, women are about as likely as men to develop diabetes. However, diabetes is a special threat to minorities. NIDDM is 50 percent higher among black men than white men and 100 percent higher among black women than white women. (About a quarter of all black women above age 55 are thought to have diabetes.) Among Hispanics the rate of diabetes is three times that of whites. The incidence is also very high among some groups of North American Indians.

Diabetes mellitus is thought to be a hereditary disease, but there is no agreement on exactly how it is passed on from one generation to the next. The precise risk of diabetes cannot be defined for any one person. Tables 21.1 and 21.2, based on several sources, give some approximations.

Table 21.1
Risk of IDDM

With this family history of IDDM:	Your risk is:
One parent	1 in 8
Two parents	1 in 4
One brother or sister (parents normal)	1 in 8
One brother or sister and one parent	1 in 4
One brother or sister and both parents	1 in 2

Table 21.2
Risk of NIDDM

With this family history of NIDDM:	Your risk is:
One grandparent	1 in 8
One parent	1 in 4
Both a parent and grandparent (or aunt or uncle)	3 in 5

(Having NIDDM does *not* increase the chances that a person's child will get IDDM.)

Figure 21.1
Factors That Cause IDDM

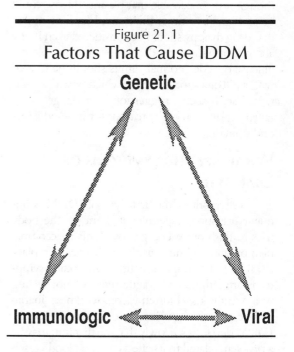

Genetic

Immunologic ⟷ Viral

CAN DIABETES BE PREVENTED?

As far as we know, IDDM cannot be prevented. Current hopes for prevention reflect the belief that an abnormal immunologic response to a viral infection causes IDDM. Someday it may be possible to immunize persons who have inherited a susceptibility to IDDM against the viruses that trigger the immune response. Or, it may be possible to block the immune response before it destroys all of the insulin-secreting cells in the pancreas. Indeed, a recent experimental study in France showed that the use of drugs that block the immune response in children who have just developed IDDM may preserve at least some of the insulin-producing cells.

NIDDM seems to be different. Most adult diabetics are overfat at the time of diagnosis. As mentioned above, their plasma glucose will fall as weight drops. It seems likely that fat control can delay, and perhaps prevent, the onset of this illness, but this is far from certain.

What is certain is that you can prevent giving yourself a disease when you don't have one. Although it is conceivable that plasma glucose could be so high (five times the normal level or more) that drug therapy should be considered even in the absence of symptoms, the notion that any plasma glucose outside "normal" limits should be treated with a pill or a shot—both of which pose risks—is nonsense. If such a suggestion is made, get a detailed explanation of the reasons for it—and a second opinion.

WHAT ARE THE SYMPTOMS OF DIABETES?

Often one of the first signs of IDDM is frequent urination, especially at night, as the body tries to flush out excess glucose. This is accompanied by unusual thirst, as the body tries to replace the fluid lost through urination. Other early symptoms are fatigue or a vague sense of not feeling well, weight loss, blurred vision, weakness, inability to concentrate and loss of coordination. Rarely, IDDM develops so slowly that the first hint may be a problem related to its effects on the blood vessels or nerves—numbness in the feet and legs, or infections that are slow to heal. Such problems are much more likely to be the first signs of NIDDM.

If symptoms are ignored and the plasma-glucose level is not controlled, IDDM may quickly become life-threatening. A very high level of plasma glucose can cause a diabetic to develop a major problem with body metabolism known as diabetic ketoacidosis. This may lead to coma or death. In the days before insulin became available, IDDM was always fatal; its young victims usually died in ketoacidosis, often within months of diagnosis.

Today, ketoacidosis is treated with intravenous fluids and large doses of quick-acting insulin, and death is rare.

A very low plasma-glucose level can also cause problems for the diabetic. This condition, known as hypoglycemia, can make a diabetic lose consciousness, convulse and even die. Hypoglycemia may be brought on when people who are taking insulin or oral hypoglycemics fail to eat enough—for instance, if they skip a meal—to balance the effects of the insulin or drugs, or when they exercise too hard. The symptoms include heavy sweating, hunger and headache. They can be countered with a quick snack or a drink containing sugar. A person who is unconscious needs an injection of glucose or a substance called glucagon. (A medical-alert bracelet explaining that the wearer has diabetes is a wise precaution for people who depend on insulin or drugs.)

Plasma-glucose levels can also be upset by stresses. These can be physical, such as illness or surgery, or emotional.

THE COMPLICATIONS OF DIABETES

Over time the chemical disruptions of diabetes produce abnormalities in blood vessels and nerves. Changes in small blood vessels, especially, characterize diabetes. It is these changes (microvascular disease) that damage the eyes and kidneys. Damage to the large blood vessels can show up as heart disease, peripheral arterial disease (circulation problems in legs and arms), and stroke. Nerve damage contributes to loss of feeling in the legs and feet.

No one can tell for sure which diabetics will go on to develop serious complications. However, such problems are more likely to show up in people who have IDDM and those who have had diabetes for many years. Even if NIDDM is untreated, ketoacidosis is rare, and blindness and amputation are infrequent. Nerve problems, however, are more common.

Heart disease (the most common cause of death among diabetics), stroke and kidney failure are often linked with other risk factors, including high blood pressure and smoking. Diabetics who

Foot Care in Diabetes

To prevent serious foot problems, diabetics have to take foot care seriously. Those who have nerve problems need to take special precautions:

- Carefully wash and dry your feet, especially between the toes, every day.
- Inspect your feet every day for blisters, cuts and scratches. Use a mirror to get a good look.
- Buy shoes that feel comfortable. Check them daily to ensure that the insides are smooth and nothing has fallen into them. Always wear socks or seamless stockings. Don't walk barefoot on the beach.
- Test the temperature of your bath water with your hand before you step into it.
- Cut toenails straight across.

smoke increase their chances of dying from heart disease by 65 percent.

Changes in the blood vessels that supply the eyes cause a disease known as *diabetic retinopathy*. At first changes can occur without causing symptoms, so regular eye exams are important. One early sign is blurred vision. Thanks to laser therapy, these changes can often be stopped before they proceed to severe vision loss. Those at special risk for diabetic retinopathy include people who have had diabetes five years or longer, those who have trouble controlling their glucose level, and diabetic women who are pregnant.

In diabetic kidney disease, or *diabetic nephropathy*, damage to the blood vessels impairs the kidneys' ability to filter the blood. This allows toxins to build up in the blood and disturbs the body's fluid balance. Eventually, the kidneys may shut down altogether, forcing the person to rely on dialysis or a kidney transplant. The chances of developing kidney disease can be increased by high blood pressure and also by urinary-tract infections—a special problem for diabetics whose nerve damage prevents the bladder from emptying completely.

Diabetic neuropathy, or nerve damage, can produce a range of symptoms. Nerve damage in the legs and feet can cause pain, prickling and burning feelings. Alternatively, it can wipe out sensation, leaving a person easy prey to injuries —from bumps and bruises, cuts, burns or pressure —that can go unnoticed and become infected. Such injuries, coupled with poor circulation due to blood vessel problems, produce sores and ulcers that refuse to heal, and make foot disease a major concern. In the worst cases, they lead to amputation.

Diabetic nerve damage can also affect digestion and blood pressure. It can cause impotence and, as noted above, urinary-tract infections. Diabetics are also more susceptible to gum disease.

HOW IS DIABETES DIAGNOSED?

The keys to a diagnosis of diabetes are:

- Symptoms, such as frequent urination and excessive thirst.
- Risk factors, such as obesity and a family history of diabetes.
- Signs of complications, such as blood vessel disease or numbness in the feet and legs.
- Laboratory tests showing glucose in the urine or elevated glucose in the blood.

Some of the problems with laboratory tests were discussed in Chapter 15. Your plasma-glucose level depends on how recently and what you have eaten and, to an extent, how old you are. These problems have been addressed by replacing plasma-glucose tests made at random with tests made when the person is fasting or at specified intervals after the person has consumed a measured amount of glucose (the so-called glucose-tolerance test).

A diagnosis of diabetes today, as outlined by the National Diabetes Data Group, requires one of the following:

- A clearly abnormal fasting glucose level (above 140 milligrams per deciliter of plasma) *on more than one occasion*.
- A clearly abnormal glucose-tolerance test (above 200 milligrams per deciliter of plasma).

• Classic symptoms of diabetes (thirst, frequent urination, rapid weight loss, etc.) with elevated glucose.

I believe that diagnosis can be simplified further. Most people with clearly abnormal glucose-tolerance tests will also have clearly abnormal fasting glucose levels on more than one occasion. Moreover, those who have abnormal glucose-tolerance tests, but whose fasting glucose levels are below 140 milligrams per deciliter of plasma rarely go on to have consistently elevated plasma-glucose levels and even more rarely develop symptoms of diabetes. Thus, the glucose-tolerance test seems unimportant. Therefore, we have only two groups in which diabetes can be diagnosed: Persons with the classic symptoms of diabetes and high plasma-glucose levels, and those without classic symptoms who have very high fasting plasma-glucose levels on many occasions.

All too often, these strict criteria are overlooked. Even today people are diagnosed and treated as diabetics on the basis of a random plasma-glucose test or a mildly elevated glucose-tolerance test.

Can Diabetes Be Treated?

When insulin was discovered in the 1920s, it was rightly hailed as a miracle drug. It did indeed prevent the untimely deaths of youngsters with IDDM. However, much to everyone's disappointment, it did not *cure* IDDM. Abnormalities in blood chemistry continued to ravage the diabetic's blood vessels and nerves, causing blindness, loss of limbs, kidney failure and infections.

More recently, hopes for a breakthrough in diabetes treatment received another setback. It had long been believed that keeping plasma-glucose levels from fluctuating too widely might prevent the devastating complications of diabetes. In a major national study designed to test this theory of "tight control," people with IDDM were divided into two groups. One group received the standard treatment, including one or two injections of insulin each day and regular self-testing of urine or blood for glucose. The test group got "intensive" treatment—insulin, either by injection three or four times a day or continuously through a tiny insulin pump worn by the patient. People in the intensive group checked their glucose levels often throughout the day, adjusting their diet or insulin dosage to keep their plasma glucose in the normal range.

Unhappily, the earliest reports out of the study stated that the test group fared worse than those getting standard treatment. The test subjects did achieve excellent control, but they paid for it with frequent bouts of hypoglycemia—an average of at least one a day—some of which were fatal. Their eye changes were just as severe as those in the standard-treatment group, and they gained much more weight. They weren't eating any more, but their bodies became more efficient at processing calories.

Thus, there is still no cure for diabetes. Treatment aims at control. While it is usually possible to control plasma glucose and prevent life-threatening episodes of ketoacidosis or hypoglycemia, the same cannot be said for the blood vessel problems that cause blindness, loss of limbs and kidney failure.

Treatment for persons with IDDM consists of daily insulin injections, a controlled diet and exercise. They also need to test the level of glucose in their blood or urine perhaps several times a day. A number of kits on the market make testing easy; paper strips or tablets change color when exposed to urine or a drop of blood. A lab test called a glycosylated hemoglobin test helps assess how well a plasma-glucose control program is working over the long term by providing a three-month average of plasma-glucose levels.

For people with NIDDM the mainstays of treatment are exercise and diet. Both help to control weight, normalize plasma-glucose levels and combat the risk factors for heart disease, including high cholesterol levels and high blood pressure. As weight drops, plasma-glucose levels tend to move toward normal. For many people with NIDDM, no other therapy is needed.

In addition to burning off calories and curbing the appetite, exercise sets off a cascade of improvements in the way the body handles glucose. It both lowers plasma glucose and increases sensitivity to insulin. And some studies have found that exercise-induced changes can persist for a day or two after a workout.

However, diabetics have to use caution in starting an exercise program. Besides being overweight and out of shape, a diabetic may be a candidate for a heart attack, a detached retina or foot damage. People with eye problems shouldn't do heavy lifting or straining, and they should avoid jarring the head. Persons with foot and leg problems should be very careful to avoid blisters and cuts; swimming or bicycling are easier on the feet than running. It's important to select a form of exercise that is both safe and enjoyable enough to do frequently, and to stick with it for life.

Diet, along with exercise, is the key to shedding the extra pounds that burden the diabetic. The recommended diet is largely the same as that suggested for fat control in persons without diabetes (see Chapters 7 and 8). The major difference for diabetics is that they must schedule their meals and snacks, exercise and any medications (insulin or oral hypoglycemic drugs) so that plasma glucose does not go too high or too low. Such a schedule must balance the glucose-lowering effects of exercise and medications against the glucose-raising effect of food. The methods by which this balance is achieved are beyond the scope of this book. Indeed, such balance is the mainstay of diabetes treatment, the subject of many medical texts and much medical training.

Because losing fat is never easy, many people find it helpful to enroll in programs that offer group support, behavior therapy and nutritional counseling. Diabetics who would like to consult with a nutritionist or dietitian can get names from local chapters of the American Diabetes Association, American Heart Association or American Dietetic Association, or from a local hospital or medical school.

In the cases of NIDDM in which fat control alone fails to bring plasma-glucose levels under control, insulin injections or drugs to lower plasma glucose may be required. As noted, oral hypoglycemic drugs have drawbacks. They may lower plasma glucose too much or not enough, and can cause skin rashes, liver problems and anemia. Many patients prefer to use insulin if diet and exercise alone are not enough.

CAN SCREENING DETECT DIABETES?

We have already discussed the difficulty of defining diabetes with laboratory tests. It is true that just about everyone who develops IDDM and most of those who develop NIDDM will have an abnormal level of plasma glucose in the urine before experiencing symptoms. However, most people who have a mildly "abnormal" level of plasma glucose will never develop any symptoms.

A urine test for glucose is an alternative to a blood test and has some advantages:

- It is inexpensive.
- You can do it yourself.
- Usually glucose appears in the urine only after plasma glucose is greatly elevated, so minor elevations don't trigger a false alarm.

The question then becomes, "What is the advantage of finding diabetes before it causes symptoms?" In NIDDM, it does little good to make a diagnosis without symptoms. This is because:

- The best therapy is diet and exercise to maintain ideal body fat. You should be doing this anyway.
- If you are obese, you already know that you need to shed some pounds—so the preceding goes double for you.
- Going beyond diet and exercise to the use of drugs, either insulin or the oral hypoglycemics, is seldom indicated in the absence of symptoms.

Then what about IDDM? Should we do a fasting plasma-glucose test on everyone who has a family history? Or should we wait until the first symptoms appear and treat it at that time? The first episode, with its excessive thirst, frequent urination and weight loss, is almost always caught and treated before anything dire results. But it seems logical that at least once in a while there might be an episode of serious, even fatal, ketoacidosis that could have been prevented by a screening program.

Still, screening to detect IDDM before it causes symptoms has several drawbacks. For one, the disease is not all that common, and the chance of detecting a high plasma glucose between the time it develops and the time symptoms occur is extremely low. Also, a large-scale screening program would be very costly. Finally, there is no evidence that using insulin treatment before symptoms appear slows the damage to blood vessels and nerves. Its only purpose would be to prevent ketoacidosis. On the other hand, being labeled a diabetic has clear disadvantages; it may be argued that a young person is better off not knowing he or she has the disease until insulin treatment must begin to avoid ketoacidosis.

WHAT SHOULD YOU DO ABOUT DIABETES?

If screening isn't for everyone, what should you do? My recommendation is as follows.

If you do not have a family history of IDDM, your only concern should be diet and exercise. These should be high on your agenda anyway—and doubly so if you are obese.

If you do have a family history of IDDM, you have a choice. You may do nothing more than diet and exercise. The chance that you will be hurting yourself if you do nothing more is very small. Or you can take advantage of the fact that when plasma glucose is high, some of it comes out in the urine. You can test your own urine cheaply and easily with "dipsticks" available at the drug store. Once every month or so will be enough. (Of course, you can test yourself any time you are feeling ill.) Don't make yourself sick by worrying that you may develop the disease. Approach it as you would a blood-pressure test. And don't panic if your urine shows some glucose; some people have glucose in the urine even though their plasma glucose is not very high. However, if the urine does show glucose, it is well worth the cost of a blood test to find out what the plasma-glucose level is.

FOR MORE INFORMATION

The American Diabetes Association is a voluntary organization that provides information on many aspects of diabetes and on support groups, and publishes a newsletter. Its National Service Center is located at 1660 Duke Street, P.O. Box 25757, Alexandria, VA 22314 (703) 549-1500.

"Noninsulin-Dependent Diabetes" is one of several publications available through the National Diabetes Information Clearinghouse, a program of the National Institute of Diabetes and Digestive and Kidney Diseases. The address of the Clearinghouse is Box NDIC, Bethesda, MD 20892 (301) 496-3583.

The American Dietetic Association is a good source of referrals for help in developing a weight-loss program. It is located at 430 North Michigan Avenue, Chicago, IL 60611 (312) 899-0040.

SECTION VI

THE LIFEPLAN
RECORD

❑ The LifePlan Record

THE LIFEPLAN
RECORD

*T*his LifePlan Record serves a variety of functions. It is a place to record important events from the past and the status of your health as indicated by LifeScore. It will make this information easily available not only to you, but to health professionals as well.

Discuss your LifePlan Record with your doctor. It will allow him or her to become familiar with your medical history quickly. It will also make it clear that you are willing and able to take responsibility for your health and would like help in meeting that goal.

PROBLEM LIST

Calculating your LifeScore should have given you a clear idea of which risks threaten your health and what you can do about them. Any lifestyle problems—smoking, obesity, excessive drinking, lack of exercise and so on—should be at the top of your list. If you have a chronic disease, such as diabetes or hypertension, list it as well. Be sure to include any allergies, especially to medications. If an immunization is out of date, it should be listed here until it is made current. Include any other aspect of your health history that you consider to be of particular importance, even though it may not be a problem at present. For example, it will help to indicate a history of tuberculosis or breast cancer, even though there are no signs of that disease now. However, most of what happened in the past and is over (appendectomy, measles, etc.) should be recorded in the sections that follow.

Cross out problems as they are resolved, and record the dates on which they ceased to be problems.

1. _____

2. _____

3. _____

4. _____

5. _____

6. _____

7. _____

8. _____

9. _____

10. _____

11. _____

12. _____

13. _____

14. _____

15. _____

16. _____

17. _____

18. _____

19. _____

20. _____

IMMUNIZATIONS

If you have been immunized against a disease that is listed, just give the date of the immunization. For an adult, the dates of all "baby shots" are not crucial as long as you know whether you had them. But it is very important to know the date of your last tetanus booster, because you need one every 10 years.

If you have actually had an illness listed, put the date you were ill preceded by the letter "I" — for example, "I — 1967."

The most common immunization to be listed under "Other" will be that for smallpox (variola). This immunization is no longer required or recommended. Others will be typhoid, typhus, rabies, or one of the many vaccines available for special circumstances. There are more than 50 different vaccines available.

Mumps: _____

Rubella: _____

Polio: _____

Tetanus: _____

Diphtheria: _____

Pertussis: _____

Measles: _____

Other: _____

_____

_____

DRUGS

List any drugs you take regularly. Give the dosage and how often you take the drug—for example, "Hydrochlorothiazide 50 mg. (milligrams) twice a day." If you do not know the dosage, it's time you found out.

_____

_____

_____

_____

_____

_____

_____

WOMEN

If you have ever sneaked a peek at your medical record, you might have been puzzled by the "G _____ P _____ Ab _____" notation. **Gravida** means pregnancy and **para** means delivery. In medical terms, **abortion** means any interrupted pregnancy, so it includes miscarriages as well as those intentionally interrupted. Thus, a history of three pregnancies, with two being successful and one a miscarriage, would be abbreviated as $G_3P_2Ab_1$. The LifePlan Record uses words rather than letters; enter your history in the blanks provided.

Menarche means the onset of menses (menstrual periods) and **menopause** indicates the end of regular menses. Enter the ages at which these events occurred.

List your contraception method and how long you have used it.

Gravida _____ Para _____

Abortions _____ Menarche _____

Menopause _____ Contraceptive method _____

HOSPITALIZATIONS

Listing the hospital and its address as well as the date and problem will help in getting hospital records if they are ever needed.

Date	Reason	Hospital

SERIOUS ILLNESSES

Giving the name of the doctor and his or her address will help in obtaining records if they are ever needed.

Date	Reason	Hospital

FAMILY HISTORY

Record any positive responses from the Family Health section of LifeScore.

_____

_____

_____

_____

_____

_____

EXPOSURES

List your X-rays by date, type and where they may be found.

Date:	Type:	Available From:

REVIEW OF SYSTEMS

Doctors have traditionally asked a long series of questions about possible symptoms as part of a "complete history and physical." This has been termed the "review of systems" (ROS) because these questions are usually organized by body system. Unfortunately, the value of such a review is often lost—most of the symptoms reported prove to be unimportant.

A better method is to use **Take Care of Yourself** (Addison-Wesley, 1990) to understand symptoms and their significance. Below are some symptoms that might be important. If you have any of these, consult the book for more information. List only those that the book indicates need attention or about which you still have some questions. These can be discussed during a visit to a health professional.

System	Symptoms
Skin	Rashes, sores, bumps, lumps
Bones, joints and muscles	Swelling, pain, stiffness, weakness, cramps
Heart and blood vessels	Shortness of breath, chest pains, palpitations
Lungs and throat	Wheezing, shortness of breath, chronic cough, chronic hoarseness
Stomach and intestines	Abdominal pain, vomiting, diarrhea, very dark or bloody stools
Kidneys, bladder	Painful or frequent urination, blood in urine, very dark urine, incontinence
Female reproductive system	Heavy or painful periods, vaginal discharge or sores, breast lumps
Male genitalia	Penile discharge or sores
Head, ears, eyes, nose	Headaches, fainting, seizure, decreased vision or hearing, chronic runny nose
General	Depression, nervousness, marked weight gain or loss, allergies, chronically swollen glands

LifeChart

Pick one day a year to review your records and to enter that year's information. New Year's Day is a good choice for many people.

YEAR	1990 ▼	1991 ▼	1992 ▼	1993 ▼	1994 ▼

I.LifeScore:

Enter your scores from Chapter 1.

	1990	1991	1992	1993	1994
Exercise					
Body Fat					
Nutrition					
Smoking					
Alcohol					
Accidents					
Mind ↔ Body					
Family Health					
Medical Screening Tests					
Total LifeScore					

II.Screening:

If the entry has a numerical value, such as blood pressure or cholesterol measurement, enter the number. If the test result is reported simply as negative or positive, record **-** or **+**. For yes or no, you may use a **"Y"** or **"N."**

Recommended:

Blood pressure					
Cholesterol					
Mammography					
Physician examination of breasts					
Pap smear					

Optional:

Breast self-examination					
Dental examination					
Hearing and vision tests					
Occult blood in stool					
Ophthalmoscopy for glaucoma					
Physical examination					
Rectal examination					
Sigmoidoscopy					
Testicular self-examination					

III.Other:

Teeth cleaning					

LifeChart

1995 ▼	1996 ▼	1997 ▼	1998 ▼	1999 ▼	2000 ▼	2001 ▼	2002 ▼	2003 ▼

INDEX